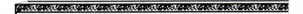

William J. Woods, PhD
Diane Binson, PhD
Editors

Gay Bathhouses
and Public Health Policy

Gay Bathhouses and Public Health Policy has been co-published simultaneously as *Journal of Homosexuality*, Volume 44, Numbers 3/4 2003.

Gay Bathhouses
and Public Health Policy

Gay Bathhouses and Public Health Policy has been co-published simultaneously as *Journal of Homosexuality*, Volume 44, Numbers 3/4 2003.

The *Journal of Homosexuality* Monographic "Separates"

Below is a list of "separates," which in serials librarianship means a special issue simultaneously published as a special journal issue or double-issue *and* as a "separate" hardbound monograph. (This is a format which we also call a "DocuSerial.")

"Separates" are published because specialized libraries or professionals may wish to purchase a specific thematic issue by itself in a format which can be separately cataloged and shelved, as opposed to purchasing the journal on an on-going basis. Faculty members may also more easily consider a "separate" for classroom adoption.

"Separates" are carefully classified separately with the major book jobbers so that the journal tie-in can be noted on new book order slips to avoid duplicate purchasing.

You may wish to visit Haworth's website at . . .

http://www.HaworthPress.com

. . . to search our online catalog for complete tables of contents of these separates and related publications.

You may also call 1-800-HAWORTH (outside US/Canada: 607-722-5857), or Fax 1-800-895-0582 (outside US/Canada: 607-771-0012), or e-mail at:

docdelivery@haworthpress.com

Gay Bathhouses and Public Health Policy, edited by William J. Woods, PhD, and Diane Binson, PhD (Vol. 44, No. 3/4, 2003). *"Important. . . . Long overdue. . . . a unique and valuable contribution to the social science and public health literature. The inclusion of detailed historical descriptions of public policy debates about the place of bathhouses in urban gay communities, together with summaries of the legal controversies about bathhouses, insightful examinations of patrons' behaviors and reviews of successful program for HIV/STD education and testing programs in bathhouses provides. A well rounded and informative overview."* (Richard Tewksbury, PhD, Professor of Justice Administration, University of Louisville)

Icelandic Lives: The Queer Experience, edited by Voon Chin Phua (Vol. 44, No. 2, 2002). *"The first of its kind, this book shows the emergence of gay and lesbian visibility through the biographical narratives of a dozen Icelanders. Through their lives can be seen a small nation's transition, in just a few decades, from a pervasive silence concealing its queer citizens to widespread acknowledgment characterized by some of the most progressive laws in the world."* (Barry D. Adam, PhD, University Professor, Department of Sociology & Anthropology, University of Windsor, Ontario, Canada)

The Drag King Anthology, edited by Donna Troka, PhD (cand.), Kathleen Le Besco, PhD, and Jean Bobby Noble, PhD (Vol. 43, No. 3/4, 2002). *"All university courses on masculinity should use this book . . . challenges preconceptions through the empirical richness of direct experience. The contributors and editors have worked together to produce cultural analysis that enhances our perception of the dynamic uncertainty of gendered experience."* (Sally R. Munt, DPhil, Subject Chair, Media Studies, University of Sussex)

Homosexuality in French History and Culture, edited by Jeffrey Merrick, PhD, and Michael Sibalis, PhD (Vol. 41, No. 3/4, 2001). *"Fascinating . . . Merrick and Sibalis bring together historians, literary scholars, and political activists from both sides of the Atlantic to examine same-sex sexuality in the past and present."* (Bryant T. Ragan, PhD, Associate Professor of History, Fordham University, New York)

Gay and Lesbian Asia: Culture, Identity, Community, edited by Gerard Sullivan, PhD, and Peter A. Jackson, PhD (Vol. 40, No. 3/4, 2001). *"Superb. . . . Covers a happily wide range of styles . . . will appeal to both students and educated fans."* (Gary Morris, Editor/Publisher, Bright Lights Film Journal)

Queer Asian Cinema: Shadows in the Shade, edited by Andrew Grossman, MA (Vol. 39, No. 3/4, 2000). *"An extremely rich tapestry of detailed ethnographies and state-of-the-art theorizing. . . . Not only is this a landmark record of queer Asia, but it will certainly also be a seminal, contributive challenge to gender and sexuality studies in general."* (Dédé Oetomo, PhD, Coordi-

nator of the Indonesian organization GAYa NUSANTARA: Adjunct Reader in Linguistics and Anthropology, School of Social Sciences, Universitas Airlangga, Surabaya, Indonesia)

Gay Community Survival in the New Millennium, edited by Michael R. Botnick, PhD (cand.) (Vol. 38, No. 4, 2000). *Examines the notion of community from several different perspectives focusing on the imagined, the structural, and the emotive. You will explore a theoretical overview and you will peek into the moral discourses that frame "gay community," the rift between HIV-positive and HIV-negative gay men, and how Israeli gays seek their place in the public sphere.*

The Ideal Gay Man: The Story of Der Kreis, by Hubert Kennedy, PhD (Vol. 38, No. 1/2, 1999). *"Very Profound. . . . Excellent insight into the problems of the early fight for homosexual emancipation in Europe and in the USA. . . . The ideal gay man (high-mindedness, purity, cleanness), as he was imagined by the editor of `Der Kreis,' is delineated by the fascinating quotations out of the published erotic stories." (Wolfgang Breidert, PhD, Academic Director, Institute of Philosophy, University Karlsruhe, Germany)*

Multicultural Queer: Australian Narratives, edited by Peter A. Jackson, PhD, and Gerard Sullivan, PhD (Vol. 36, No. 3/4, 1999). *Shares the way that people from ethnic minorities in Australia (those who are not of Anglo-Celtic background) view homosexuality, their experiences as homosexual men and women, and their feelings about the lesbian and gay community.*

Scandinavian Homosexualities: Essays on Gay and Lesbian Studies, edited by Jan Löfström, PhD (Vol. 35, No. 3/4, 1998). *"Everybody interested in the formation of lesbian and gay identities and their interaction with the sociopolitical can find something to suit their taste in this volume." (Judith Schuyf, PhD, Assistant Professor of Lesbian and Gay Studies, Center for Gay and Lesbian Studies, Utrecht University, The Netherlands)*

Gay and Lesbian Literature Since World War II: History and Memory, edited by Sonya L. Jones, PhD (Vol. 34, No. 3/4, 1998). *"The authors of these essays manage to gracefully incorporate the latest insights of feminist, postmodernist, and queer theory into solidly grounded readings . . . challenging and moving, informed by the passion that prompts both readers and critics into deeper inquiry." (Diane Griffin Growder, PhD, Professor of French and Women's Studies, Cornell College, Mt. Vernon, Iowa)*

Reclaiming the Sacred: The Bible in Gay and Lesbian Culture, edited by Raymond-Jean Frontain, PhD (Vol. 33, No. 3/4, 1997). *"Finely wrought, sharply focused, daring, and always dignified . . . In chapter after chapter, the Bible is shown to be a more sympathetic and humane book in its attitudes toward homosexuality than usually thought and a challenge equally to the straight and gay moral imagination." (Joseph Wittreich, PhD, Distinguished Professor of English, The Graduate School, The City University of New York)*

Activism and Marginalization in the AIDS Crisis, edited by Michael A. Hallett, PhD (Vol. 32, No. 3/4, 1997). *Shows readers how the advent of HIV-disease has brought into question the utility of certain forms of "activism" as they relate to understanding and fighting the social impacts of disease.*

Gays, Lesbians, and Consumer Behavior: Theory, Practice, and Research Issues in Marketing, edited by Daniel L. Wardlow, PhD (Vol. 31, No. 1/2, 1996). *"For those scholars, market researchers, and marketing managers who are considering marketing to the gay and lesbian community, this book should be on required reading list." (Mississippi Voice)*

Gay Men and the Sexual History of the Political Left, edited by Gert Hekma, PhD, Harry Oosterhuis, PhD, and James Steakley, PhD (Vol. 29, No. 2/3/4, 1995). *"Contributors delve into the contours of a long-forgotten history, bringing to light new historical data and fresh insight . . . An excellent account of the tense historical relationship between the political left and gay liberation." (People's Voice)*

Sex, Cells, and Same-Sex Desire: The Biology of Sexual Preference, edited by John P. De Cecco, PhD, and David Allen Parker, MA (Vol. 28, No. 1/2/3/4, 1995). *"A stellar compilation of chapters examining the most important evidence underlying theories on the biological basis of human sexual orientation." (MGW)*

Gay Ethics: Controversies in Outing, Civil Rights, and Sexual Science, edited by Timothy F. Murphy, PhD (Vol. 27, No. 3/4, 1994). *"The contributors bring the traditional tools of ethics and political philosophy to bear in a clear and forceful way on issues surrounding the rights of homosexuals." (David L. Hull, Dressler Professor in the Humanities, Department of Philosophy, Northwestern University)*

Gay and Lesbian Studies in Art History, edited by Whitney Davis, PhD (Vol. 27, No. 1/2, 1994). *"Informed, challenging . . . never dull. . . . Contributors take risks and, within the restrictions of scholarly publishing, find new ways to use materials already available or examine topics never previously explored." (Lambda Book Report)*

Critical Essays: Gay and Lesbian Writers of Color, edited by Emmanuel S. Nelson, PhD (Vol. 26, No. 2/3, 1993). *"A much-needed book, sparkling with stirring perceptions and resonating with depth . . . The anthology not only breaks new ground, it also attempts to heal wounds inflicted by our oppressed pasts." (Lambda)*

Gay Studies from the French Cultures: Voices from France, Belgium, Brazil, Canada, and The Netherlands, edited by Rommel Mendès-Leite, PhD, and Pierre-Olivier de Busscher, PhD (Vol. 25, No. 1/2/3, 1993). *"The first book that allows an English-speaking world to have a comprehensive look at the principal trends in gay studies in France and French-speaking countries." (André Bèjin, PhD, Directeur, de Recherche au Centre National de la Recherche Scientifique (CNRS), Paris)*

If You Seduce a Straight Person, Can You Make Them Gay? Issues in Biological Essentialism versus Social Constructionism in Gay and Lesbian Identities, edited by John P. De Cecco, PhD, and John P. Elia, PhD (cand.) (Vol. 24, No. 3/4, 1993). *"You'll find this alternative view of the age old question to be one that will become the subject of many conversations to come. Thought-provoking to say the least!" (Prime Timers)*

Gay and Lesbian Studies: The Emergence of a Discipline, edited by Henry L. Minton, PhD (Vol. 24, No. 1/2, 1993). *"The volume's essays provide insight into the field's remarkable accomplishments and future goals." (Lambda Book Report)*

Homosexuality in Renaissance and Enlightenment England: Literary Representations in Historical Context, edited by Claude J. Summers, PhD (Vol. 23, No. 1/2, 1992). *"It is remarkable among studies in this field in its depth of scholarship and variety of approaches and is accessible." (Chronique)*

Coming Out of the Classroom Closet: Gay and Lesbian Students, Teachers, and Curricula, edited by Karen M. Harbeck, PhD, JD, Recipient of Lesbian and Gay Educators Award by the American Educational Research Association's Lesbian and Gay Studies Special Interest Group (AREA) (Vol. 22, No. 3/4, 1992). *"Presents recent research about gay and lesbian students and teachers and the school system in which they function." (Contemporary Psychology)*

Homosexuality and Male Bonding in Pre-Nazi Germany: The Youth Movement, the Gay Movement, and Male Bonding Before Hitler's Rise: Original Transcripts from Der Eigene, the First Gay Journal in the World, edited by Harry Oosterhuis, PhD, and Hubert Kennedy, PhD (Vol. 22, No. 1/2, 1992). *"Provide[s] insight into the early gay movement, particularly in its relation to the various political currents in pre-World War II Germany." (Lambda Book Report)*

Gay People, Sex, and the Media, edited by Michelle A. Wolf, PhD, and Alfred P. Kielwasser, MA (Vol. 21, No. 1/2, 1991). *"Altogether, the kind of research anthology which is useful to many disciplines in gay studies. Good stuff!" (Communique)*

Gay Midlife and Maturity: Crises, Opportunities, and Fulfillment, edited by John Alan Lee, PhD (Vol. 20, No. 3/4, 1991). *"The insight into gay aging is amazing, accurate, and much-needed. . . . A real contribution to the older gay community." (Prime Timers)*

Male Intergenerational Intimacy: Historical, Socio-Psychological, and Legal Perspectives, edited by Theo G. M. Sandfort, PhD, Edward Brongersma, JD, and A. X. van Naerssen, PhD (Vol. 20, No. 1/2, 1991). *"The most important book on the subject since Tom O'Carroll's 1980 Paedophilia: The Radical Case." (The North America Man/Boy Love Association Bulletin, May 1991)*

Monographs "Separates" list continued at the back

Gay Bathhouses
and Public Health Policy

William J. Woods, PhD
Diane Binson, PhD
Editors

Gay Bathhouses and Public Health Policy has been co-published simultaneously as *Journal of Homosexuality*, Volume 44, Numbers 3/4 2003.

Harrington Park Press
An Imprint of
The Haworth Press, Inc.
New York • London • Oxford

Cover Design by Paul Cotten.
Historical cover photographs by Mick Hicks.
Man in towel cover photograph by BTS.

Published by

Harrington Park Press®, 10 Alice Street, Binghamton, NY 13904-1580 USA

Harrington Park Press® is an imprint of The Haworth Press, Inc., 10 Alice Street, Binghamton, NY 13904-1580 USA.

Gay Bathhouses and Public Health Policy has been co-published simultaneously as *Journal of Homosexuality*, Volume 44, Numbers 3/4 2003.

The development, preparation, and publication of this work has been undertaken with great care. However, the publisher, employees, editors, and agents of The Haworth Press and all imprints of The Haworth Press, Inc., including The Haworth Medical Press® and Pharmaceutical Products Press®, are not responsible for any errors contained herein or for consequences that may ensue from use of materials or information contained in this work. Opinions expressed by the author(s) are not necessarily those of The Haworth Press, Inc. With regard to case studies, identities and circumstances of individuals discussed herein have been changed to protect confidentiality. Any resemblance to actual persons, living or dead, is entirely coincidental.

Cover design by Lora Wiggins

Library of Congress Cataloging-in-Publication Data

Gay bathhouses and public health policy / William J. Woods, Diane Binson, editors.
    p. ; cm.
    "Co-published simultaneously as Journal of Homosexuality, Volume, 44, no. 3/4, 2003."
    Includes bibliographical references and index.
    ISBN 1-56023-272-2 (hard : alk. paper)–USBN 1-56023-273-0 (soft : alk. paper)
    1. Bathhouses–Government policy–United States. 2. Gay men–Health and hygiene–Government policy–United States. 3. Gay men–Sexual behavior–Government policy–United States. 4. Medical policy–United States.
    [DNLM: 1. Homosexuality, Male. 2. Bath–utilization. 3. Health Policy. 4. Sex Behavior. 5. Sexually Transmitted Diseases–prevention & control. HQ 76.25 G2857 2003] I. Woods, William J., PhD. II. Binson, Diane III. Journal of homosexuality.

RA794.G39 2003
613'.086'6420973–dc21
                                              2003005401

Indexing, Abstracting & Website/Internet Coverage

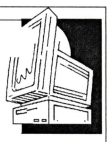

This section provides you with a list of major indexing & abstracting services. That is to say, each service began covering this periodical during the year noted in the right column. Most Websites which are listed below have indicated that they will either post, disseminate, compile, archive, cite or alert their own Website users with research-based content from this work. (This list is as current as the copyright date of this publication.)

Abstracting, Website/Indexing Coverage . . . . Year When Coverage Began

- *Abstracts in Anthropology* **1982**

- *Academic Abstracts/CD-ROM* **1989**

- *Academic ASAP <www.galegroup.com>* **2000**

- *Academic Search: Database of 2,000 selected academic*
  serials, updated monthly: EBSCO Publishing **1995**

- *Academic Search Elite (EBSCO)* **1993**

- *Alternative Press Index (print, online & CD-ROM from NISC)*
  <www.altpress.org> **1996**

- *Applied Social Sciences Index & Abstracts (ASSIA)*
  (Online: ASSI via Data-Star) (CD-Rom: ASSIA Plus)
  <www.csa.com> **1987**

- *This periodical is indexing in ATLA Religion Database, published*
  by the American Theological Library Association
  <www.atla.com> **1986**

- *Book Review Index* **1996**

- *Cambridge Scientific Abstracts <www.csa.com>* **1993**

(continued)

- *CNPIEC Reference Guide: Chinese National Directory
   of Foreign Periodicals* 1995
- *Contemporary Women's Issues* 1998
- *Criminal Justice Abstracts* 1982
- *Current Contents/Social & Behavioral Sciences
   <www.isinet.com>* 1985
- *EMBASE/Excerpta Medica Secondary Publishing Division
   <www.elsevier.nl>* 1986
- *e-psyche, LLC <www.e-psyche.net>* 2001
- *Expanded Academic ASAP <www.galegroup.com>* 1989
- *Expanded Academic Index* 1992
- *Family Index Database <www.familyscholar.com>* 2001
- *Family & Society Studies Worldwide
   <www.nisc.com>* 1996
- *Family Violence & Sexual Assault Bulletin* 1992
- *Gay & Lesbian Abstracts <www.nisc.com>* 1999
- *GenderWatch <www.slinfo.com>* 1999
- *Higher Education Abstracts, providing the latest in research
   and theory in more than 140 major topics* 1997
- *HOMODOK/"Relevant" Bibliographic Database,
   Documentation Centre for Gay & Lesbian Studies,
   University of Amsterdam* 1995
- *IBZ International Bibliography of Periodical Literature
   <www.saur.de>* 1996
- *IGLSS Abstracts <www.iglss.org>* 2000
- *Index Guide to College Journals* 1999
- *Index Medicus (National Library of Medicine)
   <www.nlm.nih.gov)* 1992
- *Index to Periodical Articles Related to Law* 1986
- *InfoTrac Custom <www.galegroup.com>* 1996
- *Leeds Medical Information* 1994
- *LEGAL TRAC on INFOTRAC web
   <www.galegroup.com>* 1990

(continued)

- *MasterFILE: Updated database from EBSCO Publishing* 1995
- *MEDLINE (National Library of Medicine)*
  <www.nlm.nih.gov> 1992
- *MLA International Bibliography (available in print,*
  on CD-ROM, and the Internet) <www.mla.org> 1995
- *National Library of Medicine "Abstracts Section"* 1999
- *OCLC Public Affairs Information Service <www.pais.org>* 1982
- *OmniFile Full Text: Mega Edition (only available electronically)*
  <www.hwwilson.com>. 1987
- *PASCAL, c/o Institute de L'Information Scientifique*
  et Technique <www.inist.fr> 1986
- *Periodical Abstracts, Research I (general and basic reference indexing*
  and abstracting database from University Microfilms
  International (UMI)). 1993
- *Periodical Abstracts, Research II (broad coverage indexing*
  and abstracting database from University Microfilms
  International (UMI)) 1993
- *PlanetOut "Internet site for key Gay/Lesbian Information"*
  <www.planetout.com/> 1999
- *Psychology Today*. 1999
- *RESEARCH ALERT/ISI Alerting Services*
  <www.isinet.com> 1985
- *Sage Family Studies Abstracts (SFSA)* 1986
- *Social Sciences Abstracts & Social Sciences Full Text*
  <www.hwwilson.com>. 1999
- *Social Sciences Citation Index <www.isinet.com>* 1985
- *Social Sciences Full Text (only available electronically)*
  <www.hwwilson.com>. 1991
- *Social Sciences Index (from Volume 1 and continuing)*
  <www.hwwilson.com>. 1991
- *Social Science Source: Coverage of 400 journals in the*
  social sciences area; updated monthly 1995
- *Social Scisearch <www.isinet.com>*. 1985

(continued)

- *Social Services Abstracts <www.csa.com>* 1982
- *Social Work Abstracts <www.silverplatter.com/catalog/swab.htm>* 1994
- *Sociological Abstracts (SA) <www.csa.com>* 1982
- *Studies on Women Abstracts <www.tandf.co.uk>* 1987
- *SwetsNet <www.swetsnet.com>* 2001
- *Violence and Abuse Abstracts: A Review of Current*
  Literature on Interpersonal Violence (VAA) 1995

Special Bibliographic Notes related to special journal issues (separates) and indexing/abstracting:

- indexing/abstracting services in this list will also cover material in any "separate" that is co-published simultaneously with Haworth's special thematic journal issue or DocuSerial. Indexing/abstracting usually covers material at the article/chapter level.
- monographic co-editions are intended for either non-subscribers or libraries which intend to purchase a second copy for their circulating collections.
- monographic co-editions are reported to all jobbers/wholesalers/approval plans. The source journal is listed as the "series" to assist the prevention of duplicate purchasing in the same manner utilized for books-in-series.
- to facilitate user/access services all indexing/abstracting services are encouraged to utilize the co-indexing entry note indicated at the bottom of the first page of each article/chapter/contribution.
- this is intended to assist a library user of any reference tool (whether print, electronic, online, or CD-ROM) to locate the monographic version if the library has purchased this version but not a subscription to the source journal.
- individual articles/chapters in any Haworth publication are also available through the Haworth Document Delivery Service (HDDS).

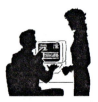

ABOUT THE EDITORS

William J. Woods, PhD, is an assistant adjunct professor in the Department of Medicine, Center for AIDS Prevention Studies, at the University of California San Francisco. He is currently engaged in several prevention intervention trials to reduce risk of HIV and sexually transmitted infections among young men leaving prison and men who have sex with men. He has published several papers related to HIV/STI prevention in bathhouses and sex clubs.

Diane Binson, PhD, is an assistant adjunct professor in the Department of Medicine, Center for AIDS Prevention Studies, at the University of California San Francisco. Her research interests center on the contextual determinants of HIV-related sexual risk behavior among gay men, particularly men who go to public sex environments. She has written several articles related to bathhouses, sex clubs and public cruising areas, as well as on methodological issues related to assessing sexual behavior in surveys.

Gay Bathhouses and Public Health Policy

CONTENTS

Public Health Policy and Gay Bathhouses   1
William J. Woods, PhD
Diane Binson, PhD

A Theoretical Approach to Bathhouse Environments   23
Diane Binson, PhD
William J. Woods, PhD

The History of Gay Bathhouses   33
Allan Bérubé

Number and Distribution of Gay Bathhouses
in the United States and Canada   55
William J. Woods, PhD
Daniel Tracy
Diane Binson, PhD

The San Francisco Bathhouse Battles of 1984:
Civil Liberties, AIDS Risk, and Shifts in Health Policy   71
Christopher Disman

Legal Aspects of Regulating Bathhouses:
Cases from 1984 to 1995   131
Scott Burris

Sex and the Baths: A Not-So-Secret Report   153
Michael Helquist
Rick Osmon

Beyond the Baths: The Other Sex Businesses   177
Michael Helquist
Rick Osmon

Designing an HIV Counseling and Testing Program
    for Bathhouses: The Seattle Experience with Strategies
    to Improve Acceptability   203
    Freya Spielberg, MD, MPH
    Bernard M. Branson, MD
    Gary M. Goldbaum, MD
    Ann Kurth, CNM, PhD
    Robert W. Wood, MD

Comparing Sexual Behavioral Patterns
    Between Two Bathhouses: Implications for HIV
    Prevention Intervention Policy   221
    Matt G. Mutchler, PhD
    Trista Bingham, MPH, MS
    Miguel Chion, MD, MPH
    Richard A. Jenkins, PhD
    Lee E. Klosinski, PhD
    Gina Secura, MPH

Contributors   243

Index   247

Public Health Policy and Gay Bathhouses

William J. Woods, PhD
Diane Binson, PhD

University of California San Francisco

SUMMARY. Public health policy on bathhouses has been limited and poorly documented. This volume is intended to expand policy-makers' and prevention-professionals' knowledge and awareness about gay bathhouses. The present paper provides a context and an overview for the volume by describing the bathhouse environment and how it differs from other public sex environments, and by describing public policies that have been implemented. *[Article copies available for a fee from The Haworth Document Delivery Service: 1-800-HAWORTH. E-mail address: <docdelivery@ haworthpress.com> Website: <http://www.HaworthPress.com> © 2003 by The Haworth Press, Inc. All rights reserved.]*

KEYWORDS. Gay bathhouses, public health policy, HIV, STI

Correspondence may be addressed to William J. Woods, Center for AIDS Prevention Studies, University of California San Francisco, 74 New Montgomery Street, Suite 600, San Francisco, CA 94105 (E-mail: bwoods@psg.ucsf.edu).

[Haworth co-indexing entry note]: "Public Health Policy and Gay Bathhouses." Woods, William J., and Diane Binson. Co-published simultaneously in *Journal of Homosexuality* (Harrington Park Press, an imprint of The Haworth Press, Inc.) Vol. 44, No. 3/4, 2003, pp. 1-21; and: *Gay Bathhouses and Public Health Policy* (ed: William J. Woods, and Diane Binson) Harrington Park Press, an imprint of The Haworth Press, Inc., 2003, pp. 1-21. Single or multiple copies of this article are available for a fee from The Haworth Document Delivery Service [1-800-HAWORTH, 9:00 a.m. - 5:00 p.m. (EST). E-mail address: docdelivery@haworthpress.com].

"Gay bathhouses? Weren't they all closed in the 1980s?" Anyone reading this volume may not be quite so naïve as to ask such a question, but the paucity of knowledge and awareness of gay bathhouses among policy-makers and prevention professionals has long been an obstacle for promoting public health. The contributions in this volume are intended to expand the body of literature informing public health policy regarding gay bathhouses. Because the baths and health issues relating to them have received little attention, and because of the gray zone in which these venues exist, much of the work that has been done has not been documented, or if it has, the documents have not been widely available. For that reason, a number of the papers in this volume are reprinted from earlier, more obscure sources in order that they may have a larger audience and thereby inform and improve relevant public health policy.

BATHHOUSES AND SEX CLUBS

In this volume "bathhouses" and "sex clubs" are considered a single type of venue. For simplicity and ease of reading, unless we are clearly distinguishing between them, when we use the terms "baths," "bathhouses" or "clubs," we are including both bathhouses as well as sex clubs. This is not to imply that there are never differences in these two types of venues. But what a specific venue is called, at least in the United States, appears to depend more on the region where it operates and local regulations than on its physical structure or what amenities are provided (Woods, Binson, Mayne, Gore, & Rebchook, 2001).

To provide an historical context of the baths in gay culture, a brief history of the baths written by Allan Bérubé in 1984 is reprinted in this volume (Bérubé, 1984; a modified version of this article was also reprinted elsewhere, Bérubé, 1996). To provide additional context, we describe the number and distribution of bathhouses in the United States and Canada by reviewing the gay travel guide, *Damron's Address Book*, from its first publication in 1968 to 1999 (Woods, Tracy, & Binson).

From a public health perspective, the baths first came to attention as a result of an exponential increase in sexually transmitted infections (STIs) among men in the 1970s (Darrow, Barrett, Jay, & Young, 1981; Institute of Medicine, 1986; Schreeder et al., 1980; Schreeder et al., 1982; Turner, Miller, & Moses, 1989). The spread of STIs among gay men stimulated public health to seek ways to combat it. Although there appears to have been some mention of closure as an approach (Merino, Judson, Bennett, & Schaffnit, 1979), the predominant message was to educate, test and treat. Several local health departments and community based organizations (CBOs) developed outreach programs for conducting STI testing in the bathhouses (Merino et al., 1979; Merino & Richards, 1977; Ritchey & Leff, 1975). At least one program that started in the 1970s continues to operate to this day (Paul Cotten, personal communication, 2002).

Of course, AIDS (Acquired Immune Deficiency Syndrome) was a different matter in a different time. The STI epidemics were of diseases familiar to health officers and could be treated, while AIDS was completely unknown and unexpected; it took three years just to identify the virus (now called human immunodeficiency virus, or HIV) and there are still arguments about possible routes of transmission. By early 1984, the once rare call for closure had gained a powerful voice in Randy Shilts, a reporter for the *San Francisco Chronicle*, as well as support in powerful gay circles, as Christopher Disman describes in his history of the San Francisco closure policy (in this volume). The twentieth century closed without a cure, although improvements in treatments stalled the rapid decline and death associated with the early epidemic. The tensions between the baths and public health that resulted from the closure debates continue to exist in some cities.

However, there are a number of examples of health professionals from local health departments and academic institutions who have established good relationships with owners and managers of bathhouses. Descriptions of collaborations between health departments and bathhouses can be found for efforts in Los Angeles (Bingham, 2001), Berkeley (Blea, 2001), Seattle (Spielberg, Kurth, Gorbach, & Goldbaum, 2001) and Portland (Oregon) (Van Beneden et al., 2003). Similarly, local coalitions of health professionals at CBOs and managers at clubs have been described (Carrel et al., 1993; Carrel et al., 1994; Kegebein, Bense, & Wohlfeiler, 1992; Klosinski, 2001; Klosinski, McCombs, Miller, & Carrel, 1993). There has also been some research involving the recruitment of bathhouse patrons, e.g. (Keogh, 2000; Richwald, Morisky, Kyle, & Kristal, 1988; Van Beneden et al., 2003), which required collaboration between bathhouse management and academics. Of course, these are just a few examples of documented collaborations and certainly others exist. For example, about 40% of bathhouses in the United States offer HIV testing (Woods, Binson, Mayne, Gore, & Rebchook, 2000; Woods et al., 2001) which typically requires collaboration either with the health department or with CBOs that run outreach HIV testing programs.

GAY BATHS AND OTHER PUBLIC SEX ENVIRONMENTS

Anyone familiar with the literature on HIV-risk among men who have sex with men might wonder why the focus of this volume includes only bathhouses and not public sex environments (PSEs) generally. Indeed, an argument must be made for considering the baths as a type apart from other PSEs, at least in terms of public health policy.

PSEs generally can be understood to include all places outside the home where people meet and engage in sex together. Although this is an impossibly inclusive definition, it is likely to continue to be used for its singular advantage: it is convenient shorthand in talking about a large and diverse group of venues. However, most considerations of PSEs reduce their focus to a few "types" of places.

A typical example of this kind of reduction is when PSEs are further distinguished based on whether the venue is a business, called "commercial sex environments" or "CSEs." While this distinguishes two groups of venues, several problems remain. Are we to consider CSEs a type of PSE (i.e., a subset) or are they two separate categories? Is a commercial venue necessarily a CSE, or does opportunity for sex have to be part of the commerce? For example, the gay gym is a commercial establishment, but when is it a CSE? In many gay gyms, sex is prohibited but men still manage to have sex there. Other gay gyms turn a blind eye to sex between customers in specified areas of the gym, but the places in the gym used for sex also continue to serve their intended purposes. And then there are the gay gyms in name only, i.e., bathhouses that provide gym equipment and are regulated as gyms or health clubs (Woods et al., 2001). Except for this third example, whether to include the gay gym as a CSE is arguable. Yet, for public health policy, there are important differences among these three types of gay gyms that have nothing to do with the fact that they are commercial establishments.

There are three useful distinguishing characteristics of PSEs that are worth noting both for future research and for public policy. The first distinguishing characteristic is whether the place where sex will occur requires a "transformation," i.e., the place was not intentionally created as a sex space. Many PSEs have no intention of providing a space for sex between men, and so the place has to be transformed into a sex space (see Leap, 1999). The introduction to cruising on the Web site called "cruisingforsex.com" says that any place where men meet other men can be transformed into a PSE. Some places are more conducive to such transformations than others (e.g., see Humphries, 1970) and some of these gain reputations, attracting larger numbers of men to these places. However, there are a number of places outside the home that were intentionally constructed to create a safe space for sex where this kind of transformation is not required.

A second useful distinguishing characteristic has to do with the primary purpose of the place, i.e., whether it's primary purpose is to provide a place for sex. This further divides venues into two groups, those that are intentionally constructed to provide a safe place for sex and those that are not. For example, the primary purpose of a bar is to serve alcohol, even if it has a "backroom" (i.e., usually a dark to pitch-black area separated from the rest of the business where men can have sex together). Of course, it must be acknowledged that in most jurisdictions, even those venues whose primary purpose is to provide places for sex exist in a gray zone in which some other official or legal purpose might stand as the primary business purpose. For example, a gay bathhouse might be registered legally as a bathhouse, and in that sense its primary purpose, in the eyes of the law, is not sex between patrons (Weinberg & Williams, 1975).

The third characteristic has to do with exclusivity, i.e., the venue operates as a club that can discriminate in its membership. Of course, this discrimination primarily restricts by age and gender (i.e., adult male), but some clubs have other restrictions as well, such as particular sexual interests or clothing. This exclusivity dramatically reduces the likelihood that someone would enter who was not comfortable with and willing to participate in the sex space. Thus, PSEs can be distinguished usefully according to whether the sex space was created intentionally, whether the venue operates primarily to provide a sex space, and whether it operates with exclusivity, i.e., requires membership. As seen in Table 1, PSEs vary along these dimensions. These variations suggest the opportunity to address HIV prevention strategically, and may be related to real distinctions in the kinds of risk activity and the degree to which men engage in these activities while frequenting these different venues. This combination of circumstances might create an environment where prevention can be practical, direct and sexually explicit without risk of offending a population not intended to be targeted (i.e., women, children, and exclusively heterosexual men).

But are these distinctions important in terms of where risk behavior actually occurs? Yes. Analysis of data from the Urban Men's Health

TABLE 1. Types of PSEs by Dimensions of the Way Sex Space Is Provided

	Intentional	Primary	Exclusive
Public Venues*	No	No	No
Traditional Bathhouse	No	No	No
Gay Motel	Yes & No	No	No
Gay Resort	Yes & No	No	No
Gay Gym	Yes & No	No	Yes & No
Backroom (Gay Bar)	Yes	No	No
Adult Bookstore	Yes	Yes & No	No
Adult Movie House	Yes	Yes & No	No
Gay Bathhouse	Yes	Yes	Yes
Gay Sex Club	Yes	Yes	Yes

*For example, parks, beaches, alleys, and t-rooms.

Survey (UMHS), a probability sample of urban MSM in four U.S. HIV epicenters showed that there were significant differences in risk behavior between men who go to baths and men who go to other PSEs (Binson et al., 2001). Similar results were found with a cohort sample of gay men in Amsterdam (de Wit, 1997). Thus, combining all these venues together creates a serious problem by giving the appearance that these environments are similar (when in fact there are a number of significant differences) and it suggests that a one-size-fits-all prevention policy is adequate. Thus, in terms of prevention policy, gay baths are a particular case. In fact, data from Matt Mutchler and his colleagues, who describe in this volume their formative work in two Los Angeles area bathhouses, remind us that policy might best be driven by consideration of individual venues rather than broad categories.

THE BATHHOUSE ENVIRONMENT

A few ethnographic and sociological accounts of bathhouses are available from sources prior to AIDS (Brown, 1979; Rumaker, 1979; Styles, 1979; Weinberg & Williams, 1975), and descriptions have been retrospectively written in the post-AIDS era (Brodsky, 1993; Tattleman, 1999). In fact, much of what is known about the baths and sex clubs comes from these sources. At bathhouses (as opposed to sex clubs) men usually rent a locker or room and remove their street clothes in exchange for a towel they wrap around their waist or otherwise carry around with them. Sex may occur in any number of places: rented rooms, showers, steamrooms, or other public areas, such as orgy rooms or dark mazes. Some public areas might be equipped with glory holes, which are holes in a wall that vary in size, but are generally large enough and at waist level so that one man can pass his penis through the hole. Of course venues vary from one to the next in terms of which types of places are available. At sex clubs, on the other hand, men typically wear their street clothes (although some clubs provide facilities to check clothes) or fetish attire. Many of the same type spaces for sex are available as are found in the traditional gay bathhouse, though sex clubs typically do not have private rooms to rent or water amenities like hot tub, sauna, steamroom and shower (Leap, 1999; Lindell, 1996). Because of these differences, sex clubs can occupy smaller physical settings and operate with lower overhead. Despite these few structural differences, they share many similarities, especially when considering risk for the transmission of HIV and other sexually transmitted infections. Primarily, both bathhouses and sex clubs facilitate easy introduction to many men looking for sex and an easy place to engage in both oral and anal intercourse.

These descriptions provide little hard data on where the riskiest sex takes place, and the extent to which the bathhouses facilitate riskier or safer sex. Two journalist described prevention and education in the San Francisco baths and other sex venues in 1984 (Helquist & Osmon, 1984a, 1984b). In fact, the spark for this volume originated with the idea simply to reprint these two articles, first published in a San Francisco gay monthly now called *Bay Times*. Other investigators at the time, including social scientists, journalists and police, explored the baths and sex clubs, but none of these took as thorough and systematic an approach as Helquist and Osmon. Their work, reprinted in this volume, provides a detailed picture of the gay bathhouse environment in the midst of the early AIDS epidemic.

An important component of any sex space is the participants and the meanings they attribute to sex in the baths (Elwood & Williams, 1998; Keogh, 2000). For instance, in Elwood and Williams' study, men perceive the bathhouse to be risky, in part, because they think other patrons were more likely to be HIV-positive. Further, the baths were seen as a fantasy setting, a place to get away or escape from the stress and tension of their day-to-day lives. Keogh and Weatherburn concluded that the fantasy nature of these environments allowed men to take on social or fantasy roles that were not their own in the real world. Contrary to stereotype, some men reported having sex with men they had seen or known from previous visits or other situations. In both studies, communication was described as tending to be less verbal, relying on visual or tactile cues instead.

Keogh and Weatherburn further identified several common elements to patron stories of UAI: Their study respondents were always the insertive partner, but at the same time the passive partner (i.e., in terms of who seemed to be in control of the situation and so they were somehow unable to control their situation), and they attributed sexual promiscuity and/or seropositive status to the partners. Men who did not engage in anal intercourse in these venues were concerned with maintaining personal hygiene in public places, while those who did engage in anal intercourse in these settings, even in circumstances of total anonymity, characterized the experience as emotionally or socially intimate.

A number of studies suggest that, although a high proportion of men who engage in high-risk sex go to the baths, only a minority of men report engaging in high-risk behavior while there (Binson et al., 2001; Klosinski, 1995; Richwald et al., 1988; Van Beneden et al., 2002; Woods, Mayne, & Kegeles, 1996). Nevertheless, there was little scientific debate as to whether or not the bathhouses played a role in the early and rapid spread of AIDS among gay men. Several early case-control studies identified "number of partners" as an important variable associated with AIDS (e.g., Darrow, Jaffe, & Curran, 1983; Jaffe et al., 1983; Marmor et al., 1982), sometimes measuring sex in the baths. Measuring the proportion of a participant's sexual partners in the past year who were from a bathhouse, Jaffe and his colleagues found bathhouses to be significantly related to illness (i.e., AIDS), though not as strongly related as number of partners. Similarly, the Darrow group found that number of partners was more important in explaining AIDS cases than was meeting partners at the baths. Darrow reaches the same conclusion in an analysis of the San Francisco Cohort data, which he reported in a letter to the San Francisco Department of Health in 1984 (see Disman, this volume; Murray, 1988, reports that these data were never published).

Other epidemiological papers reported associations of HIV with unprotected receptive anal intercourse as well as number of partners (e.g., Anderson & Levy, 1985; Curran et al., 1985; Goedert et al., 1984; Kingsley et al., 1987; Moss et al., 1987). Some investigators commented on the lower risk of insertive or active anal intercourse and the lack of evidence for oral transmission. Using data from the San Francisco Men's Health Study, Grant and his colleagues (Grant, Wiley, & Winkelstein, 1987) estimated infectivity of HIV. They suggested that the predominance of HIV infection among gay men was due primarily to their having more sexual partners than heterosexual women, and not because of differences in rectal and vaginal mucosa. Thus, although the association between HIV infection and bathhouses was never robust, the strong association of HIV with numbers of partners continued to hold.

Given that the baths facilitated men having larger numbers of partners than they might otherwise have been able to accrue, a few investigators attempted to address this facilitative role of the baths. While many investigators used the word "promiscuous" to describe multiple partners, the papers do not take a moral tone or judgment and they seemed to be aware that men would have engaged in this behavior at a time when it was impossible to know the risk of acquiring HIV. One projection from the early data suggested that the rapid spread of AIDS in the gay community may have been due more to the behavior of only a few men who had very many partners, rather than to a large number of men who had many partners (Peto, 1986). On the other hand, the same model showed an even higher prevalence of infection among those who practiced serial monogamy with an annual change in partners.

A related area of investigation is the rapid turnover of multiple sexual encounters, referred to as "concurrency" (Garnett & Johnson, 1997). Theoretically, concurrency is a booster of HIV transmission (Potterat et al., 1999; Rosenberg, Gurvey, Adler, Dunlop, & Ellen, 1999; Watts & May, 1992), though as yet there is no empirical data establishing a relationship of concurrency to HIV transmission in these settings. The two analyses reported by Darrow suggest that number of partners and not bathhouses (an indicator of social networking) were responsible for AIDS cases (Darrow et al., 1983; and Darrow's 1984 letter mentioned previously). Also, projections by Peto (1986) suggest that at least one alternative to concurrency, serial monogamy, can sometimes be a greater problem in the longer-term.

Reviewers for the Institute of Medicine summed up the epidemiological evidence in 1989. They concluded that the direct relationship of bathhouses to HIV transmission was unlikely, but they played a role at one time in facilitating exactly the kind of behavior that was most suitable to widespread transmission of HIV, i.e., UAI (Turner et al., 1989). So, defenders of the bathhouses, claiming that it is not *where* you do it but *what* you do (Bolton, Vincke, & Mak, 1992; Murray, 1988), have some support from the epidemiological literature. However, the related issues of number of partners and concurrency (especially in the immediate succession) have not been addressed satisfactorily. Because patron studies to date have been based on convenience samples, probability sampling of patrons will greatly enhance and improve our understanding of the sexual behavior and risk that occur in the bathhouses, and thereby better inform public health policy and prevention efforts.

PUBLIC HEALTH POLICY

Structural policy can be thought of as any policy that affects the bathhouse environment, generally as a result of external factors. Thus public health policies are structural by their nature, as well as external, determining at a larger society level the ways bathhouses are regulated and operated. Some structural policies attempt to eliminate bathhouses through closure (eradication policy), while others attempt to modify bathhouses by regulating various aspects of the environment. These later policies typically include the bathhouse management in the policy-making, and so can be thought of as collaborative policies.

Eradication Policy

As we have shown, early in the AIDS epidemic in the U.S., the gay community and public health officials recognized the centrality of gay bathhouses in the spread of HIV. To close bathhouses or leave them open as sites of education and prevention framed the public policy debate early in the epidemic. The legacy of that debate continues to shape the landscape of these spaces today. Although San Francisco and New York City generated much attention for their efforts to close local bathhouses, the extent to which other localities attempted to implement a closure policy is less well documented. In fact, it is difficult to say with certainty what other cities considered or implemented a closure policy. An *Advocate* article reports that Georgia closed the Atlanta clubs through an act of the state legislature (Walter, 1986). Bolton, Vincke and Mak (1992) included Las Vegas (Nevada) as a city that closed its bathhouses, but they provided no date and no reference for this claim. They also state that Stockholm was the only European city to close its bathhouse, a claim confirmed by Henriksson and Mansson (Henriksson & Mansson, 1995). Keogh and his colleagues (1998), however, indicate that other European cities debated the policy, and suggest that at least some also implemented closure. Bathhouses are also plentiful in other major English-speaking countries, such as Canada and Australia, and in some Latin American (e.g., Brazil) and East Asian (e.g., China) countries. Nevertheless, despite the attention of the 1984 debates, we are not aware of any reference to closure policy being discussed or implemented in any of these other countries. Scott Burris provides in this volume a thorough and intriguing legal perspective of the closure policy, from a paper he first presented in New York on December 11, 1995, at the Henry J. Kaiser Family Foundation's workshop titled: "Public Policy Aspects of Regulating Bathhouses and Sex Clubs."

Collaborative Policy

One way to organize collaborative policy is to draw on the person-environment theory of Rudolf Moos (Moos, 1994), who defines the environment in terms of four domains: supra personal, institutional context, physical setting, and policies and services. Using his latter three domains, we will organize the extant examples of collaborative policies. We explore the application of this theoretical approach to the baths in more detail in another paper in this volume (Binson & Woods).

Institutional Context. Institutional context relates to management and size of a particular facility. An excellent example of a policy influencing this domain can be found in Los Angeles. Although the health department in Los Angeles County did not attempt to implement a closure policy, sometime in the mid-1980s or later, several lawsuits were instigated targeting individual bathhouses to force closure. In 1992 the county District Attorney initiated a process to resolve the situation and settle the lawsuits by convening a series of meetings between owners and AIDS service and prevention/education organizations to develop a protocol for the bathhouses targeted in the lawsuits (Carrel et al., 1993; Carrel et al., 1994; Klosinski et al., 1993). This policy focused on promoting collaboration among these groups to develop behavioral interventions that would reduce risk behavior among patrons. The result was a staff-training program developed and implemented by the AIDS Project Los Angeles (APLA), a local CBO. The terms of the settlement required all bathhouse staff to participate (Klosinski et al., 1993). Though this policy applied only to those businesses named in the lawsuits, APLA invited other clubs to participate and many did (Lee Klosinski, APLA, personal communication, 1997). An additional benefit of this collaboration occurred during a recent syphilis outbreak in Los Angeles, where APLA was able to coordinate a dialogue among the bathhouses, the health department and other interested parties to respond quickly and effectively to the outbreak (Klosinski, 2001).

Another example of institutional context was a group in San Francisco that organized in response to a resurgence of gay sex venues in the late 1980s. After some police harassment and threats from the fire department and the health department, a group of owners, health educators, and concerned community members organized the Coalition for Healthy Sex (Kegebein et al., 1992) in 1990. City officials from the health department later became key members and leaders of the group. The purpose of the coalition was to assure the safety of the environments, to support a continued commitment to safer sex, and to ensure that places for people to meet and enjoy sex continued to exist. Though the organization dissolved within the decade, its impact continues to influence the perception and implementation of San Francisco's policy regulating sex clubs.

Physical Setting. The physical setting includes characteristics of the venue having to do with the physical structure or architecture of the facility. The attempts to close bathhouses in San Francisco and New York City led to two public policies regulating the types of spaces permitted in the bathhouses. As mentioned, San Francisco's Public Health Department took its initial step to close the city's bathhouses (and other assorted sex venues) in 1984 (Bayer, 1989; also see the two Helquist & Osmon papers and the Disman paper in this volume). The end result, however, was a court order establishing, first, that the public health director can proscribe any sexual behavior he considered a risk for transmission, and, second, that the city can require that all patron behavior be observable by venue staff. Much of the San Francisco policy that resulted from the court order remains in effect to this day. The only change has been to what sexual behaviors are proscribed by the health department, i.e., initially all sexual contacts were proscribed, now only unprotected anal intercourse is proscribed.

The current bathhouse regulations in New York City also resulted from an attempt by that city's health departments to close local bathhouses. In 1985 New York State passed a law intended to close bathhouses, but implementation was left to the local jurisdiction (Bayer, 1989). The health department successfully closed some of the bathhouses. For example, the St. Marks, which received the bulk of the city's attention, was closed, while the Mount Morris Baths, which opened circa 1895, remains open to this day. Thus, some bathhouse owners were successful in limiting the interpretation of the law, and as a result New York City policy permits bathhouses to operate but they must ensure that patrons do not have sex at the venue. This policy resulted in removing open spaces where staff might observe patrons having sex (e.g., orgy rooms, mazes), and posting signs on doors to all rented rooms that indicate that occupancy by more than one person is strictly prohibited. Thus, all sex must take place behind closed doors and in violation of the stated rules.

In San Francisco and New York the resulting policies regulate the physical structure of the environments that owners can create. Ironically, however, the policies are diametrically opposite. The San Francisco policy eliminates private spaces while the New York policy results in the removal of public spaces where sex might occur. What real impacts these regulations have on reducing HIV transmission have not been thoroughly investigated. However, analysis of the Urban Men's Health Survey data show that risk behavior among residents of these cities who visit the baths is not significantly different from risk behavior in cities without these regulations (Woods, Binson, Pollack, & Catania, 2003).

Policies and Services. This domain is the area where most health and safety issues would be addressed, including education (such as fliers, brochures and posters). Even before the closure policy received a lot of attention, health professionals and gay community members were developing prevention interventions for the community. Although there is some doubt about the value of information and education at this time in the U.S. epidemic, there is no question that these were important intervention aims in the early 1980s (Murray, 1988; Richwald et al., 1988). As early as 1982, The Sisters of Perpetual Indulgence (a San Francisco nonprofit group) prepared, published and distributed a flier called "Play Fair!" The flier addressed preventing STIs and included a special section on Kaposi's sarcoma and pneumocystis pneumonia (part of the flier is reproduced in Figure 1). Similarly, in 1984, the Harvey Milk Lesbian & Gay Democratic Club of San Francisco prepared and published a flier, called "Can We Talk?" Their flier addressed risk behavior for transmission of "the AIDS virus" (part of the flier is reproduced in Figure 2), and was distributed through various local CBOs. Both fliers were found in gay venues throughout the city, and gave gay men very basic information about avoiding infection, and stand as a clear indication that the community itself organized an early and swift response to this new threat. It is not clear to what extent these two fliers were distributed in the bathhouses, if at all, but four sources identify bathhouses as places where fliers (not necessarily these fliers) were seen between 1983 and 1986 (Helquist & Osmon, 1984a, 1984b; Murray, 1988; Richwald et al., 1988).

FIGURE 1. Play Fair, part of flier, copyright 1982 by The Sisters of Perpetual Indulgence, reprinted here by permission.

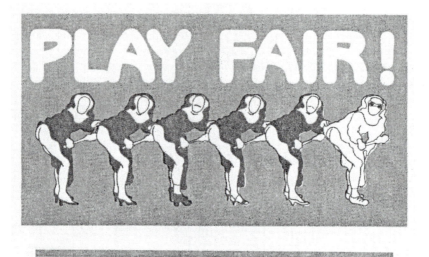

Q: What is an STD?

A: STD stands for "Sexually Transmitted Disease". These are all infections caused by bacteria, viruses and parasites that can be passed from person to person in the course of getting your rocks off. Sisters have listed some of the most common STDs below. There are others which are not as common, but are becoming more so, weekend by weekend.

KAPOSI'S SARCOMA and PNEUMOCYSTIS PNEUMONIA In the past 2 years some gay men in large American cities have developed severe problems with their immune systems. (The immune system helps the body fight off disease.) No one knows what is causing these problems, or whether they are sexually transmitted but they are serious and occasionally fatal. Some of these men have developed Kaposi's sarcoma —the so-called "gay cancer." Some have Pneumocystis pneumonia—"gay pneumonia." SYMPTOMS: KS: Painless, slightly raised red or purple blotches on the skin, weight loss, or swollen lymph nodes. Pneumocystis: Dry cough, fever, or run-down feeling. Some gay men have neither disease but nonetheless have weakened immune systems. If you have enlarged lymph nodes, fever, weight loss, unusual or persistent viral or fungal infections, dry cough, or unusual skin spots, don't panic, but see a doctor who is familiar with this problem. Bay Area Physicians for Human Rights can refer you.

The Helquist and Osmon articles, reprinted in this volume, give examples of the variety of other education and prevention efforts that can be employed in the baths. Indeed, it would appear from a telephone survey of U.S. bathhouses in 1996 that the prevention efforts identified before 1984 have since been implemented at least across most of the U.S.

FIGURE 2. Can We Talk?, part of flier, copyright 1984 by Harvey Milk Lesbian & Gay Democratic Club, reprinted here by permission.

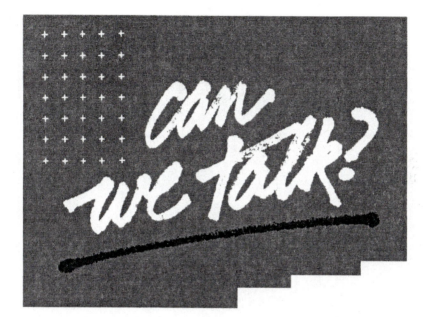

FUCKING
DON'T FUCK WITHOUT A CONDOM!

Being Fucked—There is increasing evidence that this is one of the most likely ways to get AIDS. Because the rectal lining can be easily injured during anal intercourse, germs in your partner's semen can enter your bloodstream. If you're going to fuck, use a condom. Condoms have been shown to be reliable in containing viruses. To further reduce the transmission of germs, don't use spit as a lubricant and only use lubricants from a spigot-like closed container that can't spread fecal germs.

Fucking—Use of a condom will protect the wearer against many of the sexually transmitted infections.

Dildos and Toys—If you are going to use dildos and toys, only use your own. Keep your toys clean, don't share them with others.

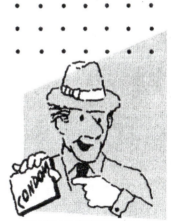

STREETS OF SAN FRANCISCO
STAR
KARL MODERN SEZ:
"DON'T LEAVE HOME
WITHOUT IT"

(Woods et al., 2001). That survey revealed that all bathhouses provide condoms to patrons for free. Lubricant was also available at all the sites, though not always for free. Furthermore, 95% of the venues provided educational materials such as posters and flyers about HIV/AIDS. However, only 40% provide HIV testing on site and half of these also provide STI testing. In short, the telephone survey found that some HIV services were nearly universal (e.g., providing condoms, lubricants, fliers) and others were less prevalent (providing HIV or STI testing). Unfortunately, the way these services are provided and advertised is not known, and the full impact of these services on the club environment and patron sexual risk behavior has not been tested. Nor was there any indication given as to whether the services provided were the result of the owner's initiative, competition with other venues, or local public health policy.

Clearly, there is much to learn about the efficacy of these services, and the other affects of collaborative policy described previously on the risk and protective behavior of men who go to the baths. Moreover, it is important to learn the value of using public health policy to improve the implementation of these programs. However, some attention has been given to on-site HIV and STI testing as prevention interventions in bathhouses (Spielberg et al., 2003; Spielberg et al., 2003; Spielberg et al., 2001; Woods et al., 1999). Freya Spielberg and her colleagues describe the development and implementation of the HIV testing program they initiated in all three bathhouses in Seattle, Washington.

Policy Summary

Public health has been accused of either debating closure or paying no attention whatsoever (Bolton et al., 1992). Despite a few examples at the local level, this seems accurate. Nevertheless, the evidence also suggests that there are a number of policies other than closure that public health could embrace to reduce the risk of HIV and STI transmission in the baths. More evaluation and research is necessary to determine what, if any, efficacy these potential policies might have. Regardless of demonstrated efficacy, public health will be in a better position if it actively pursues and maintains collaborative relationships with owners and managers of the baths, as was witnessed in the Los Angeles response to a syphilis outbreak. It is hoped that the papers in this volume will contribute significantly to greater knowledge and awareness of the possibilities for improved public policy in addressing HIV/STI risk in gay bathhouses.

ACKNOWLEDGMENTS

The authors gratefully acknowledge the generous assistance, support and encouragement of Dr. John De Cecco, without whom this effort would not have been undertaken, much less completed. Special thanks to Paul Cotten and Megan Gaffigan for their contributions to acquiring and organizing all the necessary backup documents.

The authors also wish to acknowledge contributions to completing this paper. They extend special thanks to several people who participated in making it possible to reprint parts of educational fliers first published in 1982 and 1984. Of course, among these are the Sisters of Perpetual Indulgence and the Harvey Milk Democratic Club who hold copyright and generously gave the authors their permission to reprint the fliers in whole or part. Also, Megan Gaffigan assisted with obtaining copyright permission and, with Christopher Disman, prepared the fliers for this manuscript. The authors also wish to thank Megan Gaffigan and Paul Cotten for their assistance with the literature and references, and Paul Cotten for his review of this manuscript.

REFERENCES

Anderson, R. E., & Levy, J. A. (1985). Prevalence of antibodies to AIDS-associated retrovirus in single men in San Francisco. *Lancet, 1*(8422), 217.

Bayer, R. (1989). *Private acts, social consequences: AIDS and the politics of public health.* New Brunswick, NJ: Rutgers University Press.

Bérubé, A. (1984). The history of gay bathhouses. *Coming Up!, 15-19.*

Bérubé, A. (1996). The history of gay bathhouses. In E. G. Colter, W. Hoffman, E. Pendleton, A. Redick, & D. Serlin (Eds.), *Policing public sex* (pp. 187-220). Boston: South End Press.

Bingham, T. (2001). *The Los Angeles bathhouse study: Elements of an innovative HIV-testing program.* Paper presented at the Gay men/MSM bathhouse & sex club meeting, Sacramento, CA.

Binson, D., Woods, W. J., Pollack, L., Paul, J., Stall, R., & Catania, J. (2001). Differential HIV risk in bathhouses and public cruising areas. *American Journal of Public Health, 91*(9), 1482-1486.

Blea, L. (2001). *Men's project: A collaborative effort to arrest the spread of HIV and other STIs in public sex environments in the city of Berkeley.* Paper presented at the Gay men/MSM bathhouse & sex club meeting, Sacramento, CA.

Bolton, R., Vincke, J., & Mak, R. (1992). Venues of HIV transmission or AIDS prevention? *National AIDS Bulletin, 9,* 22-26.

Brodsky, J. I. (1993). The Mineshaft: A retrospective ethnography. In J. P. De Cecco & J. P. Elia (Eds.), *If you seduce a straight person, can you make them gay? Issues in biological essentialism versus social constructionism in gay and lesbian identities.* New York: The Haworth Press, Inc.

Brown, R. M. (1979). Queen for a day: Stranger in paradise. In K. Jay & A. Young (Eds.), *Lavender culture* (pp. 69-76). New York: Harcourt Brace Jovanovich.

Carrel, J., Klosinski, L., Ramirez, R., McCombs, M., ReConco, O., Miller, S., & Richwald, G. (1993). *From litigation to health education: An emerging model for*

STD/HIV education for bathhouse personnel. Paper presented at the American Public Health Association 121st annual meeting, San Francisco, CA.

Carrel, J., Klosinski, L., Ramirez, R., Richwald, G., McCombs, M., ReConco, O., & Ferry, J. (1994). *Bathhouses: Creating safer sex environments.* Paper presented at the American Public Health Association 122nd annual meeting, Washington, D.C.

Curran, J. W., Morgan, W. M., Hardy, A. M., Jaffe, H. W., Darrow, W. W., & Dowdle, W. R. (1985). The epidemiology of AIDS: Current status and future prospects. *Science, 229*(4720), 1352-1357.

Darrow, W. W., Barrett, D., Jay, K., & Young, A. (1981). The gay report on sexually transmitted diseases. *American Journal of Public Health, 71*(9), 1004-1011.

Darrow, W. W., Jaffe, H. W., & Curran, J. W. (1983). Passive anal intercourse as a risk factor for AIDS in homosexual men. *Lancet, 2*(8342), 160.

de Wit, J. B., de Vroome, E. M., Sandfort, T. G., van Griensven, G. J. (1997). Homosexual encounters in different venues. *International Journal of STDs and AIDS, 8*(2), 130-134.

Elwood, W. N., & Williams, M. L. (1998). Sex, drugs, and situation: Attitudes, drug use, and sexual risk behaviors among men who frequent bathhouses. *Journal of Psychology & Human Sexuality, 10*(2), 23-44.

Garnett, G. P., & Johnson, A. M. (1997). Coining a new term in epidemiology: Concurrency and HIV. *AIDS, 11*(5), 681-683.

Goedert, J. J., Sarngadharan, M. G., Biggar, R. J., Weiss, S. H., Winn, D. M., Grossman, R. J., Greene, M. H., Bodner, A. J., Mann, D. L., Strong, D. M. et al. (1984). Determinants of retrovirus (HTLV-III) antibody and immunodeficiency conditions in homosexual men. *Lancet, 2*(8405), 711-716.

Grant, R. M., Wiley, J. A., & Winkelstein, W. (1987). Infectivity of the human immunodeficiency virus: Estimates from a prospective study of homosexual men. *J Infect Dis, 156*(1), 189-193.

Helquist, M., & Osmon, R. (1984a). Beyond the baths: The other sex businesses. *Coming Up!,* 19-24.

Helquist, M., & Osmon, R. (1984b). Sex and the baths: A not so secret report. *Coming Up!,* 17-22.

Henriksson, B., & Mansson, S. A. (1995). Sexual negotiation: An ethnography study of men who have sex with men. *Culture and Sexual Risk: Anthropological Perspectives on AIDS,* 157-182.

Humphries, L. (1970). *Tearoom trade: Impersonal sex in public places.* New York: Aldine de Gruyter.

Institute of Medicine. (1986). *Confronting AIDS: Directions for public health, health care, and research.* Washington, D.C.: National Academy of Sciences.

Jaffe, H. W., Choi, K., Thomas, P. A., Haverkos, H. W., Auerbach, D. M., Guinan, M. E., Rogers, M. F., Spira, T. J., Darrow, W. W., Kramer, M. A., Friedman, S. M., Monroe, J. M., Friedman-Kien, A. E., Laubenstein, L. J., Marmor, M., Safai, B., Dritz, S. K., Crispi, S. J., Fannin, S. L., Orkwis, J. P., Kelter, A., Rushing, W. R., Thacker, S. B., & Curran, J. W. (1983). National case-control study of Kaposi's sarcoma and Pneumocystis carinii pneumonia in homosexual men: Part 1. Epidemiologic results. *Annals of Internal Medicine, 99*(2), 145-151.

Kegebein, V., Bense, B., & Wohlfeiler, D. (1992). *Keeping San Francisco sex clubs open and safe: Community/public health partnerships.* Paper presented at the VIII International Conference on AIDS, The Netherlands.

Keogh, P. G., Weatherburn, P. (2000). Tales from the backroom: Anonymous sex and HIV risk in London's commercial gay sex venues. *Venereology, 13*(4), 150-155.

Kingsley, L. A., Detels, R., Kaslow, R., Polk, B. F., Rinaldo, C. R., Jr., Chmiel, J., Detre, K., Kelsey, S. F., Odaka, N., Ostrow, D. et al. (1987). Risk factors for seroconversion to human immunodeficiency virus among male homosexuals. Results from the Multicenter AIDS Cohort Study. *Lancet, 1*(8529), 345-349.

Klosinski, L. (2001). *Los Angeles success story.* Paper presented at the Gay men/MSM bathhouse & sex club meeting, Sacramento, CA: California State Office of AIDS, Department of Health Services.

Klosinski, L., & Carrel, J. (June 1995). *The Los Angeles Bathhouse Patron Survey; Implications for Program Design.* Paper presented at the 17th National Lesbian and Gay Health Conference and 13th Annual AIDS/HIV Forum, Minneapolis, MN.

Klosinski, L., McCombs, M., Miller, S., & Carrel, J. (1993). *A bathhouse HIV education campaign.* Paper presented at the Fifteenth National Lesbian and Gay Health Conference and Eleventh Annual AIDS/HIV Forum, Houston, TX.

Leap, W. L. (1999). Introduction. In W. L. Leap (Ed.), *Public sex/Gay space* (pp. 1-21). New York: Columbia University Press.

Lindell, J. (1996). Policing public sex. In D. Serlin (Ed.), *Policing public sex* (pp. 73-80). Boston: South End Press.

Marmor, M., Friedman-Kien, A. E., Laubenstein, L., Byrum, R. D., William, D. C., D'Onofrio, S., & Dubin, N. (1982). Risk factors for Kaposi's sarcoma in homosexual men. *Lancet, 1*(8281), 1083-1087.

Merino, H. I., Judson, F. N., Bennett, D., & Schaffnit, T. R. (1979). Screening for gonorrhea and syphilis in gay bathhouses in Denver and Los Angeles. *Health Reports, 94*(4), 376-379.

Merino, H. I., & Richards, J. B. (1977). An innovative program of venereal disease casefinding, treatment and education for a population of gay men. *Sexually Transmitted Diseases, 4*(2), 50-52.

Moos, R. H. (1994). *The social climate scales: A user's guide,* 2nd edition. Palo Alto, CA: Consulting Psychologists Press.

Moss, A. R., Osmond, D., Bacchetti, P., Chermann, J. C., Barre-Sinoussi, F., & Carlson, J. (1987). Risk factors for AIDS and HIV seropositivity in homosexual men. *American Journal of Epidemiology, 125*(6), 1035-1047.

Murray, S. O., & Payne, K. W. (1988). Medical Policy Without Scientific Evidence: The Promiscuity Paradigm and AIDS. *California Sociologist* (Winter-Summer 1988).

Peto, J. (1986). AIDS and promiscuity. *The Lancet,* 979.

Potterat, J. J., Zimmerman-Rogers, H., Muth, S. Q., Rothenberg, R. B., Green, D. L., Taylor, J. E., Bonney, M. S., & White, H. A. (1999). Chlamydia transmission: Concurrency, reproduction number, and the epidemic trajectory. *American Journal of Epidemiology, 150*(12), 1331-1339.

Richwald, G. A., Morisky, D. E., Kyle, G. R., & Kristal, A. R. (1988). Sexual activities in bathhouses in Los Angeles County: Implications for AIDS prevention education. *Journal of Sex Research, 25*(2), 169-180.

Ritchey, M. G., & Leff, A. M. (1975). Venereal disease control among homosexuals: An outreach program. *JAMA: Journal of the American Medical Association, 232*(5), 509-510.

Rosenberg, M. D., Gurvey, J. E., Adler, N., Dunlop, M. B., & Ellen, J. M. (1999). Concurrent sex partners and risk for sexually transmitted diseases among adolescents. *Sexually Transmitted Diseases, 26*(4), 208-212.

Rumaker, M. (1979). *A day and a night at the baths.* San Francisco, CA: Grey Fox Press.

Schreeder, M. T., Thompson, S. E., Hadler, S. C., Berquist, K. R., Maynard, J. E., Ostrow, D. G., Judson, F. N., Braff, E. H., Nylund, T., Moore, J. N., Gardner, P., Doto, I. L., & Reynolds, G. (1980). Epidemiology of Hepatitis B infection in gay men. *Journal of Homosexuality, 5*(3), 307-310.

Schreeder, M. T., Thompson, S. E., Hadler, S. C., Berquist, K. R., Zaidi, A., Maynard, J. E., Ostrow, D. G., Judson, F. N., Braff, E. H., Nylund, T., Moore, J. N., Gardner, P., Doto, I. L., & Reynolds, G. (1982). Hepatitis B in homosexual men: Prevalence of infection and factors related to transmission. *Journal of Infectious Diseases, 146*(1), 7-15.

Spielberg, F., Branson, B., Goldbaum, G., Lockhart, D., Kurth, A., Celum, C. L., Rossini, A., Critchlow, C. W., & Wood, R. (2003). Overcoming barriers to HIV testing: Preferences for new strategies among clients of a needle exchange, a sexually transmitted disease clinic, and sex venues for men who have sex with men. *Journal of Acquired Immune Deficiency Syndromes, 32,* 318-328.

Spielberg, F., Branson, B. M., Goldbaum, G., Henderson, K., Kurth, A., & Wood, R. W. (2003). Designing an HIV counseling and testing program for bathhouses: The Seattle experience with strategies to improve acceptability. *Journal of Homosexuality, 44*(3/4), pp. 203-219.

Spielberg, F., Kurth, A., Gorbach, P., & Goldbaum, G. (2001). Moving from apprehension to action: A qualitative study of HIV counseling and testing preferences in three at-risk populations. *AIDS Education and Prevention, 13*(6), 524-540.

Styles, J. (1979). Outsider/insider: Researching gay baths. *Urban Life, 8*(2), 135-152.

Tattleman, I. (1999). Speaking to the gay bathhouse: Communicating in sexually charged spaces. In W. L. Leap (Ed.), *Public sex/Gay space* (pp. 71-94). New York: Columbia University Press.

Turner, C. F., Miller, H. G., & Moses, L. E. (1989). *AIDS: Sexual behavior and intravenous drug use.* Washington, DC: National Academy Press.

Van Beneden, C. A., Modesitt, S., O'Brien, K., Yusem, S., Rose, A., & Fleming, D. (2002). Sexual behaviors in an urban bathhouse fifteen years into the HIV epidemic. *Journal of Acquired Immune Deficiency Syndromes, 30,* 522-526.

Walter, D. (1986). Georgia bans gay bathhouses. *Advocate* (447), 15-16.

Watts, C. H., & May, R. M. (1992). Concurrent partnerships and the spread of HIV. *Math Biosci, 108,* 89-104.

Weinberg, M. S., & Williams, C. J. (1975). Gay baths and the social organization of impersonal sex. *Social Problems, 23*(2), 124-136.

Woods, W. J., Binson, D., Mayne, T. J., Gore, R., & Rebchook, G. (2000). HIV/STD education & prevention in U.S. sex environments. *AIDS, 14*(5), 625-626.

Woods, W. J., Binson, D., Mayne, T. J., Gore, R., & Rebchook, G. (2001). Facilities and HIV prevention in bathhouse and sex club environments. *The Journal of Sex Research, 38*(1), 68-74.

Woods, W. J., Binson, D. B., Pollack, L. M., Wohlfeiler, D., Stall, R. D., & Catania, J. A. (2003). Public policy regulating gay bathhouses: Affects on HIV risk behavior. *Journal of Acquired Immune Deficiency Syndromes, 32,* 417-423.

Woods, W. J., Mayne, T., & Kegeles, S. (1996). *Few men have unprotected intercourse.* Paper presented at the XI International Conference on Acquired Immune Deficiency Syndrome in Vancouver, British Columbia, Canada.

A Theoretical Approach
to Bathhouse Environments

Diane Binson, PhD
William J. Woods, PhD

University of California San Francisco

SUMMARY. HIV prevention guidelines have aimed primarily at the individual level, although recently the field of public health has begun to focus more on structural level interventions. This paper explores an application of Rudolf Moos' person-environment theory as one model that helps to provide an understanding of the dynamic relationship between bathhouse patrons and the environment within which they engage in sexual activities. Understanding how different dimensions of the environment affect behavior could be instrumental in revealing not just that a bathhouse intervention works, but *how* it works. Knowing more about how an intervention works would facilitate its application in other settings. *[Article copies available for a fee from The Haworth Document Delivery Service: 1-800-HAWORTH. E-mail address: <docdelivery@haworthpress.com> Website: <http://www.HaworthPress.com> © 2003 by The Haworth Press, Inc. All rights reserved.]*

Support for this paper was provided in part by a grant from the National Institute of Mental Health (R01 MH61162).

Correspondence may be addressed to Dr. Diane Binson, Center for AIDS Prevention Studies, University of California San Francisco, 74 New Montgomery Street, Suite 600, San Francisco, CA 94105 (E-mail: dbinson@psg.ucsf.edu).

[Haworth co-indexing entry note]: "A Theoretical Approach to Bathhouse Environments." Binson, Diane, and William J. Woods. Co-published simultaneously in *Journal of Homosexuality* (Harrington Park Press, an imprint of The Haworth Press, Inc.) Vol. 44, No. 3/4, 2003, pp. 23-31; and: *Gay Bathhouses and Public Health Policy* (ed: William J. Woods, and Diane Binson) Harrington Park Press, an imprint of The Haworth Press, Inc., 2003, pp. 23-31. Single or multiple copies of this article are available for a fee from The Haworth Document Delivery Service [1-800-HAWORTH, 9:00 a.m. - 5:00 p.m. (EST). E-mail address: docdelivery@haworthpress.com].

10.1300/J082v44n34_02

KEYWORDS. Gay bathhouses, person-environment theory, HIV, interventions

One theme that runs through many of the papers collected in this volume is the use of bathhouse settings for promoting health education and prevention programs. The goal of these programs is to encourage men to protect themselves from activities related to sexually transmitted infections (STIs). For the most part, the prevention guidelines are aimed at the individual level. They are organized and directed specifically at the bathhouse patron, to inform and encourage him to practice safe behaviors, whether it be using condoms, abstaining from high risk behavior, negotiating safer behavior with someone he's about to have sex with, reducing the number of sex partners, or seeking out HIV/STI testing.

What has been missing in how policy makers and researchers have thought about these facilities is the ways in which environments–the physical, social, normative environments–influence individual behavior. Managers and architects who design bathhouse environments no doubt have given considerable attention to how different physical constructions influence patron behaviors. Unfortunately, these "behavioral blueprints" circulate only within industry networks and as such don't reach those who design prevention policy. Additionally, although there has been a long history of academic studies that examine the relationship between the environment and human behavior, there is little trace of these perspectives in social behavioral research on AIDS (Magnusson & Toerestad, 1992; Maines, 1979; Proshansky, 1990; Tomaszewski, 1980; Walsh, Clark, & Price, 1992). Perhaps the medicalization of AIDS that reduced the behavioral paradigm to models in which individual skills, motivations, and intentions tend to dominate may explain the lack of attention to the study of the environment as an influential factor in explaining risk behavior (Sumartojo, 2000; Tawil, Verster, & O'Reilly, 1995).

STUDYING THE ENVIRONMENT

One can conceptualize the environment at several different levels, depending on the research question. For example, urbanologists focus on the design of cities and how the physical landscape of buildings and open space influence sociability among urban residents (Jacobs, 1961).

Other writers focus within institutions or organizations, for example, schools (Anthony, 1987; Minami, 1995), or work space and the correlation to worker satisfaction and productivity (Wineman, 1982), or the structure of a hospital ward and the set of social relationships in the ward (Holahan, 1976). However, even when looking at institutions or organizations, one could focus on how the external environment influences the internal environment and how the change in the internal environment affects individual behavior.

Similarly, the study of bathhouse environments might focus on the external or internal environment. For example, one could define the external bathhouse environment as society's political and/or economic forces. In particular, the political environment could be defined as the community's laws and statues in order to study how the legal system was used as a tool to influence the shape and uses of bathhouses. Or, we could define the political and economic environment as agents of social control (the police, local elected governments, health departments, and local citizens groups) and examine efforts to close bathhouses in the mid-1980s. What were the effects of this turbulent environment on bathhouses, how did they respond (or not) to the threats of closure, what were the alignments and realignments? For examples of public policy that had implications for changing the environment within the bathhouse see the section on structural policy in the introduction to this volume (Woods and Binson).

Our particular interest is in understanding how the environment within the bathhouse might influence patrons' risk or protective behaviors. Despite decades of scientific study associating sexual risk behavior with the environment, little is known or understood about how these environments facilitate risk. While there are other theories that may help explain patron risk behaviors in bathhouse settings, we've found that the person-environment theory of Rudolf Moos and colleagues is a particularly promising model to apply to the study of the bathhouse environment and its influence on patron behavior.

PERSON-ENVIRONMENT THEORY

Since the 1970s, Moos and his colleagues have studied the person-environment interaction in specific settings (e.g., geriatric, psychiatric and residential treatment facilities, educational institutions, prisons and military bases) (Moos, 1994), developing a conceptual model to describe the interaction of person-environment factors (Moos, 1997; Moos & Lemke,

1996). Moos conceives of the environment as a dynamic system composed of four principal domains: supra personal (i.e., aggregate staff and client characteristics), institutional context (i.e., management, size), physical features, and policies and services (Moos & Lemke, 1996). These four interacting domains form the environment's "social climate," what Moos calls the "personality" of an environment (Moos, 1994).

Moreover, Moos' model goes beyond a unilateral approach to further the understanding of the interaction effects of the environment and individual characteristics, i.e., the ways in which the environment differentially affects individuals' behavior. According to this theory, it is the social climate, interacting with a person's individual characteristics that conditions or determines behavioral outcomes. Figure 1 illustrates the application of the complete model to the bathhouse environment. The shaded areas in the figure represent aspects of the theory relevant to the environment, which generally are the factors affecting the social climate, and the interaction of the environment with the individual patron. Individual characteristics and behavior are unshaded. However, the individual's behavior is affected by the interaction of the individual ("person

FIGURE 1. Moos' Person-Environment Theoretical Framework Applied to the Risk Environment/Bathhouse Setting

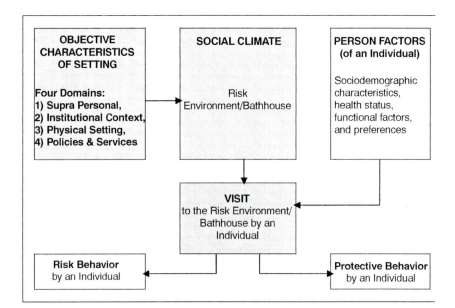

factors") with the environment ("social climate"), which leads to individual patron behavior (in this case, either risk or protective behavior).

BATHHOUSE SOCIAL CLIMATE

Using ethnographic reports (Brodsky, 1993; Brown, 1979; Rumaker, 1979; Styles, 1979; Tattleman, 1999; Weinberg & Williams, 1975) and preliminary observations of several bathhouses in different regions of the U.S., it is possible to suggest a description of the social climate of bathhouses according to Moos' theory. Table 1 is a listing of examples of dimensions within the four domains that form the bathhouse environment.

To start, the theory recognizes all environments as dynamic. "The aggregate of the members' attributes, the supra personal domain, in part defines the subculture that develops in a group, and this subculture in turn can influence the behavior of individual members" (p. 29) (Moos & Lemke, 1996). Thus, changes in the make-up of the group affect social climate. A bathhouse could be considered extremely dynamic, since the turnover of members (the supra personal domain) is constant. This appears to play an important role in the sexual tension in the atmosphere, and potentially to the degree to which risk behavior is prevalent.

The second domain, institutional context, is primarily related to management and size of a facility (Moos & Lemke, 1996). Of note about a bathhouse environment is how little interaction there is between bathhouse staff and the patrons. Most patrons encounter staff only at two times during their stay, when checking in and again when checking out. There is also the occasional passing in the hall, as staff go about clean-

TABLE 1. Four Domains of the Bathhouse Environment

SUPRA PERSONAL	INSTITUTIONAL CONTEXT	PHYSICAL SETTING	POLICIES & SERVICES
Aggregate staff and patron demographics Staff and patron interactions Patrons interaction with other patrons	History of the establishment Size and layout of the building Number of staff	Types of spaces Area for socializing Atmosphere: Clean/Dirty Dark/Bright Music/Art/Wall decoration HIV fliers/posters	Rules re: Drugs Talking/silence What norms for HIV risk HIV/STI testing Counseling available DPH/CBO involved Other special events

ing rooms or public areas, as well as a visit to the front desk to exchange towels. But generally, the patrons go about using the facility with little or no intrusion from staff. An exception would be facilities that have staff "monitors" who roam in search of rule violations. Just as Moos found (Moos & Lemke, 1996), facility size is important because it generally has great influence on the physical amenities and services an institution can afford to offer. The size of the facility can contribute significantly to risk behavior not only due to monitoring, but also to the number and diversity of patrons it will accommodate and draw.

Moos' third domain, physical setting, includes amenities, resources and structural characteristics. In the bathhouse environment these would include things like showers, steamroom, sauna, as well as specialized private rooms (e.g., with a bed or a television), dark areas, mazes, and glory holes. Some bathhouses have swimming pools, outdoor areas, or other special areas. In general, though, the physical setting is designed to enhance a sexualized atmosphere. The patron is provided with numerous opportunities to interact with men, and the setting characteristics are designed to foster and enhance those interactions. Once beyond the front lobby (and sometimes even there) (Rumaker, 1979), the sexualized atmosphere bombards the senses. Almost any interaction has a sexual potentiality.

The final domain of Moos' theory, policies and services, is the area where most health and safety issues would be addressed. Much like the institutional context (and very unlike the physical setting), this domain goes on behind the scenes or in a passive way. While much of this is significant in terms of costs or commitment from the bathhouse management, most patrons have little direct interaction with these features. Many bathhouses across the United States have some level of health services available in the bathhouse, usually, at a minimum, addressing sexually transmitted infections (Woods, Binson, Mayne, Gore, & Rebchook, 2001).

STRUCTURAL INTERVENTIONS AND BATHHOUSE POLICY

There has been discussion lately in public health and HIV prevention about the need to design HIV/STI interventions at the structural level (Sumartojo, 2000; Tawil et al., 1995). Individual-level interventions tend to locate the cause of risk, and, therefore, the target of change, within the individual. Structural-level interventions, on the other hand, focus on changing environments. For example, to examine the determi-

nants of risky sex using an individual-level focus, one would think of
education or skills or a psychological problem as the probable root
cause of risk (Cohen & Scribner, 2000). The mechanisms of change in
an intervention, then, would be to provide more education or more
counseling or both. In contrast, structural-level interventions aim outside the individual and most are designed to alter the context within
which individuals live, behave, interact, and assemble. While the goal
might be to change individual behavior, the mechanism to change behavior is beyond the individual. Typically these mechanisms have been
described as a change in law, public policy or regulation at various levels of government or changes in the physical or social environment
within organizations (e.g., bathhouses), or changes in norms at the soci-
etal, community, or organizational level. That is, structural interventions seek to change the environment with the potential of reaching a
greater number of individuals than an individual-level intervention.

BATHHOUSE INTERVENTIONS RECONSIDERED

It's useful to think about the kinds of interventions that have been implemented in bathhouse settings in the context of Moos' model of social
climate. As we mentioned earlier, many of the prevention programs introduced in bathhouses over the last 20 years have been directed at individuals to encourage them to reduce their risk behavior. These have
included distribution of condoms, safe-sex workshops, sexual behavior
guidelines, health-related pamphlets, and opportunities for HIV/STI
testing, to name a few (Woods et al., 2001). Moos' theory provides a
framework for conceptualizing the environment within the bathhouse in
terms of four domains. Its interesting to step back and view these interventions from the perspective of Moos' theory of social climate and to
ask oneself how does incorporating these interventions into the bathhouse environment affect the social climate? And if the social climate
has changed, what is the effect on patron behavior? For example, does
having condoms available and well distributed throughout the club influence men by the very nature of seeing condoms everywhere they
look? Does the availability of condoms encourage men to change their
behavior, even those who do not use them because they decide instead
to engage in less risky behavior? Is there perhaps a "tipping point"
whereby having two, three, or more prevention programs changes the
bathhouse social climate and reduces patron risk behavior (Binson,
Woods, & Mayne, 1998)? It is likely that there are benefits for individu-

als who participate in prevention programs. But, the more promising and, perhaps, more important question is does a transformed social climate result in less risk behavior and more protective behavior not only for those who participate, but also for those who do not? Do the individual level interventions in these settings also embody a structural efficacy? In the theoretical ideal, public policy could direct prevention interventions (at both external and internal levels) to transform the bathhouse social climate (the shaded areas in Figure 1). One measure of the efficacy of such transformations can be evaluated by measuring the change in patrons' risk and protective behavior.

The person-environment theory is one model that helps to provide an understanding of the dynamic relationship between bathhouse patrons and the environment within which they engage in sexual activities. One aspect of this theory that is particularly promising is the possibility of explaining how interventions work. Breaking the environment into component parts (domains) allows us to begin to see how different dimensions of the environment might affect behavior. Being able to tease out the ways in which interventions affect the social climate and in turn patron behavior would help us understand not just that an intervention works, but *how* it works. Knowing more about how an intervention works would facilitate its application in other settings.

REFERENCES

Anthony, K. H. (1987). Environment-behavior research applied to design: The case of Rosemead High School. *Journal of Architectural & Planning Research, 4*(2), 91-107.

Binson, D., Woods, W. J., & Mayne, T. J. (1998). *HIV prevention: Some better than others.* Published abstract, 12th World AIDS Conference, Geneva.

Brodsky, J. I. (1993). The Mineshaft: A retrospective ethnography. In J. P. De Cecco & J. P. Elia (Eds.), *If you seduce a straight person, can you make them gay? Issues in biological essentialism versus social constructionism in gay and lesbian identities.* New York: The Haworth Press, Inc.

Brown, R. M. (1979). Queen for a day: Stranger in paradise. In K. Jay & A. Young (Eds.), *Lavender culture* (pp. 69-76). New York: Harcourt Brace Jovanovich.

Cohen, D. A., & Scribner, R. (2000). An STD/HIV prevention intervention framework. *AIDS Patient Care & STDs, 14*(1), 37-45.

Holahan, C. J. (1976). Environmental change in a psychiatric setting: A social systems analysis. *Human Relations, 29*(2), 153-166.

Jacobs, J. (1961). *The death and life of great American cities.* New York: Random House.

Magnusson, D., & Toerestad, B. (1992). The individual as an interactive agent in the environment. In W. B. Walsh, K. H. Clark, & R. H. Price (Eds.), *Person-environment psychology: Models and perspectives*. Hillsdale, NJ: Lawrence Erlbaum Associates.

Maines, D. R. (1979). Ecological and negotiation processes in New York subways. *Journal of Social Psychology, 108*(1), 29-36.

Minami, H., & Tanaka, K. (1995). Social and environmental psychology: Transaction between physical space and group-dynamic processes. *Environment & Behavior, 27*(1), 43-55.

Moos, R. H. (1994). *The social climate scales: A user's guide*, 2nd edition. Palo Alto, CA: Consulting Psychologists Press.

Moos, R. H. (1997). *Evaluating treatment environments: The quality of psychiatric and substance abuse programs*, 2nd edition. New Brunswick, NJ: Transaction Publishers.

Moos, R. H., & Lemke, S. (1996). *Evaluating residential facilities: The multiphasic environmental assessment procedure*. Thousand Oaks, CA: Sage Publications.

Proshansky, H. M. (1990). The pursuit of understanding: An intellectual history. In I. Altman, & Christensen, K. (Eds.), *Environment and behavior studies: Emergence of intellectual traditions* (pp. 9-30). New York: Plenum Press.

Rumaker, M. (1979). *A day and a night at the baths*. San Francisco, CA: Grey Fox Press.

Styles, J. (1979). Outsider/insider: Researching gay baths. *Urban Life, 8*(2), 135-152.

Sumartojo, E. (2000). Structural factors in HIV prevention: Concepts, examples, and implications for research. *AIDS, 14*(Suppl1), S3-S10.

Tattleman, I. (1999). Speaking to the gay bathhouse: Communicating in sexually charged spaces. In W. L. Leap (Ed.), *Public sex/Gay space* (pp. 71-94). New York: Columbia University Press.

Tawil, O., Verster, A., & O'Reilly, K. R. (1995). Enabling approaches for HIV/AIDS prevention: Can we modify the environment and minimize the risk? *AIDS, 9*(12), 1299-1306.

Tomaszewski, R. J., Strickler, D. P., & Maxwell, W. A. (1980). Influence of social setting and social drinking stimuli on drinking behavior. *Addictive Behaviors, 5*(3), 235-240.

Walsh, W. B., Clark, K. H., & Price, R. H. (1992). Person-environment psychology: An introduction. In W. B. Walsh, K. H. Clark, & R. H. Price (Eds.), *Person-environment psychology: Models and perspectives*. Hillsdale, NJ: Erlbaum Associates.

Weinberg, M. S., & Williams, C. J. (1975). Gay baths and the social organization of impersonal sex. *Social Problems, 23*(2), 124-136.

Wineman, J. D. (1982). Office design and evaluation: An overview. *Environment & Behavior, 14*(3), 271-298.

Woods, W. J., Binson, D., Mayne, T. J., Gore, R., & Rebchook, G. (2001). Facilities and HIV prevention in bathhouse and sex club environments. *The Journal of Sex Research, 38*(1), 68-74.

The History of Gay Bathhouses

Allan Bérubé

SUMMARY. Public policy regarding bathhouses has been criticized as being based on political expediency rather than on medical or social science. To affect that shortcoming, we include here a brief history of gay bathhouses. The history of the baths is rarely told, but whenever it is told it necessarily reflects the times in which it was written. For that reason, we include a history written in 1984, at the time that much of what was known about AIDS, routes of transmission and the role of the bathhouses was very much in flux. This history not only gives a context for the current discussion, but also allows the reader to see the history from that distant point in time. This paper was first published in December 1984 as an article in *Coming Up!*, a lesbian and gay community newspaper published monthly in San Francisco (California). It was later edited and reprinted in a book titled *Policing Public Sex* (1996). The version of the paper presented here is from the original 1984 article (pp. 15-19); several images appeared with the article that are not reproduced here. As with all the reprinted papers in this volume, no editorial changes were made to the paper and only minor typographical errors were corrected.

KEYWORDS. Gay bathhouses, history

For centuries, society has stigmatized homosexual men and women as sinners, criminals and diseased because of their sexuality. Baths and bars were the first institutions in the United States that contradicted

---

This paper reprinted here by permission of the San Francisco *Bay Times*. Correspondence may be addressd: 64 Carrier Street, Liberty, NY 12754.

[Haworth co-indexing entry note]: "The History of Gay Bathhouses." Bérubé, Allan. Co-published simultaneously in *Journal of Homosexuality* (Harrington Park Press, an imprint of The Haworth Press, Inc.) Vol. 44, No. 3/4, 2003, pp. 33-53; and: *Gay Bathhouses and Public Health Policy* (ed: William J. Woods, and Diane Binson) Harrington Park Press, an imprint of The Haworth Press, Inc., 2003, pp. 33-53.

10.1300/J082v44n34_03

these stigmas and gave Gay Americans a sense of pride in themselves and their sexuality. As such, gay bars and baths are an integral part of gay political history.

Before there were any openly gay or lesbian leaders, political clubs, books, films, newspapers, businesses, neighborhoods, churches or legally recognized gay rights, several generations of pioneers spontaneously created gay bathhouses and lesbian and gay bars. These men and women risked arrest, jail sentences, loss of families, loss of jobs, beatings, murders, and the humiliation that could lead to suicide; in order to transform public bars and bathhouses into safety zones where it was safe to be gay. In a nation which has for generations mobilized its institutions toward making gay people invisible, illegal, isolated, ignorant and silent, gay baths and bars became the first stages of a movement of civil rights for gay people in the United States.

For the gay community, gay bathhouses represent a major success in a century-long political struggle to overcome isolation and develop a sense of community and pride in their sexuality, to gain their right to sexual privacy, to win their right to associate with each other in public, and to create "safety zones" where gay men could be sexual and affectionate with each other with a minimal threat of violence, blackmail, loss of employment, arrest, imprisonment, and humiliation.

EARLY HISTORY OF GAY BATHHOUSES IN THE UNITED STATES

The transformation of Turkish baths, Russian baths, public baths, health resorts and spas into gay institutions began in the late 19th and early 20th centuries in the United States. In California as in other states, all sex acts between men were illegal as "crimes against nature." Thus, men having sex with each other had no legal right to privacy. Records of California state appeals court cases around the turn of the century contain many cases of men who were arrested after landlords, housekeepers, neighbors, policemen, and YMCA janitors drilled tiny holes in walls, peeped through keyholes, transoms, and windows or broke down doors to discover men having sex with each other. Because *all* sex acts between men were considered public and illegal, gay men were forced to become sexual outlaws [see Figure 1]. They became experts at stealing moments of privacy and at finding the cracks in society where they could meet and not get caught.

FIGURE 1. Sidebar to Original Article (p. 16)

A 1929, Bathhouse Raid

As the police, moral reformers and the public became more aware that some Turkish baths were becoming "favorite spots" for homosexuals, police entrapment and raids became more common. In April, 1929, an eyewitness account of a raid in the Lafayette Brothers' Turkish Baths in New York City was published in a German gay magazine (reprinted in Jonathan Katz' *Gay/Lesbian Almanac*, 1983). The raid took place during a city-wide politically-motivated crackdown on "suspicious" people. In this raid, the night manager, who had apparently protected the homosexual patrons on his shift, was arrested with the patrons.

The 26-year-old eyewitness, apparently a European, described the baths as "very well known . . . especially as a place where likeminded people meet." He entered the baths at 9pm, paid $1 at the door, undressed and entered the steam room, where he had sex with another man. "At about ten-thirty I go up to the dormitory and look for a bed. Chance brings me together with a young, racy Sicilian. Unfortunately, we hadn't noticed that there were eight detectives among the customers of the baths. . . . Now it's midnight, and I'm already asleep, my friend at my side.

"All at once there's a whistle, someone yells 'Hallo,' and everyone has to go to the front room. The bath is locked shut. Various people were struck down, kicked, in short, the brutality of these officials was simply indescribable. A Swede standing next to me was struck on the eye with a bunch of keys, and then he got hit in the back so that two of his ribs broke. There was a telephone call, and then policemen, even more detectives, an inspector, and the captain of the detectives arrived. 'Put on your clothes.' Everyone, from the night manager to the most recent arrival, was put in the paddy wagon, taken to the station, and jailed. By noon on Sunday we appeared before the magistrate's court at 2nd Avenue and 2nd Street and were charged with things we hadn't done. All of the forty-five people who were there were fined ten dollars, or two days in the workhouse, except for four who were sentenced to six months, three weeks, two weeks and one month . . .

"This is the crudest treatment I've ever been through," the young man concluded. "I would place the blame for this on the terrible furtiveness and phony shame which prevails here in America . . ."

These "cracks in society" expanded as the rapidly growing cities of the late 19th and early 20th centuries created more and more public places where men could be anonymous and intimate with each other. These included public parks at night; certain streets and alleys; empty box cars in train yards; remote areas of beaches; YMCA rooms, steam rooms and shower stalls; public rest rooms in department stores, train stations, bus depots, parks, subway stations and public libraries; balconies of silent movie theaters; cheap hotel rooms; parked automobiles; and bathhouses. These locations were attractive because they offered the protection of anonymity, a degree of privacy, and the possibility of meeting men interested in sex. They were dangerous because men who went there could be arrested, blackmailed, beaten, robbed, or killed.

Despite these dangers, a growing number of men risked having sex in these semi-public places. In San Francisco, early popular spots included the Ferry Building, Union Square, Market Street from the Embarcadero to 5th Street, the corner of Powell and Market, the Embarcadero, YMCA, the men's rooms in Macys and the Emporium, the streets in the Tenderloin, the balconies of the Unique Theater and other movie houses on Market Street, the all-night cafeterias and their toilets on Market Street between 5th and 3rd Streets, the Harman Baths, Sutro Turkish Baths, and the changing booths at Sutro Baths near the Cliff House.

Bathhouses evolved in gay institutions not by themselves, but in the context of the slowly developing sexual landscape in the nation's cities. Men–both heterosexual and homosexual–chose to meet each other in the bathhouses as alternatives to other places, usually for reasons of safety and privacy.

Historical records beginning in the 1890s document the 4 major stages in which bathhouses evolved into homosexual institutions.

1. *Ordinary Bathhouses*: Places where men would occasionally have sex but where it was unusual.

2. *Favorite Spots:* These bathhouses–and YMCAs–developed reputations as "favorite spots" for men to have sex with each other. Word got out that a certain manager, masseur, employee or police officer would look the other way when they were on duty, or that homosexuals were known to gather there at certain hours, usually in the afternoon or late at night. Some private bathhouse owners tried to prevent their places from becoming popular homosexual spots and called in the police or hired thugs and private guards. Others did not discourage their specialized clientele, paid off the cop on the neighborhood beat, told the managers and employees to keep things discreet, and increased their profits.

3. *Early Gay Bathhouses:* Mostly evolved in the 1920s and 1930s. Physically, they were no different than other Turkish or Russian baths, except that sex was permitted in closed and locked cubicles. These places were subject to raids by vice squads, in which the employees, managers and owners could be arrested with their patrons. The owners sometimes tried to protect their patrons from arrest, blackmail and violence if at all possible without hurting their businesses.

4. In the 1950s and 1960s, the first *Modern Gay Bathhouses* began to open. These places were meant to be exclusively gay and catered to the sexual and social needs of gay men. With the beginning of the gay liberation movement in the 1970s, these bathhouses went through dramatic changes. Today there are approximately 200 gay bathhouses in the United States, from Great Falls, Minnesota and Toledo, Ohio to New York City, Los Angeles and San Francisco.

Many of the advantages of modern gay bathhouses were already recognized in the newspaper, medical and legal reports describing the earliest "favorite spots":

1. *Safety:* Patrons felt they were more protected from blackmail at
the baths than in other public places; the baths seemed to offer an alternative to sex in the public parks; and there was additional safety in numbers and in their identification as homosexual baths, because those who
would be offended by the behavior there would not go there or would
leave.

2. *Democracy and Camaraderie:* Some accounts describe "the early
gay bathhouses" as refuges from society's prejudice against homosexuals, as oases of freedom and homosexual camaraderie. The clientele
was primarily homosexual and from a variety of occupations and
classes, temporarily "democratic" in their nakedness. Members of the
staff, too, were sometimes homosexual making these early baths one of
the first identifiably gay social and sexual institutions.

3. *Privacy:* Sex took place in an establishment separated from the
general citizenry. This created the first urban zone of privacy, as well as
safety, for gay men.

4. *Erotic Facilities:* Cabins, steam rooms, dressing rooms, pools and
hot air rooms were all available for meeting other patrons. At primarily
homosexual establishments, patrons could feel secure that other patrons
would not be offended by physical intimacy between men.

5. *A Social Environment:* Old friendships could be renewed, "new
intimacies" were "ever in the air." Patrons socialized with each other in
the common areas.

6. *Protection:* The management and employees often tried to protect
the patrons from violence and blackmail: the police generally allowed
the bathhouses to stay open because they were discreet "outlets for the
vast homosexual life of the city" and because some of the "best citizens" went there.

THE EARLY HISTORY OF GAY BATHHOUSES
IN SAN FRANCISCO

In San Francisco, the first references to sex between men in the City's
Turkish baths began in the 1890s. By the late 1920s and early '30s, a
few of these "favorite spots" in San Francisco began to turn into predominantly gay bathhouses. These are the earliest gay bathhouses in
San Francisco that anyone alive today remembers. One was known as

the Palace Baths near the Palace Hotel; another was known as Jack's Baths on 3rd near Mission Street.

When these gay bathhouses emerged in the 1920s and 1930s, they offered homosexual men a new option: they could meet and have sex in a gay bathhouse, in addition to having sex with heterosexual men in a public bathhouse. Many men who came out before there were any gay baths looked down on having sex with other gay men. They had learned to prefer "servicing" straight men in semipublic places.

It was a later generation of gay men who, partly by using the gay bathhouses, learned to enjoy having sex with and loving other gay men. At a time when no one was saying "gay is good," the creation of an institution in which gay men were encouraged to appreciate each other was a major step toward gay pride. Since then, several generations of gay men–partly because of the opportunities provided them by gay bathhouses and, later, gay bars–have learned to prefer sexual partners who are also gay. The bathhouses, thus, are partly responsible for this major change in the sexual behavior and self-acceptance of gay men.

These first gay baths in San Francisco went through dramatic changes during World War II. Thousands of servicemen went to the baths in San Francisco before shipping overseas.

Many were afraid they would never return from the Pacific, and felt they deserved one last chance to enjoy other men in the freedom of the baths. The baths were an important alternative to picking someone up in Union Square, the main gay cruising park in the city, because they offered a safe and private place at a time when hotel rooms downtown were impossible to find. They were also a useful alternative to the gay bars that began to open in San Francisco during the war, because many of the bars were declared "off-limits to military personnel."

During the 1950s, two major changes took place that affected the baths in San Francisco. For the first time, baths like the Club Turkish Baths in the Tenderloin had opened with the intent of catering to a homosexual clientele. These were the City's first modern gay bathhouses. But this happened at a time when an anti-homosexual panic was sweeping the country, inspired by McCarthyism and bathhouses as well as bars became the primary targets of anti-gay crackdowns and panics. The protective anonymity at the baths helped many gay men survive the crackdowns of the 1950s.

Despite the stepped-up attacks on gay baths and bars during the 1950s, which one local newspaper called a "war on homosexuals," more baths–and bars–slowly opened as explicitly gay institutions. In May of 1954, possibly the first guide to San Francisco's gay bars and baths was printed. It was a mimeographed sheet handed out at a Mattachine Society meeting–San Francisco's first Gay organization. Warning that it was "Confidential and Unofficial," it listed Jack's Baths, the Club Baths on Turk, the Palace Baths on 3rd Street and the San Francisco Baths on Ellis. In the 1960s, a second generation of modern gay baths opened, including Dave's Baths on Broadway (which moved from Sansome and Washington and claimed to be the first gay-owned bathhouse in San Francisco), the Baths on 21st Street, and the Ritch Street Baths.

By the late 1960s and throughout the 1970s, gay bathhouses went through dramatic changes. They established themselves as a major gay institution that could both shape and respond to the rapid social, sexual and political changes that were taking place. Some of these important changes included:

- San Francisco's Embarcadero YMCA, along with many YMCAs in other cities, had earned reputations as "favorite spots" for sexual activity at least as early as World War II. By the 1960s, according to men who were early frequenters of the Y, sexual activity there began to decline. Many of these men attribute this decline to the opening of gay baths during the same period.
- In March 1966, as gay bathhouses continued to open in San Francisco, the Assistant Police Chief announced a " 'crackdown'. . . on public baths . . . suspected of tolerating . . . homosexual problems." Undercover police arrested a Methodist minister at the 21st Street Baths for "making sexual advances to a policeman," as well as a clerk who refused to call the police after the arrest of his patron. The crackdown was short-lived and the minister's trial ended in a hung jury.
- When the "Summer of Love" in 1967 created a new communal ethic among the hippie generation, "orgy rooms" were installed in some bathhouses where group sex became more popular.
- In January 1976, Representative Willie Brown's "consenting adult sex bill" went into effect in California. As a result, gay bathhouses and the sex that went on in them became legal for the first time.
- In January 1978, to test whether this new law applied to bathhouses, officers from Northern Station raided the Liberty Baths on Post Street and arrested three patrons for "lewd conduct" in a public place. This was the first bathhouse raid since the 1966 crackdown, but Police Chief Charles Gain denied that the police were beginning a new crackdown. The District Attorney's Office dropped the charges against the three men. "There's no question this was a private place," the DA's office said.
- In the late '70s, with the new technology that allowed the projection of video tapes onto large screens, bathhouses began installing

video rooms where patrons could masturbate alone or with each other while watching gay sex videos that many could not afford to have at home. In fact, masturbation became a more acceptable practice in the bathhouses partly as a result of these videos.

- In the 1960s, '70s and '80s, several bathhouses, including Dave's, the Barracks, Liberty Baths and the Bulldog Baths, encouraged gay artists who were their employees or patrons to decorate the walls with erotic murals. For some artists, these murals were the first opportunity to create and display their art for an exclusively gay audience.
- In the 1970s, fantasy environments were installed that recreated the erotic situations that still were illegal, public and dangerous outside the walls of the baths. Glory holes recreated the toilets. Mazes recreated park bushes and undergrowth. Steam rooms and gyms recreated the YMCA and Video rooms recreated the balconies and back rows of movie theaters. Cells recreated and transformed the environment of prisons and jails, where generations of gay men have ended up for risking sex in toilets, parks, and the YMCA.
- In the 1970s, some bathhouses featured entertainers that appealed to a gay male audience. The best known was Bette Midler, who began her career performing to gay men at the Continental Baths in New York City. In San Francisco, one bathhouse opened a "Starlite Cabaret," which featured local singers and bands. Country Western bands also began playing on "Western Night" at the baths.
- Several bathhouses began to feature weekly "Movie Nights," when they presented current Hollywood films. At the same time, Hollywood produced two major films situated in gay bathhouses: "The Ritz" and "Saturday Night at the Baths."
- Many gay bathhouses threw parties for their members on major holidays: Lesbian and Gay Pride Day, Halloween, New Year's Eve, Christmas, Valentine's Day. These parties were a tremendous service to the gay men whose families had rejected them and for whom holidays represented a particularly depressing time of year. Holiday parties at the baths, especially for the men who frequented them regularly, could become a social event with familiar people that affirmed their sexuality. They offered a welcome alternative to loneliness and isolation.
- Also in the '70s, the City Clinic began to conduct free VD testing, usually by gay health workers, in many of the baths on a regular basis.

- In the 1970s, as the gay press in San Francisco began to come of age, newspapers like *Kalendar, Bay Area Reporter*, the *Sentinel, The Crusader, Databoy, The Voice, Coming Up!* and others were distributed for free in the bathhouses as well as the bars.
- Throughout the 1970s and 1980s, gay bathhouses offered their patrons a variety of new services: snack bars and cafes, dance floors for disco and country-western dancing, theme nights such as Buddy Night and Western Night. They also served the gay community by sponsoring benefits for community organizations.

The 1980s witnessed even more dramatic changes at the baths. With the increased popularity of exercise and bodybuilding, gyms and workout rooms were installed. In the last year, safe sex posters, brochures, cards and condoms have been displayed and given out, and safe sex forums have been held on the premises. In the last few months, orgy rooms, mazes and glory holes have been boarded up. Several bathhouses introduced "jack-off" nights, and some made their facilities available to private gay male jack-off clubs.

THE URBAN POLITICS OF GAY BATHHOUSE RAIDS, CLOSURES AND SURVEILLANCE IN HISTORICAL PERSPECTIVE

Since they were first discovered by city officials in the United States, gay bathhouses and bars have been kept under surveillance by undercover police officers. Yet police departments have also tolerated gay baths and bars as practical solutions to the difficult law enforcement problems of controlling sex in public places. During periodic "anti-vice drives clean-up campaigns," and "morals drives," bars and bathhouses have been harassed, raided and shut down by police, state liquor agents, district attorneys, military police and arsonists [see Figure 2]. During these drives, plainclothes police officers have compiled secret reports on the sexual behavior inside bars and baths–"sexual behavior" that has included dancing, caressing, kissing, and invitations to one's home. Plainclothes officers have used entrapment techniques to entice gay men and women into illegal sexual activities. The city and state used this sexual "evidence" to close gay bars and baths in an attempt to deny homosexuals any legal places to congregate.

Since the 19th century, these campaigns against gay bars and baths have developed in urban politics as a strategy toward attaining specific political goals, new laws, election to office, larger police budgets, moral

FIGURE 2. Matrix of Three Raids on Gay Establishments (p. 17)

	The Baker Street Club San Francisco, 1918	World War II Morals Drive San Francisco, 1943	Toronto Bathhouse Raids Canada, 1981
goals	To round up all men associated with the Baker Street club and their friends.	To protect servicemen stationed in the Bay Area from homosexuals who were known to gather in public areas.	The raids followed a successful anti-gay campaign that drove a pro-gay mayor out of office and ushered in an anti-gay administration. As a secret undercover operation, the goals of the raids were never clearly stated: But it seems likely they were an attempt to test whether the recently politically active gay community could be discredited and destroyed by attacking the bathhouses.
target	The Baker Street Club, its lessees and patrons, their friends.	Bars frequented by homosexual patrons. Union Square (the city's main "cruising" park for gay men).	All 6 gay bathhouses in Toronto.
agents	San Francisco Police Department Morals Squad, Army Police, Army Intelligence, the courts.	The San Francisco Police Department Morals Squad, a joint Army and Navy Vice Control Board functioning within the 12th Naval District and the Northern California Sector of the Western Defense Command, District Provost Marshal, District Morale Officer, San Francisco Health Department, State Board of Equalization.	Toronto Municipal Police Officers, Toronto Municipal Police. Intelligence Bureau, Attorney General's Office.
description	In 1918, two men who had met at the YMCA leased two flats at 2525 Baker street where they held private parties for gay men and offered rooms for gay men to have sex in private. In February, the San Francisco Police Department Morals Squad and U.S. Army Police put the Baker Street Club flats under surveillance. They planted a cook inside as a spy to collect evidence of sexual activity.	In May 1943, a joint Army and Navy Vice Control Board was formed to crack down on vice, venereal disease and liquor license violations in Northern California "to protect servicemen." Targeted bars were placed under surveillance and many had their licenses suspended. During the first wave, nearly all of the six or seven gay bars in San Francisco were harassed or had their licenses suspended. Patrons quickly moved	On the evening of February 5, 1981, Toronto Police raided 4 of the 6 gay bathhouses in the city. Undercover police intelligence officers had placed all the bathhouses under surveillance for a 6-month period. Starting at 11:00 pm, undercover police officers entered the bathhouses and arrested 304 men in a 3-hour, city-wide raid. Patrons were rounded up in ways designed to terrify and humiliate them.

description			
On February 16, officers entered the premises and began what newspapers called a "siege of the two flats." For a period of 10 days, as men entered the house, they were locked up in rooms as prisoners and questioned until they signed confessions, gave the names of their friends and surrendered personal letters and address books. Eleven men were arrested at the house, including an auditor for the Standard Oil Company, various salesmen and clerks, two singers, a broker, a soldier and a retired merchant. Using the names extracted from the arrested men, the San Francisco Morals Squad began a campaign to round up a second wave of homosexuals who could provide them with even more names. Their goal was to round up all the homosexuals they could identify. They began to hunt down men in other cities and on military bases. Eventually, in this second wave, 20 more men were arrested, including the 2 cops on the beat in the Baker Street neighborhood.	to other bars that would accept their business. Within a week or so, two bars in Chinatown became the new gay spots. When police discovered that the gay bar crowd had relocated to Chinatown, they sent in plainclothesmen to conduct surveillance. During a second wave of the drive they pressured the management of Li Po's to refuse admittance to gay patrons and the bar lost all of its weekend business. Police raided the Rickshaw and arrested 24 patrons. Two lesbians fought back during the raid and a small riot ensued. Police also arrested dozens of men in Union Square. For two weeks the gay bar crowd had nowhere to go. Finally, on a Saturday night, over 50 gay men showed up at the Top of the Mark, and converted it into a gay bar. The Top of the Mark thus earned the reputation as a "favorite spot" for homosexuals for the rest of the war.	At one bathhouse, men clad only in towels were lined up in the snow on the street while they were questioned. In another, patrons were herded into shower rooms and lined up naked against the walls. Several patrons reported that one police officer told his prisoners in the shower room, "Too bad the showers aren't hooked up to gas." A city-commissioned report following the raids revealed that arresting officers scrutinized the genitals and anuses of the arrested men. The day after the raids, a crowd of 3,000 angry demonstrators marched on the police station that had conducted the raid. Then they marched to the Ontario Legislature, where they tried to break down the doors in a riot reminiscent of the rage expressed at San Francisco's City Hall the night of Dan White's sentencing. More arrests followed from the demonstration. On June 16, angered by the massive protests of the original raids, police raided the remaining 2 bathhouses. Two thousand angry demonstrators once again marched on the police station.	

FIGURE 2 (continued)

	The Baker Street Club San Francisco, 1918	World War II Morals Drive San Francisco, 1943	Toronto Bathhouse Raids Canada, 1981
social/financial costs	**The Gay Community:** At least 31 men arrested, some of whom lost their jobs, went to jail, or jumped bail to flee the city; 2 attempted suicides. **The City:** Several months of trials in Superior Court; a seven-week grand jury investigation; city and military surveillance of the Club for several weeks; a wave of anti-homosexual hysteria that needed to be controlled.	**The Gay Community:** At least 50 arrests, several injuries during a street brawl, suspended licenses or loss of business at approximately 10 bars that accepted gay patrons. **The City:** The creation of a floating and growing population of gay bar patrons looking for new places to congregate: the cost of mobilizing state, city and military agents to conduct weeks of surveillance and mass arrests; an undetermined number of trials and Board of Equalization hearings.	**The Gay Community:** A total of 304 men were arrested in the February and June raids. Police called the employers of many of these men to ask if they knew their employees had been arrested. As a result, many of the men lost their jobs. One bathhouse went out of business as a result of the damages to its property. **The City:** Estimates of total costs to taxpayers of the police operations and court proceedings ranged as high as $10 million. These included over $35,000 of damages to the premises of the bathhouses when police broke down doors, walls and lockers during the raid. A massive mobilization of police was required to monitor and control three large protest demonstrations. An official investigation was commissioned by the city, in which the police were strongly condemned for their actions, the right of men to engage in consensual sex in private was confirmed, the practice of conducting police surveillance of public parks and rest rooms was attacked, and the city was urged to take emergency steps to rebuild a climate of trust and cooperation between the city and the gay community.

44

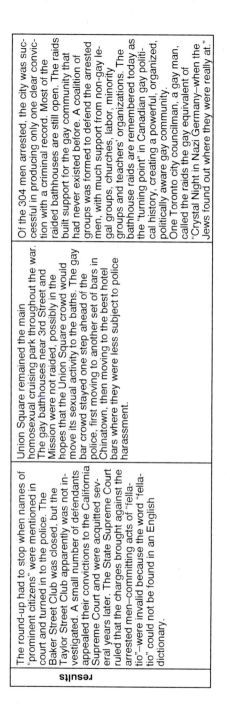

results			
	The round-up had to stop when names of "prominent citizens" were mentioned in to the police. The Baker Street Club was closed, but the Taylor Street Club apparently was not investigated. A small number of defendants appealed their convictions to the California Supreme Court and were acquitted several years later. The State Supreme Court ruled that the charges brought against the arrested men—committing acts of "fellatio"—were invalid because the word "fellatio" could not be found in an English dictionary.	Union Square remained the main homosexual cruising park throughout the war. The gay bathhouses near 3rd Street and Mission were not raided, possibly in the hopes that the Union Square crowd would move its sexual activity to the baths. The gay bar crowd stayed one step ahead of the police, first moving to another set of bars in Chinatown, then moving to the best hotel bars where they were less subject to police harassment.	Of the 304 men arrested, the city was successful in producing only one clear conviction with a criminal record. Most of the raided bathhouses are still open. The raids built support for the gay community that had never existed before. A coalition of groups was formed to defend the arrested men, with much support from non-gay legal groups, churches, labor, minority groups and teachers' organizations. The bathhouse raids are remembered today as the "turning point" in Canadian gay political history, creating a powerful, organized, politically aware gay community. One Toronto city councilman, a gay man, called the raids the gay equivalent of "Crystal Night in Nazi Germany—when the Jews found out where they were really at."

45

crusades. Their success at preventing homosexuals from gathering in public or in stopping gay sexual acts have at best been short-lived.

On the surface, the goals of the early anti-bath and anti-bar campaigns in San Francisco were to protect the public morals, health and safety by:

- rounding up all homosexuals and driving them out of the city once and for all;
- eliminating all sex between men in public, semi-public and even private places; and
- preventing homosexual men and women from meeting or socializing in public.

No campaign against San Francisco's gay bars or gay bathhouses has succeeded in attaining these three goals. Bars and baths remained open; homosexuals always stayed one step ahead of the police in finding new places to meet or have sex; gay men and lesbians were forced to become more politically aware and organized. These campaigns have always failed to achieve their stated goals because the social costs became too high, or the real goals were eventually achieved: a new anti-gay law, a larger budget, or election to public office.

While the general public may quickly forget them, the stories of how gay men and women survived or were destroyed in these bathhouse and bar raids have passed down from one generation to another, told and re-told as part of the unique history and culture of the lesbian and gay communities [see Figure 3]. As a result, gay men and women carry with them a lingering mistrust of government and its attempts to intervene in their lives. Any government attempt to once again eliminate all bars or all bathhouses, no matter how well-motivated, cannot help but take its place in the long history of government attacks on homosexuals and their meeting places that has created this mistrust and kept it alive.

In addition, such a drastic measure as the closure of all gay bathhouses cannot avoid the unexpected social costs that have plagued city governments, the gay community and the general public during similar campaigns in the past.

A HISTORICAL PERSPECTIVE ON THE BATHHOUSE CLOSURE, SAN FRANCISCO, 1984

San Francisco has never attempted to close every gay bathhouse and sex club in San Francisco before. But from 1954 to 1965, the SFPD, the DA's Office, State ABC agents, the *Examiner* and the Grand Jury all

FIGURE 3. Sidebar to Original Article (p. 18)

Jack's Baths in the 1930s & '40s

A man who frequented the baths in the 1920s and 1930s remembers that Jack's Baths "may have been intended as a 'real' Turkish (style) Baths," but it quickly developed into a gay bathhouse. "Sometime in the mid-thirties, a Jack G____ opened a Baths on Post St., between Polk and Van Ness. It had as many small cubicles (each with cot, chair, closet, a locking door) as possible; a steam room, warm room, masseurs, showers, T-room, though no pool. . . . By midnight on Friday and Saturday nights, the Baths was filled to beyond capacity. . . . Someone spread the rumor that the U.C. football team came over from Berkeley every Monday evening; the place was mobbed, though it is doubtful if any of these athletes did appear. In those days, however, many 'men' (young, handsome, available, but still MEN), came for servicing."

Jack's Baths is remembered by many servicemen who went there before fighting in the Pacific. Bob Ruffing, who served in the Navy, learned about Jack's by asking a bartender at the Claridge Room, a discreet gay bar on Maiden Lane that was popular with sailors. Trying to be non-committal, the bartender ignored Bob's question, then cautiously said, "Some of the people come in here and tell me about something called Jack's." "I finally found out from him where Jack's was," Bob recalls, "and went there immediately. It's the same Jack's that exists now on Post. That was the best one then."

Bob still fondly remembers what Jack's Baths was like during the war. "It was *good*," he told me. "Very, very busy. They didn't have an orgy room, just regular rooms. There wasn't much general activity; pickups in the hallways and stuff like that, or you'd leave your door open. It was all very quiet, but still very active. I think it was all gay, or at least people who went there knew it was gay. There was never any question about being careful when making passes at certain people."

During one of his visits to Jack's Baths in 1944, Bob met another Navy man whom he was fond of, "it seemed like a good thing," Bob remembers. "We saw each other several times, outside of Jack's Baths. We went back out to the Pacific. It seemed so good to each of us that we decided to get together after the war to give it a whirl. And it turned out to be a 15-year love affair, the major love affair of my life. So nice things can come out of baths."

Bob remembers how the baths changed in San Francisco as a result of the political climate of the 1950s. "I used my real name when I went to Jack's during the war," he told me. "It wasn't raided during the war. I'm sure that the military knew it was there, just as they knew whorehouses were there and they served a purpose. No, there was no question of any raid then. That all came afterward. They raided the baths a few times. When you went to the baths [in the 1950s] you just automatically—at least I did—invented another name, never signed your own name, because when they would raid the bars or the baths, they'd publish the complete list of people who were taken in, in the paper, in the *Examiner*. That was a nasty period, the '50s and early '60s."

joined forces in an attempt to shut down all gay bars. By 1955, these agencies succeeded in pressuring the California Legislature to pass a law allowing the revocation of a bar's liquor license if it had the reputation as a "resort for sexual perverts."

The anti-gay bar drive began in 1954 because, according to Police Chief Michael Gaffey, "a small army of homosexuals had invaded the city, many of them apparently driven here after other cities had been closed to them by similar raids." During these years, massive drives against gay and lesbian bars swept most large American cities as the bars developed into the major gay institution in the United States. These national anti-homosexual campaigns created a growing population of gay refugees moving from city to city looking for safe places to live.

During a major crackdown in San Francisco following the passage of the "resorts for sex perverts" law, gay men and women were driven to Oakland, San Mateo and San Jose. Police chiefs in these neighboring communities complained of a "huge influx" of "undesirables" and began conducting surveillance and raids of local bars whose weekend crowds had suddenly swelled with Gay San Franciscans.

By 1958, 15 of San Francisco's 20 gay bars had had their licenses challenged and hundreds of bar patrons had been arrested. In 1959, one bar owner's appeal reached the California State Supreme Court, which ruled that homosexuals had a right to gather in public and that gay bars could remain licensed. But arrests and bar raids continued in the early 1960s, with police sending in undercover agents looking for "lewd acts" on the premises. By 1965, after hundreds of bar patrons had been arrested, public opinion began to turn against the police and in support of leaving gay bars alone. While many public officials still wanted to eliminate gay bars, the new pragmatic approach was summed up by the Assistant District Attorney: "It's better to have homosexuals in one resort rather than spread throughout the city."

An unexpected consequence of this 10-year attempt to close all gay bars was to transform the gay community into a politically aware minority in local politics. During the gay community's campaign to defend the bars, the Tavern Guild was formed, a gay press emerged and was distributed through the bars and baths, defense committees were set up, those arrested learned to plead not guilty in court, the Council on Religion and the Homosexual was formed. By 1965, city officials finally realized that gay bars were a permanent part of the city and could not be eliminated without tremendous social, financial and human costs. More than 120 lesbian and gay bars now operate in San Francisco.

It is impossible to predict exactly what social, financial and health costs will result from the current bathhouse closure in San Francisco. However, in the two weeks since the closure of the baths, a pattern is already taking shape, which indicates that, as in past campaigns against the bars, the unexpected social and financial costs to the city threaten to become extremely high:

Goals: To stop the spread of AIDS by preventing gay men from engaging in "high risk" sexual contact with each other.

Targets: Gay bathhouses, sex clubs and adult bookstores.

Agents: San Francisco Health Department, Mayor's Office, private undercover detectives, San Francisco Police Department, the courts.

Social/Financial Costs

(1) Dispersion of Gay Bathhouse Patrons:

Outside San Francisco: A bathhouse owner in Oakland reports that the weekend after the bathhouse closure, his business increased 142%, indicating that, as in the 1956 crackdown on gay bars, some bathhouse patrons prefer to relocate their sexual activity to other bathhouses remaining open. This places the burden of changing the sexual behavior of San Francisco residents onto our neighboring city governments.

To Old Sexual Territories: Historically the development of gay bathhouses has offered gay men and the police a practical solution to the danger and the law enforcement problems associated with sex in public places. Elimination of gay bathhouses should therefore recreate the pre-bathhouse sexual landscape. Reports have already appeared in the gay press, and stories are spreading through the gay community, that street arrests have stepped up on Polk Street and South of Market, and that mounted police have increased surveillance of Buena Vista Park. This suggests that sexual activity that had occurred in the baths is now occurring with more frequency in the parks and streets, and that the burden of controlling this behavior is now placed on the Police Department. If this is the case, then men who were previously law-abiding in their sexual activity are now being driven to criminal behavior. Bathhouse closure removes the legal alternative to "outlaw" sex and encourages the practice of sex outside the law.

Another "old territory" for sexual activity is the YMCA. Since the degree of sex activity in the YMCAs declined as gay bathhouses opened, it might be expected that sexual activity in the YMCAs would increase as bathhouses are closed. This predictable consequence has already taken place. On November 1, signs went up at the Central YMCA in response to increased sexual activity in the steam room and dry room following the bathhouse closure. "The Central YMCA is not a bathhouse," the signs read. "We will not function as one." The next day the steam room and dry room were closed. On November 3, they were reopened, but with the introduction of continual surveillance of the facilities.

(2) Financial Costs:

According to the Health Department's supplemental budget request, the initial expense of hiring detectives to conduct the surveillance that led to closure was $35,000, and an additional $25,000 has been requested for continued surveillance. To this must be added the costs of sending undercover San Francisco Police officers into the baths to compile the Mayor's secret bathhouse sex report in March. Additional immediate costs include court costs following sex arrests; filing the city's suit against the bathhouses; processing the bathhouse and sex club closures through the state appeals courts, with the possibility that, as in the past, the bathhouses will ultimately remain open.

(3) Political Consequences:

As, might be expected, bathhouse closure has already forced portions of the gay community to organize themselves around defending the baths, as the gay community has done in the past to defend the bars in San Francisco and the baths in Toronto. New gay organizations already include the Northern California Bathhouse Owners' Association, the Adult Entertainment Association, the Community Partnership (a coalition of gay community groups) and the Committee to Preserve Our Sexual and Civil Liberties. In addition, anti-gay organizations, including the Moral Majority, the Cops for Christ and a group in San Antonio, Texas, have begun to use the bathhouse closure to fuel their anti-gay campaigns.

CONCLUSIONS

As a historian whose research has focused on the social effects of attacks against gay institutions in the past, it is clear to me that the attempted closure of the baths will only relocate the sexual activity that has taken place in the baths. In addition, the unexpected social, financial and health costs to the gay community, the city and the general public will be high. Bathhouse closure will create more problems than it will solve [see Figure 4].

To avoid unexpected social problems and still take strong measures to halt the spread of AIDS, I suggest that:

FIGURE 4. Sidebar to Original Article (p. 19)

"Pashy Steamrooms Pander to Pansies"

[*Broadway Brevities,* a 1933 New York tabloid]

"The pansy men of the Nation–New York, Philadelphia and San Francisco–are just nuts about Turkish bathing. Steam joints of the aforementioned cities are the gathering places of perverts . . .

"In most instances the proprietors are not aware of the goings-on in their establishments, but now a few of the places which cater to the public demand for steam baths are glad to enjoy the patronage of pansies provided their actions do not result in police proceedings. . . . Seldom in the vapor-laden interior of a Turkish bath is a contact successfully accomplished without the connivance of a wily manager who gains thereby in fat tips from his degenerate patrons . . .

"In Frisco may be found a bath where queers gather, who boast of this neat hide-and-seek joint, and although the management aims toward eliminating such patronage, the practice is carried on surreptitiously . . . to the accompaniment of warnings by and for queer patrons. . . . [Homosexuals say to each other:] 'It's an all right place, but one must be careful of the manager, he's rough' . . . and who wouldn't be! Many a pansy, caught in the act of approach, has been tossed from this place by a gang of wise-money boys who patronize the establishment in hours of relaxation from guiding the destinies of their rackets. A martyr among homos is the lad who died of a fractured skull a few years ago. Cracked on the head with a gin bottle while 'bathing,' he was accused posthumously of having attempted unnatural sex acts upon his assailants."

"Vapour-Bath Establishments"

Edward Stevenson, a gay New Yorker living in Europe, included a description of U.S. gay bathhouses in his 1908 book *The Intersexes.* "Resorts in the way of steambaths," he wrote, "are plentifully known–to the initiated. With many such resorts there is no police-interference, though their proceedings and patronage, night by night, day by day are perfectly plain. A special factor in homosexual uses of vapour-bath establishments (in larger cities) is the fact that in America these are kept open, and much patronized, during all night-hours, and first morning ones; indeed, some are never closed at all; in many examples a double staff of attendants being employed. In most such baths, each client has always a separate dressing-room, usually with a couch. What 'goes on' is under the guest's own lock and key, and without surveillance. New York, Boston, Washington, Chicago, St. Louis, San Francisco, Milwaukee, New Orleans, Philadelphia, are 'homosexual capitals.' "

1. *Bathhouses should be used as a community resource to promote safe sex and safe sex education.* Bathhouses have undergone dramatic changes over the last 100 years, changes that gay men have sometimes risked and lost their lives to bring about. They have become an integral part of the gay community. In the last year they have changed even more dramatically by taking measures to encourage safe sex practices and education. The baths should be allowed to continue these rapid changes in order to serve the community's needs during the present health crisis. They should entice gay men into them, especially if they

now engage in high-risk sex, so they can be exposed to more safe sex education. They should function as erotic environments where safe sex activity can be encouraged and where men can enjoy sexual intimacy and affection in an environment that is safe, clean and pro-gay.

2. *Bathhouses should be preserved as zones of safety, privacy and peer support as long as gay men are attacked for their sexuality.* Harvey Milk once called our society "fiercely heterosexual," a dangerous place to be gay. Since his murder six years ago last month, things have not changed. Gay men and lesbians are still assaulted and attacked every day for their sexuality. A national survey recently discovered that over 90% of gay men and lesbians have been physically attacked or otherwise victimized because they were gay. Gay bathhouses still represent one of the very few places where gay men can escape the anti-gay hostility that still is out of control in our city and our nation.

3. *A working relationship of cooperation and trust between the city and the gay community is critical in the fight against AIDS.* Bathhouse closure, together with the sex arrests and political backlash that are likely to follow, will make city agencies and the gay community adversaries once again. This will increase mistrust and lack of compliance with government health programs. Until recently, a remarkable aspect of the fight against AIDS has been the cooperative relationship between the government and the gay community that is unprecedented. The breakdown of that relationship will endanger lives and obstruct the health measures necessary to halt the spread of AIDS.

To defend its case for closure, the Health Department has already begun to stigmatize segments of the gay community. It has called bathhouse owners "merchants of death" and bathhouse patrons "Evel Knievels of medicine." It has also revived the old rhetoric of crime and disease that was used to attack the bars. Part of the old anti-gay rhetoric was that "sick" people went to the bars to spread the "disease" of homosexuality. In its press statement announcing closure of the baths, the Health Department similarly portrayed the bathhouse as "not fostering gay liberation" but instead "fostering disease and death." This inflammatory rhetoric and scapegoating only adds to the gay community's fears that it is once again under attack.

Recently, reports that the Centers for Disease Control considered establishing an HTLV-3 name registry have also increased gay men's fears of government persecution. As a result of these fears, a UC Berkeley epidemiological study that the gay community desperately needs may now be doomed for lack of volunteers. The bathhouse closure further increases the mistrust of health authorities. Fears have even been expressed that confidential bathhouse membership lists might be used to discriminate against these men.

My research over the past five years has revealed that the gay community's fears that the government will compile massive lists of names, enforce quarantines and establish detention camps for homosexuals are justified. Both the Army and Navy after World War II compiled lists of over 10,000 men suspected of being homosexual. In 1956, the FBI compiled a 53-page list of homosexuals in San Francisco and their friends. The federal government still has these lists. Several times during World War II, the Navy Department considered a plan to set up detention camps where homosexuals identified by the military would be interned for the duration of the war, not to punish them, but allegedly to protect the nation.

As a historian, it is clear to me that yet another government campaign to dismantle gay institutions, even in the well-motivated attempt to stop the spread of AIDS, will only backfire. Instead, the city should join the gay community in using these institutions creatively. The city's goals should include positive steps toward: (1) dispelling fears that the city is attacking the gay community, (2) rebuilding a working relationship of trust and cooperation with the gay community, and (3) decreasing scapegoating and restoring morale. Bathhouse closure, surveillance of sexual activity, sex arrests, the compiling of lists of names, and scapegoating will only undermine these goals.

Instead of wasting its time defending its bathhouses, its bars and its very right to exist, the gay community must be allowed to devote all of its resources, including the bathhouses, toward promoting the research, health programs and safe sex educational measures that will save lives.

Number and Distribution of Gay Bathhouses in the United States and Canada

William J. Woods, PhD
Daniel Tracy
Diane Binson, PhD

University of California San Francisco

SUMMARY. Although gay bathhouses have been the subject of debate and some public health policy for decades, the relative number and geographic distribution of these establishments has not been described. As a result, it is easy to miss or ignore them in making public policy in response to disease prevention. No straightforward methodology for such a description is available, so we used a series of gay travel books, first published in 1965 by the Damron Company, to estimate this distribution in the United States and Canada. Each of the annual guides published from 1968 to 1999 were reviewed for listings of bathhouses and sex clubs. The results suggest that bathhouses and other similar establishments exist in most states and provinces and in most large and many moderate-sized cities. Furthermore, the largest numbers of listings for bathhouses were in the same six cities across the decades, three in the U.S. and three in Canada. The greatest change in the number of listings

---

Correspondence may be addressed to William J. Woods, Center for AIDS Prevention Studies, University of California San Francisco, 74 New Montgomery Street, Suite 600, San Francisco, CA 94105 (E-mail: bwoods@psg.ucsf.edu).

[Haworth co-indexing entry note]: "Number and Distribution of Gay Bathhouses in the United States and Canada." Woods, William J., Daniel Tracy, and Diane Binson. Co-published simultaneously in *Journal of Homosexuality* (Harrington Park Press, an imprint of The Haworth Press, Inc.) Vol. 44, No. 3/4, 2003, pp. 55-70; and: *Gay Bathhouses and Public Health Policy* (ed: William J. Woods, and Diane Binson) Harrington Park Press, an imprint of The Haworth Press, Inc., 2003, pp. 55-70. Single or multiple copies of this article are available for a fee from The Haworth Document Delivery Service [1-800-HAWORTH, 9:00 a.m. - 5:00 p.m. (EST). E-mail address: docdelivery@haworthpress.com].

was seen in the three U.S. cities where a public policy of closure was attempted. Nevertheless, the numbers of venues in these three cities have been increasing again since the early 1990s, although nothing near the numbers of listings in the late 1970s and early 1980s. *[Article copies available for a fee from The Haworth Document Delivery Service: 1-800-HAWORTH. E-mail address: <docdelivery@haworthpress.com> Website: <http://www. HaworthPress.com> © 2003 by The Haworth Press, Inc. All rights reserved.]*

KEYWORDS. Gay bathhouses

Within the body of academic literature, the gay bathhouse has received sporadic attention over the past three decades. First entering the field as a sociological symbol of gay liberation (Delph, 1978; Lee, 1976; Styles, 1979; Weinberg & Williams, 1975), the gay bathhouse has more recently been transformed into an epidemiological landmark for the transmission of HIV (human immunodeficiency virus) (Bayer, 1989; Rofes, 1998; Rotello, 1997; Shilts, 1987; Turner, Miller, & Moses, 1989). Current dialogue has focused largely on the debate concerning bathhouses and public health policy. Whereas some have advocated for the closing of bathhouses as a strategy of preventing further HIV transmissions among men who have sex with men (MSM) (Bayer, 1989; Rotello, 1997; Shilts, 1987), others argue that the bathhouse can be utilized as a site for HIV- and STD-prevention education (see Bérubé, 1984; Helquist & Osmon, 1984a; Helquist & Osmon, 1984b, all reprinted in this volume).

The first descriptions of the baths in the literature were a variety of ethnographic studies. Some of these studies served solely to describe the physical space of bathhouses and the activities that took place within them (Rumaker, 1979). One important, early, methodological paper described the transition from nonparticipant to participant observer in the gay baths, rather than specific venues (Styles, 1979). Other researchers identified characteristics of gay baths conducive to sexual activity (Weinberg & Williams, 1975).

Also at that time and into the early 1980s, epidemiological studies indicated that frequenting bathhouses was a common characteristic of men who reported repeated infections with sexually transmitted infections (STIs) (Darrow, Barrett, Jay, & Young, 1981; Judson, Miller, & Schaffnit, 1977; Ostrow, Shaskey, Steffen, & Altman, 1980; Schreeder et al., 1980; Schreeder et al., 1982; Szmuness et al., 1975). Initially these data were interpreted and utilized by public health officials in conflicting ways: some used these data to support the development of interventions to reach out to men in these environments and argued that bathhouses provided an ideal space for the implementation of such interventions (Judson et al., 1977; Merino, Judson, Bennett, & Schaffnit, 1979; Merino & Richards, 1977; Ostrow et al., 1980). Nevertheless, at least some gay men at the time supported the idea that these places should be shut down to prevent further transmission of venereal diseases (see Merino et al., 1979). With the introduction of the AIDS epidemic in the early 1980s, the vibrancy of this debate was heightened tremendously, and some efforts to shut down bathhouses succeeded in some cities (see Bayer, 1989; Shilts, 1987; Disman, in this volume), at least temporarily.

The work of some historians illustrates the significance of the role played by bathhouses and similar environments on the dynamics of gay communities. Some of these authors suggest that the baths played a significant role in the individual development of gay men as well as that of the gay community (Chauncey, 1994; Bérubé, in this volume).

Although the baths have clearly played a significant role in the existence and growth of gay male communities and networks, there has never been an effort to describe the extent to which bathhouses have actually existed. And although ethnographies and studies have described particular bathhouses, this body of literature has long been missing a description of the number and distribution of gay bathhouses across the continent.

There is a reasonable explanation for this lack of detailed description. Identifying and enumerating these places would never have been easy. There does not appear to have been a national association to represent these businesses, and even regional or local associations seem to have been short-lived; personal communications about such groups always refer to collaborations among some of the local or regional clubs for a brief period to address specific needs. Further, depending on local law and differences in what the business is actually providing, the businesses may fall under different jurisdictions (e.g., health or police departments) or not be registered as bathhouses at all.

A cursory review of a publication called *Saunaguide*, published in Germany, confirms that bathhouses exist in many cities, large and not so large, and on every habitable continent (Bedford, 2000). Nevertheless, the purpose of this study was to address this lack of quantification by providing both a reasonable estimate of the number of bathhouses that have existed in the U.S. and Canada and a description of their geographic distribution across time. This estimate cannot be exact for all the reasons mentioned above, but it can give a better picture than what has been available to date. Furthermore, by looking at available data throughout the last three decades of the 20th century, a reasonable estimate of their number and distribution can be gleaned.

We used the *Damron Address Book* to estimate the number and distribution of gay bathhouses in the U.S. and Canada in large part because it is the oldest and most complete resource available on North American cities. First published in 1965, the *Damron Address Book* has been updated annually at least since 1968. It came into existence through the work of Bob Damron, a gay man active within the San Francisco gay community from the 1960s until his death in 1989. Published during a time when one's knowledge of existing establishments catering to gay men came primarily from word of mouth, the *Damron Address Book* was the product of the compiled knowledge of Bob Damron and his social network. From its inception, it listed the names and addresses of gay bars, cafés, and, more importantly for our purposes, bathhouses. It has since grown tremendously in size and readership, and the *Damron Address Book* (renamed the *Damron Men's Travel Guide* in 1999) exists now as one of the most well-known gay directories in publication. Businesses have never had to pay to be listed, and anyone could contact the company to add a listing. The company attempted to verify listings annually, prior to publication.

METHODS

We had access to the archives of the Damron Company in San Francisco for this research. The record was complete from 1968, although the very first volume had a 1965 copyright date, and there was a revised edition with a 1966 copyright date. Because the first two extant volumes were not numbered, and the 1968 volume was the "fourth edition," it was not exactly clear how the earliest editions were counted or numbered, and just how many editions were published between 1965 and 1968. But the numbering of the guide suggested that there was at least one other addition published before 1968, though our efforts to find the missing volume(s) were not successful.

Generally, the address books were divided alphabetically by U.S. states followed by listings of Canadian establishments by province, with cities listed alphabetically within states and provinces. Later editions included Mexico and the Caribbean; recently, European cities were incorporated into the publication. Within each city subsection there were listed various businesses and attractions that might be of interest to gay males (and more recently lesbians, although the company now publishes a separate book for women). Over the years the format of the publication changed. Prior to the 1990 edition, all listings were provided in alphabetical order with cruisy areas (such as alleys, parks and toilets) separated out at the end of the city listing. In the 1990 edition categories were introduced to subdivide the overall listings into separate sections. For example, the 1994 edition included the following categories: info lines and services, accommodations, bars, restaurants and cafes, gyms and health clubs, bookstores/retail shops, travel/tour operators, men's clubs, erotica, cruisy areas), with some differences from year to year in the category types or titles.

Early editions of the *Damron Address Book* had no advertisements (with one exception, a single ad for a book at the back of the 1968 edition), and were dedicated solely to the listing of establishments. They began including ads in 1974 (10th edition), and immediately these were plentiful, with individual bathhouses and bathhouse chains among the major advertisers.

The charge for our data collection was to review all listings in the extant editions from 1965-1999 (although for this paper, we only include the contiguous years from 1968 to 1999), identifying and recording any item that might be a bathhouse or sex club. To collect the data we were inclusive, writing down all information provided by the guide about a given item, as long as something about the item suggested a possible venue of interest. For example, if the item was described as a bath or it was coded with a "P" (or, in later editions, "PC," both indicating private club), we included it in our data. The idea was to be inclusive so that we would have everything listed in the guide and during analysis we could make more precise definitions and exclude any venue that failed to meet the definition. However, all cruisy areas were excluded, since the primary purpose of those venues is not to provide a safe place for gay men to meet for sex. For example, a bathhouse listed under a cruisy area would not be a gay bathhouse, since a gay venue would have been listed in the general listings, even as far back as 1965. Also, we did not include adult movie theaters and adult bookstores. While later editions of the guide did categorize "Men's Clubs" (1990 on), identifying appropriate listings was not a straightforward task even in those years. As a result of these differences in format, the methodology for reviewing the guides varied slightly for different periods: the first 25 editions (early methodology, reflecting years 1965 to 1989), the editions 26-28 (middle methodology, reflecting years 1990 to 1992), and editions 29-35 (late methodology, reflecting years 1993 to 1999).

The early methodology included any venue that was listed as a "bath" or "baths," or included the word in its name. We also included any venue that was coded with "health club," "sauna" or "spa," or had any of those terms in its name. Although many baths had the word "club" in their titles, we did not include such a venue in our data unless there was more in the listing to indicate it was not a bar, since many bars also used the word "club" in their names. For example, if a venue had the word "club" in the name and was coded "P" (for "private"), we did not include the venue in the data. However, if the listing included codes such as steam room or spa, we did include it. Many sex clubs look like bars in the listings and did not have steam rooms or spas that would distinguish them. However, listings that coded as after-hours locations (AH) or that indicated "no booze" were included.

The middle methodology changed because the guide started to break listings up into numerous categories. Between 1990 and 1993, bathhouses and sex clubs were listed under the category "Gym/Health Club." Rather than review all listings, we restricted our search to listings under these categories. In general, we used the additional information provided with the listings under this category to distinguish whether the venue was only a gym for physical exercise, or if it was also a sex venue. For example, a listing might say "gym only" or be coded as gay friendly (GF), in such cases venues were excluded. On the other hand, a listing might say "private rooms available" or be coded for leather (L), in such cases those venues would be included.

The third and last methodology was changed to accommodate the added category of "Men's Clubs." The category "Gym/Health Club" continued, but most of the baths and sex clubs were listed under "Men's Clubs." However, some venues continued to be listed under "Gym/Health Club," so it was necessary in this methodology to review both categories. We used a similar strategy to distinguish items for inclusion or exclusion under "Gym/Health Club" that was used in the middle methodology. However, any venue listed under "Men's Clubs" was included in the data.

These methodologies allowed for the occasional inclusion of what would probably be an isolated motel or resort, because of the inclusion of items that list "spa" or "sauna." When possible, these items were excluded, though a few may have remained due to insufficient evidence that they were not a bathhouse.

The three authors reviewed the available address books to record the listings that met inclusion criteria. Because the review itself was time consuming and required many hours sitting at the conference table of an active business organization, most of the data were not double-checked, though there were periodic checks and reviews to improve reliability or to check on apparent errors. The data on the identified listings were hand recorded on structured forms, including volume, page, business name, address, phone number, and up to 14 codes (e.g., "PC" and "GF"). Data from the structured forms were entered into Microsoft Excel spreadsheets. The spreadsheet was exported to Microsoft Access for analysis. The publisher and editor of the *Damron Address Book* reviewed the paper for accuracy in reflecting procedures and history of the publications.

RESULTS

The primary question was: How many clubs were there in the United States and Canada? There were 4,685 listings that met the inclusion criteria across the 32 guides, and these were broken down by year (Figure 1). The pattern suggests that there was a precipitous increase in the number of listings from the early 1970s to the early 1980s, followed by a steady decline from 1982 until 1991. A new increase began in 1990, though not as dramatic as the first rise.

Table 1 lists alphabetically the U.S. states (including the District of Columbia and Puerto Rico) and Canadian provinces indicating several types of information about listings identified in each of the 32 books reviewed. The column "numbers of listings in 1999" gives an estimate of the current status of clubs in the various states and provinces. The other three columns provide the big picture look for each individual state/province across the 32 books by listing the specific years listings appeared, the total number of years and the average number of listings per year (given as a range). Sixteen states and two provinces had listings in 1968 as compared with 24 states and six provinces in 1999, and with 43 states and 6 provinces having listings in any year. In states or provinces with small numbers, it is important to remember that there were a number of businesses that opened in the late 1970s and early 1980s that did not survive the dramatic changes in sexual behavior of gay men that followed the identification of HIV. On the other hand, some of the numbers may also represent newer businesses opening in the later 1990s. Nine of the 50 states and half the Canadian provinces never had a single

FIGURE 1. Number of Club Listings in the USA and Canada by Year (1968-1999)

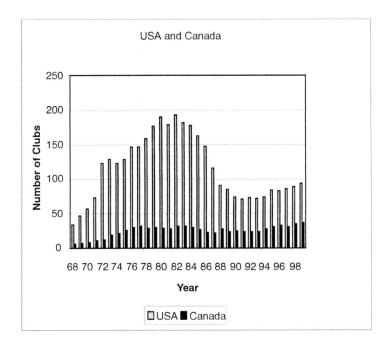

listing in the 32 address books reviewed. Also of note, the southern tier of U.S. states included several states with rather a large number of listings, e.g., Texas, Louisiana, Missouri, Georgia and Florida.

Because it would make sense that the larger cities would contribute more to the number of bathhouses than smaller cities or towns, we broke down the number of listings by city and year. Six cities consistently had more listings than other cities across the 32 years of data; the three largest were in the United States (Los Angeles, New York, San Francisco) followed by three Canadian cities (Vancouver, Toronto and Montreal). Figure 2 shows the distribution of listings for the six cities with the most listings across all years of data. The figure shows that throughout the years, Los Angeles always had the most listings, and by a large number. Further, though San Francisco and New York were fairly similar in number of listings throughout the years, San Francisco

TABLE 1. State/Province Listings in *Damron Address Book* by Number and Specific Years

	# of Listings in 1999	Specific Years with Listings	# of Years with Listings	Average # of Listings per Year (Range)
US State/DC & PR				
Alabama				
Alaska	0	79	1	1
Arkansas				
Arizona	2	68, 74-99	27	1 - 3
California	23	68-99	32	15 - 66
Colorado	3	68-99	32	1 - 7
Connecticut	0	77-86	10	1 - 2
Delaware				
District of Columbia	3	70-99	30	1 - 5
Florida	10	68-69, 71-99	31	1 - 10
Georgia	2	70-89, 92, 97-99	24	1 - 3
Hawaii	2	73-99	27	1 - 3
Idaho				
Iowa	0	79-81, 85-86	5	1
Illinois	3	68, 71-99	30	1 - 7
Indiana	3	68-99	32	1 - 3
Kansas				
Kentucky	0	69-78, 82-83	12	1
Louisiana	2	68, 71-99	30	1 - 5
Maine				
Massachusetts	1	68-69, 72-93, 95-99	27	1 - 4
Maryland	0	69-86	18	1 - 4
Michigan	1	73-99	27	1 - 8
Minnesota	0	68-89, 94-96	25	1 - 6
Missouri	2	71-99	29	1 - 5
Mississippi	0	74, 85	2	1
Montana	0	68-80, 82, 84, 90-92	18	1 - 2
Nebraska	0	78, 86-87	3	1
New Hampshire	0	73	1	1
New Jersey	0	69-86	18	1 - 6
New Mexico	1	76-77, 81-85, 99	8	1 - 2
Nevada	2	68-99	32	1 - 3
New York	10	68-99	32	4 - 22

TABLE 1 (continued)

	# of Listings in 1999	Specific Years with Listings	# of Years with Listings	Average # of Listings per Year (Range)
North Carolina	0	73-88	16	1 - 2
North Dakota				
Ohio	5	68-99	32	1 - 8
Oklahoma	0	81, 83-86, 93-94	7	1
Oregon	1	68-99	32	1 - 5
Pennsylvania	3	69-99	31	2 - 7
Puerto Rico	1	69-99	31	1
Rhode Island	1	79-99	21	1 - 2
South Carolina	0	86	1	1
South Dakota				
Tennessee	0	80-81, 83-85, 87	6	1
Texas	7	68-70, 72-99	31	1 - 9
Utah	1	71, 74-80, 84-91, 95-99	21	1 - 2
Virginia	0	72-73, 82-83, 91-92	6	1
Vermont	0	87	1	1
Washington	5	68-99	32	2 - 7
Wisconsin	0	71-90	20	1 - 4
West Virginia	0	80, 82	2	1
Wyoming				
Canadian Province				
Alberta	3	73-99	27	1 - 6
British Columbia	5	68-73, 75-99	31	1 - 9
Manitoba	2	69-99	31	1 - 3
New Brunswick				
Newfoundland and Labrador				
Northwest Territories				
Nova Scotia	1	82-96, 98-99	17	1 - 2
Prince Edward Island				
Ontario	11	68-99	32	3 - 18
Quebec	15	71-99	29	1 - 16
Saskatchewan				
Yukon				

Note: Highlighted states/provinces had no bathhouse listings in any year.

FIGURE 2. The Distribution of Club Listings in the Six Cities with the Most Listings

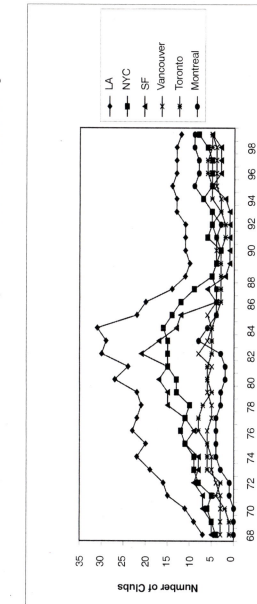
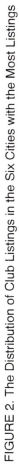

is the only one of the three major U.S. cities to ever have fewer listings than all three major Canadian cities.

Also of note is that the variability in number of listings per year was almost entirely due to changes in the U.S. cities. That is, the pattern mentioned above, of striking increases up to the early 1980s, followed by a steady decline from 1982 until 1991, reflected only the U.S. listings. Although there were some rises and falls in the distribution of Canadian listings, a better description of the Canadian experience would be quite different. The overall best description might be a slow growth until about 1978, followed by relative stability in the number of listings throughout the remaining years of the century.

Some additional data were gleaned through the data collection process and are included here for its informative value. As soon as ads began to appear in the address books (1974), the baths were the primary advertisers, both in that they comprised a sizeable proportion of all ads (though not measured, it was enough to be striking) and they tended to be half or full page ads. When collecting the data it was clear that many bathhouses that opened were part of chains, such as Club Bath Chain (CBC), that advertised both locally and nationally. From 1974 (i.e., from the first year ads appeared) until 1984, CBC ran two-page ads either on the inside front or back cover spread. After 1984 ads for the bathhouse chains in *Damron* almost disappeared. They continued to be listed, but ads were primarily local and not as chains. There were exceptions (e.g., Flex and Midtowne Spa continued to list their clubs in other cities in the local ads), but the change was noticeable in our review. Venues that continued to be listed in a national ad were part of the "Independent Gay Health Clubs" (IGHC), which included other kinds of venues, veiling the bathhouse nature of many of the listings. Two-page ads for IGHC first appeared in 1985.

DISCUSSION

This study was interested primarily in estimating the extent to which bathhouses existed and how they were distributed across the United States and Canada in the later third of the 20th century. The estimates provided by our review of the *Damron Address Book* show that they were distributed far more widely than the attention they receive might suggest. Nevertheless, the data do support the often-reported fact that the baths increased in number prior to the AIDS epidemic and that many swiftly closed following the identification of the disease among gay men, at least that was the case in the United States.

The Canadian experience with the baths is clearly different, despite having a similar history of police harassment of bathhouses (e.g., Hannon, 1982; Higgins, 1999) and a relatively similar AIDS trajectory (World AIDS Campaign, 2001). A different public policy approach to the baths, however, may have made a substantial difference in the relative stability of these businesses. While, to our knowledge, none of the Canadian cities had a policy to close any of these businesses as a response to the AIDS epidemic, all three major U.S. cities attempted to close some or all of the bathhouses and sex clubs within their jurisdiction (see Bayer, 1989; Klosinski, McCombs, Miller, & Carrel, 1993).

Bolton, Vincke and Mak (1992) compared the 1984 edition of a European travel guide for gay men with the1992 edition to identify changes in the number of sauna listings. They found results similar to ours, that is, the number of saunas in some of the larger cities declined, but in most cities the number of saunas operating in 1992 were the same as had been operating in 1984.

It is important to remember when reviewing the figures that the data have numerous limitations. The Damron Company relied on informants to tell them when businesses opened and closed. While this system seemed to work well enough to make their address book indispensable to some gay travelers, it is, without doubt, not a perfectly reliable source. It was clear in data collection that they included some businesses that they thought would open, though perhaps they never did, or did not last long enough to be listed in the next book. Other times, businesses might have opened in one year, but not appeared in the address book for one or more years because no one informed the company. Although the listings were free, there was an effort on the part of the company to contact businesses and confirm their continued operation. The current editor acknowledges that the reliability of the listings in the late 1980s was not good, in part because the company, like much of the gay community, was decimated by the AIDS epidemic and so they were less active in checking on the accuracy of listings. Unfortunately, this is the same period where the U.S. data takes its greatest dip. However, the dip is likely to be real, given that these were mirrored in the largest U.S. cities, where we know that efforts were made to close the businesses (Bayer, 1989; Walter, 1986), and where Damron had easiest access to information. While absolute numbers or quantifiable changes in number of listings from one year to the next are not recommended, the larger picture described through this record is likely to be accurate and reliable.

Thus the study provides a picture of the early increase in the number of gay baths in the early years of the gay movement. The listings suggest that while the AIDS epidemic had a large impact on the U.S. businesses, the Canadian businesses remained fairly stable since their early growth. The U.S. businesses have rebounded during the 1990s and appear to be achieving a level of stability similar to their Canadian counterparts. While larger cities appear to accommodate a number of businesses, baths can be found in most moderate sized cities, even in states with anti-sodomy laws (e.g., Texas). That cities and states that tried to close these businesses were partly successful and that four-fifths of the states and half of the provinces have bathhouses suggests that these venues are here to stay at least for the foreseeable future. In light of recent studies suggesting that sexual risk behavior and sexually transmitted infections are increasing among gay men (Centers for Disease Control and Prevention, 1999; Katz, 1997; Yang, 2000), it becomes imperative that prevention efforts consider ways to address public health concerns related to these businesses.

ACKNOWLEDGMENTS

The authors gratefully acknowledge the generous contribution of the Damron Company, especially Gina Gatta, President and Editor-in-Chief, and Ian Philips, Managing Editor. They not only provided access to the company's archival collection, but they provided space in their offices for the time consuming data collection process and their emotional support provided encouragement in completing the project. They also reviewed a draft of the manuscript. Nevertheless, the study and this paper are independent of Damron Company, and the company is not responsible for any errors in the study. The authors are also grateful to Michael Helquist for introducing them to Gina Gatta, and to Christopher Disman and Tor Neilands for their input into the early analysis plans, and to Paul Cotten, Greg Rebchook and Susan Kegeles for their reviews of the manuscript. The authors also offer thanks to Megan Gaffigan for her assistance with the literature and references.

REFERENCES

Bayer, R. (1989). *Private Acts, Social Consequences: AIDS and the Politics of Public Health*. New Brunswick, NJ: Rutgers University Press.
Bedford, B. (2000). *Saunaguide & gay bathhouses international*. Berlin: Bruno Gmunder Verlag.

Berube, A. (1984). The history of gay bathhouses. *Coming Up!*, 15-19.

Bolton, R., Vincke, J., & Mak, R. (1992). Venues of HIV transmission or AIDS prevention? *National AIDS Bulletin, 9*, 22-26.

Centers for Disease Control and Prevention. (1999). Increases in unsafe sex and rectal gonorrhea among men–San Francisco, 1994-1997. *Morbidity and Mortality Weekly Report, 48*(3), 45-48.

Chauncey, G. (1994). *Gay New York: Gender, urban culture, and the making of the gay male world 1890-1940.* New York: Basic Books.

Darrow, W. W., Barrett, D., Jay, K., & Young, A. (1981). The gay report on sexually transmitted diseases. *American Journal of Public Health, 71*(9), 1004-1011.

Delph, E. W. (1978). *The silent community: Public homosexual encounters.* Beverly Hills: Sage.

Hannon, G. (1982). Raids, rage and bawdyhouses. In E. Jackson & S. Persky (Eds.), *Flaunting It!: A decade of gay journalism from The Body Politic* (pp. 273-294). Vancouver and Toronto: New Star Books and Pink Triangle Press.

Helquist, M., & Osmon, R. (1984a). Sex and the baths: A not so secret report. *Coming Up!*, 17-22.

Helquist, M., & Osmon, R. (1984b). Beyond the baths: The other sex businesses. *Coming Up!*, 19-24.

Higgins, R. (1999). Baths, bushes, and belonging: Public sex and gay community in pre-Stonewall Montreal. In W. L. Leap (Ed.), *Public Sex/Gay Space* (pp. 187-202). New York: Columbia University Press.

Judson, F. N., Miller, K. G., & Schaffnit, T. R. (1977). Screening for gonorrhea and syphilis in the gay baths: Denver, Colorado. *American Journal of Public Health, 67*(8), 740-742.

Katz, M. H. (1997). AIDS epidemic in San Francisco among men who report sex with men: Successes and challenges of HIV prevention. *Journal of Acquired Immune Deficiency Syndromes and Human Retrovirology, 14*(Suppl 2), S38-46.

Klosinski, L., McCombs, M., Miller, S., & Carrel, J. (1993). *A bathhouse HIV education campaign.* Paper presented at the Fifteenth National Lesbian and Gay Health Conference and Eleventh Annual AIDS/HIV Forum, Houston, TX.

Lee, J. A. (1976). Forbidden colors of love: Patterns of gay love and gay liberation. *Journal of Homosexuality, 1*(4), 401-418.

Merino, H. I., Judson, F. N., Bennett, D., & Schaffnit, T. R. (1979). Screening for gonorrhea and syphilis in gay bathhouses in Denver and Los Angeles. *Health Reports, 94*(4), 376-379.

Merino, H. I., & Richards, J. B. (1977). An innovative program of venereal disease casefinding, treatment and education for a population of gay men. *Sexually Transmitted Diseases, 4*(2), 50-52.

Ostrow, D. G., Shaskey, D., Steffen, G., & Altman, N. (1980). Epidemiology of gonorrhea infections in gay men. *Journal of Homosexuality, 5*, 285-288.

Rofes, E. (1998). Context is everything: Thoughts on effective HIV prevention and gay men in the United States. *Journal of Psychology & Human Sexuality, 10*(3-4), 133-142.

Rotello, G. (1997). *Sexual ecology: AIDS and the destiny of gay men.* New York: Penguin Putnam.

Rumaker, M. (1979). *A day and a night at the baths.* San Francisco, CA: Grey Fox Press.

Schreeder, M. T., Thompson, S. E., Hadler, S. C., Berquist, K. R., Maynard, J. E., Ostrow, D. G., Judson, F. N., Braff, E. H., Nylund, T., Moore, J. N., Gardner, P., Doto, I. L., & Reynolds, G. (1980). Epidemiology of Hepatitis B infection in gay men. *Journal of Homosexuality, 5*(3), 307-310.

Schreeder, M. T., Thompson, S. E., Hadler, S. C., Berquist, K. R., Zaidi, A., Maynard, J. E., Ostrow, D. G., Judson, F. N., Braff, E. H., Nylund, T., Moore, J. N., Gardner, P., Doto, I. L., & Reynolds, G. (1982). Hepatitis B in homosexual men: Prevalence of infection and factors related to transmission. *Journal of Infectious Diseases, 146*(1), 7-15.

Shilts, R. (1987). *And the band played on: Politics, people and the AIDS epidemic.* New York: St. Martin's Press.

Styles, J. (1979). Outsider/insider: Researching gay baths. *Urban Life, 8*(2), 135-152.

Szmuness, W., Much, I., Prince, A. M., Hoofnagle, J. H., Cherubin, C. E., Harley, E. J., & Block, G. H. (1975). On the role of behavior in the spread of hepatitis B infection. *Annals of Internal Medicine, 83*(4), 489-495.

Turner, C. F., Miller, H. G., & Moses, L. E. (1989). *AIDS: Sexual behavior and intravenous drug use.* Washington, DC: National Academy Press.

Walter, D. (1986). Georgia bans gay bathhouses. *Advocate* (447), 15-16.

Weinberg, M. S., & Williams, C. J. (1975). Gay baths and the social organization of impersonal sex. *Social Problems, 23*(2), 124-136.

World AIDS Campaign. (2001). *Men who have sex with men and HIV/AIDS.* Geneva: UNAIDS.

Yang, S. (2000). AIDS strategy needed, officials say. *WebMD Medical News.*

The San Francisco Bathhouse Battles of 1984: Civil Liberties, AIDS Risk, and Shifts in Health Policy

Christopher Disman

San Francisco

SUMMARY. In the mid-1980s, controversy emerged in a number of American cities over the roles gay bathhouses and sex clubs might play in the spread of AIDS, and in raising safe-sex awareness. In 1984, San Francisco became the first city where political debates broke out over AIDS-related policies for bathhouses and sex clubs. These debates were dominated by questions of public health and gay civil liberties. A variety of proposals were put forward during 1984 to try to reconcile these two concerns, or to give one a higher priority than the other. Certain officials in San Francisco's government, and members of its gay/lesbian/bisexual community, strongly disagreed over whether the businesses should be closed, should make their own AIDS-prevention efforts, or should continue operating under new regulations. Policies implemented for the city's baths were disconnected from the known AIDS risk of different sexual behaviors, and from research findings on AIDS and the local baths. Political and judicial decisions concerning San Francisco's bath-

Correspondence may be addressed: 584 Castro Street, #622, San Francisco, CA 94114-2594.

[Haworth co-indexing entry note]: "The San Francisco Bathhouse Battles of 1984: Civil Liberties, AIDS Risk, and Shifts in Health Policy." Disman, Christopher. Co-published simultaneously in *Journal of Homosexuality* (Harrington Park Press, an imprint of The Haworth Press, Inc.) Vol. 44, No. 3/4, 2003, pp. 71-129; and: *Gay Bathhouses and Public Health Policy* (ed: William J. Woods, and Diane Binson) Harrington Park Press, an imprint of The Haworth Press, Inc., 2003, pp. 71-129. Single or multiple copies of this article are available for a fee from The Haworth Document Delivery Service [1-800-HAWORTH, 9:00 a.m. - 5:00 p.m. (EST). E-mail address: docdelivery@haworthpress.com].

houses and sex clubs that were made in 1984 had continuing influences on
these businesses through the later 1980s and the 1990s. *[Article copies available
for a fee from The Haworth Document Delivery Service: 1-800-HAWORTH. E-mail
address: <docdelivery@haworthpress.com> Website: <http://www.HaworthPress.
com> © 2003 by The Haworth Press, Inc. All rights reserved.]*

KEYWORDS. Bathhouse, AIDS, sex club, San Francisco, civil liberties, public health, gay

INTRODUCTION

There are no gay bathhouses in San Francisco in 2001, but there are a
number of businesses in the city that men can pay to go to, to meet other
male patrons for sex. Historical and semantic confusions have muddied
the question of how the city's bathhouses closed between their heyday
in the 1970s, and their absence in the 1990s as the city's sex clubs
reemerged. Many statements have been made which exaggerate the authority of officials in San Francisco's City government to close these
businesses, and which oversimplify the drawn-out story of how the
businesses closed or changed.

One of the most prominent statements representing these misunderstandings came at the end of the 1993 HBO film adaptation of *And the
Band Played On,* based on the late Randy Shilts's 1987 book about the
initial years of the AIDS epidemic. Shilts was a gay reporter for the *San
Francisco Chronicle,* who had often written articles about AIDS and
the city's baths.[1] After the action of the HBO film closes, journalistic
frames of text summarize aspects of the epidemic that the film focuses
on. The mistaken text of one frame begins, "San Francisco's gay bathhouses were closed in 1985."

The accuracy of the statement that the city's gay bathhouses were
closed at all hinges on the questions of who closed each one, how will-
ingly, and when. It also hinges on the definition of the term *bathhouse*
as it's distinguished from informal terms for other kinds of businesses
that provide space for sex between patrons. I've used the blanket term
"the baths" for all these businesses.[2] In 1984, a City official did order
the closure of most of San Francisco's baths, but most of these businesses defied the order. One judge ordered them closed again and another judge let them reopen, and then the city's regulation/closure story

dragged on from 1985 to 1989, shifting in focus by the 1990s from San Francisco's bathhouses to its sex clubs.

I've referred here to San Francisco's City government, and San Francisco's gay/lesbian/bisexual community, simply as "the City" and "the community."[3] In 1984, the baths emerged as a point of friction among certain City officials and community members, over what were the most appropriate methods to fight AIDS. Local arguments over the baths centered on whether closing them would be legally feasible for the City or epidemiologically necessary, and not on whether they were the primary locations in San Francisco where men were contracting AIDS.

Many members of the community argued that regulating the baths would be more effective than closing them, and that they should be used to educate patrons how AIDS was transmitted, at a time when raising AIDS awareness was still an urgently important goal. Many community members were also deeply concerned that closing the baths would lead to efforts in San Francisco and elsewhere to close down gay bars where patrons also cruised for sex partners, and to efforts to reestablish California's and other states' anti-sodomy laws.

Local debate over the baths became irreversibly enmeshed with City-government decisions in early 1984. From March to December 1984, different San Franciscans made their most strenuous efforts to close the city's baths, keep them open, or change them. That year San Francisco had the highest urban per capita prevalence of AIDS in America,[4] and the year was the most turbulent in the history of the local baths.[5]

The history of AIDS very often involves hostility and indifference. But it is relatively easy to believe that the San Francisco officials named here made sincere efforts to check the spread of AIDS, and did their best, by their own lights, to act for the welfare of men who had sex with men in the city. Community debate centered on whether these efforts really were in the community's best interests, or were unwarranted interference in gay and bisexual men's lives.

My focuses will be on AIDS-containment strategies that were publicly considered by the City in 1984 concerning former San Francisco businesses that provided space for sex between men, and on public statements about these strategies made by representatives of community organizations. At times, extraneous political pressures influenced City officials' positions on the baths, inching them towards or away from regulation or closure. Eventual policy decisions disregarded which sexual activities were considered high or low risk for AIDS, and disregarded research findings available in mid-1984, indicating that attendance at San Francisco's baths was not correlated with AIDS risk.

SAN FRANCISCO'S BATHS FROM THE 1970s TO 1984

Bay Area residents, men from across Northern California, and tourists went to the men's bathhouses, sex clubs, and back rooms of bookstores, adult theaters, and bars in San Francisco. Many of them were openly bisexual and gay, and others confined their sexual encounters with other men to these businesses, and to certain city alleys, parks, restrooms, and beaches. In early 1984 there were fourteen men's bathhouses and sex clubs in San Francisco, with average monthly attendance rates that had ranged from 3,500 to 12,000 patrons.[6] That April, the owner of a medium-sized local bathhouse said he could gross $500,000 "in a good year."[7] AIDS had already made 1984 the worst year yet for business at the baths.

Allan Bérubé's 1984 article "The History of Gay Bathhouses" is reprinted in this volume, and contributed to dialogue over the baths that year. In it, Bérubé described sexual and nonsexual facilities and social events that the baths had come to offer. They had a variety of functions: they were spaces to find other men for sex; businesses to make money; safe havens from homophobia and places to celebrate gayness; places to eat, exercise, or sit in a jacuzzi; uncomfortably critical evaluation grounds for male attractiveness; and places to sleep overnight for men who were too drunk to drive after the bars closed.

San Francisco writer Armistead Maupin mentioned the baths in several of his 1970s-80s *Tales of the City* books. In the first, 1978, book several characters go to the Club Baths at Eighth and Howard, the largest bathhouse in the city. Jon, one of the series' most sympathetic characters, is closeted in this book. He escapes a dinner party and drives from Sea Cliff to South of Market:

> At times like this, the tubs was an easy way out.
> Discreet, dispassionate, noncommittal. He could diddle away a frenzied hour or two, then return unblemished to the business of being a doctor.
> It was really his only choice.[8]

Maupin's *Babycakes* was published in 1984; like his first book, it had been serialized first in the *San Francisco Chronicle*. In *Babycakes*, an

English character named Teddy describes group sex he's had at the Hothouse, a bathhouse men especially went to for sexual fantasy and role-playing scenes. Teddy reflects that

> "One learns a lot in orgy rooms. Camaraderie. Patience. Humor. Being gentle and generous with strangers. It's not at all the depravity it's cracked up to be." He cocked his head in thought. "Just a lot of frightened children being sweet to one another in the dark."
> Michael sipped his tea.[9]

Frank Browning spoke with Maupin in the early 1990s, "at the dawn of the sex resurrection" of the sex clubs in San Francisco. He summarizes their radio interview by writing,

> The parks and the bathhouses have been places of freedom and fraternity in Maupin's life. . . . "I learned," he says with a chuckle, "that you could tell the difference between a nice guy and a bastard in the dark." In the baths, he found remarkable qualities of communication with men whose names he never knew, men with whom he did not even have sex, with whom he embraced and then moved on.[10]

The book of *And the Band Played On* offers a sharp and more or less uniform contrast from these views. Shilts repeatedly focuses on an increasing sensationalism in the baths by 1980, which he portrays as eliminating intimacy and caring from patrons' interactions.[11] The baths are described as "an amalgam of good and bad elements" in a 1983 book on gay liberation, co-authored by three women and a man, with a prefatory quotation by San Francisco's highest openly gay elected official that year, Supervisor Harry Britt. The authors mention an "ease of sexual objectification" between patrons, which chimes with Shilts's portrayals, but they also write that what "we can be proud of in the baths are the elements that we will seek in the new society [which gay liberation may realize]: friendship and caring, delight in sexual play, and an experimental approach to sexuality."[12]

The topic of sexual delight faded into the background by 1984, in most of the local debate over the baths.[13] In another 1984 article, Allan Bérubé described the bathhouse controversy in San Francisco as a "sexual panic" that had the potential to diminish the community's sexual freedom and civil liberties. He wrote that as gays and lesbians had gained political ground since the 1950s, "a tension has developed between our political movement and our sexual desires." He suggested that the community's actual political successes had introduced a note of ambivalence over whether to celebrate or downplay sexual aspects of gay/lesbian/bisexual culture.

Bérubé wrote that since accusations of lewdness had been prime ammunition in political salvos at gay rights, "We change the subject away from sex so we can defend our right to free assembly and our right to privacy" with less difficulty, as a recurring political tactic when the community was under siege.[14] Pleasure itself was a relatively rare topic in community members' defense of the baths in the mid-1980s. Community attitudes about gay sexuality often manifested either through anger at potential losses of civil liberties that safeguarded homosexual privacy, or uncertainty about the exact value of sexuality, since it had given AIDS opportunities to spread in the community.

EARLY ASPECTS OF AIDS IN SAN FRANCISCO

In the 1970s, sexually transmitted diseases (STDs) were increasingly common among men who had sex with men in San Francisco, in or out of the baths, although the ferocity of AIDS would have been very difficult to predict before the epidemic hit.[15] At least some men used condoms in some baths in the 1970s,[16] but their use was rare since nonviral STDs could be cured. A local hepatitis B epidemic in the late 1970s was something of a harbinger for AIDS.

The first AIDS cases in San Francisco surfaced in 1981, with 8 cases by August and 2 deaths. By mid-1983 the numbers had risen to 249 local cases and 72 deaths, and to 550 cases and 213 local deaths by mid-1984.[17] The City and the community began mobilizing against AIDS well before the local baths became a source of public contention, and there was considerable cooperation between them. Many community members were involved in professional work in San Francisco, including the political and medical fields. This factor greatly strengthened San Francisco's response to AIDS.[18]

Randy Shilts's journalism, his book *And the Band Played On*, and the HBO film adaptation of it have been influential in shaping public understanding of both the early AIDS epidemic, and the role of the baths in the spread of AIDS. In his book and journalism, Shilts strongly implied that the baths had to close before any effective local work could be done against AIDS. This is a very debatable contention, and it was peripheral to the mid-1980s debates over the baths in San Francisco.

In 1984, both community workers and City officials acknowledged that high-risk sex between men was spreading AIDS in bedrooms as well as the baths. Dr. Mervyn Silverman was the director of the San Francisco Department of Public Health (the DPH), and played the most important single role in the city's unfolding bathhouse debates. He believed a generally accepted estimate that "the number of people regularly frequenting the bathhouses probably represented 5 percent of the gay population," or "maybe at most 10" percent. Years later, he said that "If bathhouses were the only place that people were being infected [with HIV], closing them wouldn't have been an issue. It was very clear that 90 percent of the gay community was having the same kind of sex, maybe with fewer people, maybe a little variation on the theme."[19]

It was known by 1983 that AIDS was spread through direct contact with blood or semen, and not through casual contact. Gay and bisexual men represented about 75% of the total American cases then, and about 95% of the San Francisco cases.[20] The terms *AIDS patients* and *AIDS victims* were commonly used. San Franciscan Mark Feldman spoke at the first Candlelight Memorial March in the city in May 1983, and affirmed, "I am a *person* with AIDS . . . a human being, not a victim, and only a patient when I am in a hospital."[21]

The plural of the term Feldman coined became the name of an organization with chapters in San Francisco and other cities–People With AIDS (PWA). This term was incorporated into the Denver Principles, which were drafted by PWA activists at a 1983 conference. The principles included recommendations that no one "scapegoat people with AIDS, blame us for the epidemic or generalize about our lifestyles." PWA also recommended that people with AIDS practice only low-risk sex, and inform sex partners that they had AIDS. PWA also affirmed the rights of people with AIDS to "as full and satisfying sexual and emotional lives as anyone else."[22]

At a cancer symposium, Silverman of the DPH said that in 1983, "we began to see policemen driving down the streets of the Castro District wearing surgical masks, nurses refusing to care for AIDS patients, [and] a bus driver refusing to touch a transfer that was handed to him by a possibly gay male." Silverman said that by March 1984, San Franciscans in general had come to feel much less anxiety about AIDS because of DPH education efforts.[23] But because of the baths, local debate over political, medical, and gay-rights aspects of AIDS intensified very soon after this statement. Michael Helquist, a local gay journalist, described this period as "a very charged, very emotional, and very unpleasant time."[24]

In April 1984, different health officials announced the discoveries of LAV and HTLV-III, which turned out to be the same virus; renamed HIV in 1986. The theory of this single etiological trigger for AIDS emerged conclusively in November 1984.[25] Widely available tests for viral antibodies were expected to be forthcoming then, but there were strong community concerns about potential discrimination against people who tested positive. In a November 1984 interview, the editor of a community paper suggested to Silverman that his actions over the baths had increased local men's distrust of government, and reluctance to participate in a badly needed, federally funded epidemiological study of AIDS. Silverman acknowledged this possibility, but asserted that the DPH would protect the confidentiality of test results.[26]

THE BATHS, AIDS AWARENESS, AND RISK LEVELS

As early as July 1981, in an interview with AIDS clinician Dr. Alvin Friedman-Kien, Dr. Lawrence Mass raised the question in the *New York Native* of whether the baths could be targeted for closure if AIDS were found to spread in them. Friedman-Kien said he doubted it, unless a communicable disease were isolated for AIDS that was "being spread from a specific location *because* of that location."[27] These emphases on causation and location remained at the center of public health questions of AIDS and the baths beyond 1984. In the early 1980s, other people inside and outside the community suggested either that the baths were ideal locations to distribute condoms and raise AIDS-awareness among people at sexual risk for AIDS, or that men would continue to engage in self-destructive behaviors at the baths until they were closed.[28]

Fear of AIDS contributed to a very sharp slump in business at San Francisco's baths by mid-1983. Shilts wrote in the *Chronicle* that attendance was down by 50% at the Sutro Baths, and that this was an unusually mild annual decrease for a local bathhouse that year.[29] In 1983 the Sutro Baths published ads in community papers telling readers to use condoms, and reminding them that sexually, "It's Not *Where* You Do It, It's *How* You Do It" that created AIDS risks.[30] In mid-1983 the Hothouse was closed by its owner Louis Gaspar, who said, "I don't think it's where you have sex that causes AIDS," but "I just couldn't stay open when I felt I might be somehow responsible for people getting it."[31]

In late 1983, a community reporter paraphrased Silverman of the DPH as emphasizing that "the type of sexual activity in which one engages (not sharing bodily fluids), is far more important than the number of sexual contacts one has, in reducing the risk of contracting AIDS. He strongly urged the use of condoms."[32] In January 1984, six of the eight bathhouses in San Francisco agreed to the City's request that they distribute condoms to patrons, and were praised for it by DPH representatives.[33] But in crucial statements he made and orders he issued later in 1984, Silverman neglected these two emphases on avoiding fluid exchange and using condoms during sex.

In these early years of the epidemic, the community and health officials agreed on a strong need to continue raising awareness, especially among all men who had sex with men, of what AIDS was and how it was spread. Community papers did a much better job at discussing sex and risk than mainstream newspapers. Men who had sex with men, but had limited involvement with the openly gay and bisexual community, had correspondingly limited access to accurate information about sexual risks for AIDS. The baths were much more practical forums to reach these men than city parks with nighttime, homosexually active reputations.

A chart for risk guidelines that ran in community papers was produced in June 1984 by the San Francisco AIDS Foundation (SFAF) (Figure 1). The chart's classifications of safe, possibly safe, and unsafe activities are different in some important ways from the received HIV-risk standards of 2001. Fellatio with withdrawal before ejaculation was only listed as possibly safe, and fellatio with ejaculation was listed as definitely unsafe. Insertive and receptive anal sex with a condom were listed as possibly safe.[34] HTLV-III was discovered in saliva in 1984. Federal and local authorities issued strong reassurances that the public at large didn't need to worry about AIDS risk "if a gay waiter sneezes on your steak." But in 1985, the SFAF took out ads in community papers discussing the uncertain safety of French kissing.[35]

Also in June 1984, the community-based Bay Area Physicians for Human Rights (BAPHR) issued a wallet-sized card with the same categories of risk levels and sexual behaviors (Figure 2). A number of San Francisco baths stocked these and other AIDS-education materials, and in fall 1984, one bathhouse owner claimed to have distributed about 5,000 of BAPHR's cards.[36] But during 1984, different local baths showed uneven levels of commitment to promoting AIDS awareness.

1983: SILVERMAN AND LARRY LITTLEJOHN

Debate over the baths in San Francisco had begun, erratically, by 1983. Different people disagreed deeply about how urgent an issue the

FIGURE 1. **AIDS-Awareness Chart, San Francisco AIDS Foundation, Mid-1984.** The chart ran in gay papers in San Francisco from 1984 to 1985. Courtesy of the SFAF; scan courtesy of the Gay, Lesbian, Bisexual, Transgender Historical Society of Northern California.

Can You Pass The Safe Sex Test?
Safe Sex Protects You and Your Partner

Sex I Like To Do (Or Might Be Talked Into)

	SAFE	POSSIBLY SAFE	UNSAFE
☐ Being fucked without a condom			■
☐ Fucking without a condom			■
☐ Being fucked with a condom		☐	
☐ Fucking with a condom		☐	
☐ Getting sucked to climax			■
☐ Getting sucked - stopping before climax		☐	
☐ Sucking to climax			■
☐ Sucking - stopping before climax		☐	
☐ Masturbation/jacking off	☐		
☐ Massage/hugging/dry kissing	☐		
☐ Watersports in mouth			■
☐ Watersports on skin		☐	
☐ Rimming/scat			■
☐ Fisting			■
☐ Sharing dildos and sex toys			■
☐ Dildos and sex toys - not shared	☐		
☐ Body-to-body rubbing (frottage/tribadism)	☐		
☐ Semen or urine in mouth or anus			■
☐ Cunnilingus		☐	
☐ Contact with someone's blood			■
☐ Sharing needles			■

AIDS HOTLINES: (415) 863-AIDS / Toll-Free in N. CA (800) FOR-AIDS / TTY (415) 864-6606   Produced by the San Francisco AIDS Foundation, June 1984.

Another Message From The San Francisco AIDS Foundation

baths were in light of AIDS, and whether they ought to change or be changed. That May, longtime gay activist Larry Littlejohn wrote to urge Silverman to try to check the spread of AIDS by closing the city's baths.[37] In the 1960s Littlejohn was a president of the Society for Individual Rights, a pioneering San Francisco gay-rights group whose magazine ran reviews praising different baths.[38]

In his reply to Littlejohn, Silverman made claims that would later rebound on him, writing that it would be "inappropriate and in fact illegal for me to close down all bathhouses and other such places." Silverman also felt that closure would "insult the intelligence of many of our citizens and it would be an invasion of their privacy to take such an action." He said the primary goal of the DPH was to cooperate with other organizations "to educate the public, both gay and straight," about how AIDS could be spread.[39]

FIGURE 2. **Wallet-Sized AIDS-Awareness Card, Bay Area Physicians for Human Rights, Mid-1984.** The card was distributed at certain San Francisco baths in 1984. © and courtesy of BAPHR.

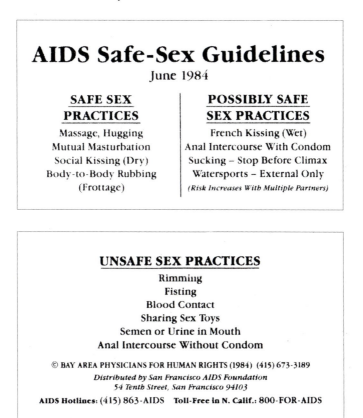

AIDS Safe-Sex Guidelines
June 1984

SAFE SEX PRACTICES	POSSIBLY SAFE SEX PRACTICES
Massage, Hugging	French Kissing (Wet)
Mutual Masturbation	Anal Intercourse With Condom
Social Kissing (Dry)	Sucking – Stop Before Climax
Body-to-Body Rubbing	Watersports – External Only
(Frottage)	*(Risk Increases With Multiple Partners)*

UNSAFE SEX PRACTICES
Rimming
Fisting
Blood Contact
Sharing Sex Toys
Semen or Urine in Mouth
Anal Intercourse Without Condom

© BAY AREA PHYSICIANS FOR HUMAN RIGHTS (1984) (415) 673-3189
Distributed by San Francisco AIDS Foundation
54 Tenth Street, San Francisco 94103
AIDS Hotlines: (415) 863-AIDS **Toll-Free in N. Calif.:** 800-FOR-AIDS

That September, Silverman replied to another letter from Littlejohn. He wrote that owners of local baths were cooperating with the DPH in risk-reduction work. Warnings about AIDS-risk behaviors had been posted, attendance had decreased, and there seemed to be less group sex at the baths. Silverman wrote, "My fear is that if the bathhouses were to close the community might perceive that the problem of AIDS is solved. This is, of course, patently incorrect." He also feared that if the baths were closed, patrons might "immediately switch to other locations where we would have less access to post warnings and provide some education." He disagreed with Littlejohn about the potential medical or social benefits of closure, given the current state of knowledge about AIDS and the "substantial civil rights issues connected to a policy to close the bathhouses."[40] These issues included national freedom-of-assembly rights, and a state guarantee of consenting adult Californians' right to engage in sexual behavior.

In October 1983, federal officials indicated that the regulation of sexual conduct involving AIDS risks was a thorny decision that local officials would have to make for themselves, since federal rights and various state and local sexual privacy rights were involved. San Francisco's mayor Dianne Feinstein and Silverman's boss, the city's chief administrative officer, both favored the closure of the city's baths. But because of City-Charter constraints on them, San Francisco's AIDS decisions rested largely with Silverman.[41] Through 1984, the brunt of the responsibility was on Silverman to decide how to use or not use the DPH's authority to try to manage the spread of AIDS among San Franciscans.

JANUARY-FEBRUARY 1984:
THE CHRONICLE, AIDS, AND THE BATHS

In the early 1980s the gay press offered almost all the coverage of AIDS that was available in nontechnical language, although from 1981 to 1984, the *San Francisco Chronicle* published more AIDS stories than the *New York Times* and *Los Angeles Times* combined.[42] In mid-1983, Randy Shilts wrote a *Chronicle* article about DPH AIDS cautions for the Gay Pride parade, when the city and its baths saw a regular, large influx of tourists. Shilts quoted Supervisor Harry Britt's speculation that people who were still going to baths despite AIDS risks were "either unaware of the problem or have a psychological investment in going that is so strong that they're willing to risk their lives."[43] This generalization implied that all patrons went to the baths for high-risk sex.

On 3 February 1984, Shilts gave his first quotations criticizing the baths from AIDS researchers and clinicians who were willing to be named. Shilts quoted local gay doctor Donald Abrams as saying he didn't favor City closure of the baths, "but they need to close because of lack of business. I'm in favor of a boycott." Shilts also quoted Dr. James Curran, head of the AIDS Activity Office at the federal Centers for Disease Control, as saying, "I'd like to see all the bathhouses go out of business."[44] Curran later objected–saying, "I didn't see a role for government in legislating behavior or legislating change," and "concerns about bathhouses should come from the gay community rather than from government."[45] In another interview Curran said he wasn't "in favor of bathhouses," but "I didn't say most of the things in the article!" Curran said about Shilts that "He means well but he doesn't ask himself why he writes what he does."[46]

In a 4 February *Chronicle* article, Shilts quoted local gay clinician Dr. Marcus Conant's rhetorical question about the baths, "What are we going to do about compulsively promiscuous men?" Shilts also quoted Harry Britt as saying, "Sexual activity in places like baths or sex clubs should no longer be associated with pleasure–it should be associated with death."[47] Britt also claimed that Shilts misrepresented him, and "wants to shut down the bathhouses and tried to get someone to say that." Shilts was quoted in the *Advocate* as insisting that "he has no opinion on whether bathhouses should close. 'I write news stories, not editorials,'" Shilts said.[48]

In the 4 February article, Shilts also ran an SFAF poster that showed two naked men embracing, and promoted lower-risk sex (Figure 3). Shilts wrote that "AIDS researchers privately have mocked these efforts," which focused on "the fun to be had with 'safe sex.'" Shilts wrote that Britt had said, "We need a new style of education campaign." A few days later, the *Chronicle*'s gossip columnist Herb Caen wrote, "MAYBE YOU MISSED that anti-AIDS poster put out by the AIDS Foundation. If so, you bettah off [*sic*]." Caen wrote, "For what I suppose are non-racist reasons the black man [in the poster] is elegantly built . . . while the white fellow is an overweight blob with a large posterior." He summed up the poster as "All quite adorable and ineffectual. What is needed is something tough, like a skull and crossbones and a few harsh words, such as 'Stop acting stupid or you gonna die, suckah.'"[49]

The distribution of the poster and other educational materials to the baths was facilitated by the Department of Public Health. Years later Silverman would say about Shilts's articles,

> I remember he talked about the [DPH's] lackluster AIDS education plan. The thing was, he didn't say, "So-and-so said it was lackluster." Lackluster was *his* word, and that's not reporting. That's commenting. It's opinion. So I finally got tired of this really biased treatment. In fact, I got so upset–obviously, none of us like to be criticized, but it's okay if at least there's balance–that I cut him off from access to me.
>
> He ended up writing me a note saying, "I'm sorry, you're right, I shouldn't do this, and I promise not to do it again." Not

FIGURE 3. **AIDS-Awareness Poster, San Francisco AIDS Foundation, Early 1984.** © and courtesy of the SFAF; photograph by Mick Hicks.

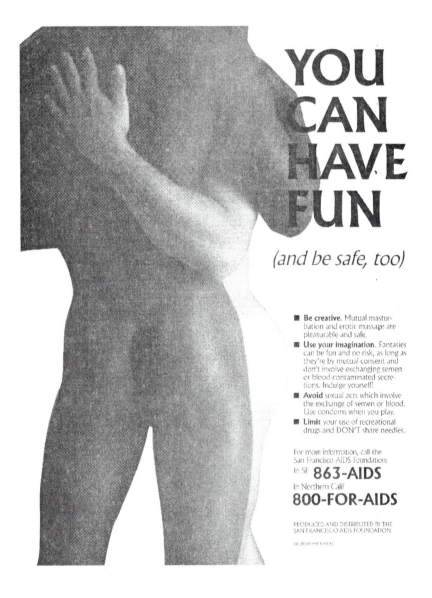

promise not to be critical, but promise not to be so biased and one-sided. I used to call his editor and say, "For God's sake, put him on the editorial page."[50]

THE LITTLEJOHN PETITION

The bathhouse debates' momentum became irreversible on 27 March 1984. At the monthly meeting of the Harvey Milk Lesbian/Gay Democratic Club, Larry Littlejohn distributed a press release stating his intention to seek 7,332 signatures on a petition for a new ballot initiative, to direct that "sexual activities among patrons of public bathhouses should be prohibited" in San Francisco.

Until then, the local bathhouse debates had mostly been conducted behind the scenes–in personal letters and private meetings, or for the readers of the gay press. The main exceptions were Shilts's quotations in the *Chronicle* and two men's July 1983 article on AIDS in the mainstream *California* magazine, describing the baths as "a perverse and inchoate symbol of gay liberation itself."[51] But Littlejohn's announcement immediately turned up the heat on community concerns and City plans–rattling the lid, so to speak, off the simmer of the discussions of the previous year, and bringing the debates to a boil.

No one seemed to doubt that over one percent of the city's population would sign Littlejohn's petition, or that a Yes vote was overwhelmingly likely, or that this vote would look to the rest of the country like an indirect but still crushing moral condemnation of gay sexuality, by the bulk of the electorate of the country's gay mecca. The initiative would have been put on the ballot in August for a November vote.[52] August became a galvanizing deadline for action, for community activists and City officials who felt concern about the community's civil rights and its public image.

In the coming months, circumstances strongly impelled or compelled many City officials and community members to go on record with a statement on whether and how the baths should be allowed to operate. To propose any relevant policy, it was necessary to address or dodge the concerns of public health and gay civil rights–often bluntly favoring one over the other. The two priorities were often seen as being difficult or impossible to reconcile. Dennis Altman's sensible, reconciling assessment is that "there can be genuine disagreement on this question that need not imply one is homophobic."[53]

In the first week of March 1984, Silverman had made a speech addressing these two priorities, and echoing many of the statements he'd written in 1983 to Littlejohn. In the speech, Silverman had said that in terms of civil liberties, closure could "lead to the passage of restrictive legislation" that would damage "the social fabric or political rights that have been made by lesbian and gay individuals." As for public health, he also said closing the baths "would, in the first place, not end the [high-risk sexual] activities that have taken place in them, and equally important, we would lose the potential of reaching" people with AIDS-education messages at these centralized venues.[54] These statements demonstrate a ten-month continuity in Silverman's anti-closure stance on the baths, from May 1983 to early March 1984. After Littlejohn's 27 March announcement and the turmoil that followed it, Silverman began what would eventually be a 180-degree shift in his positions.

COMMUNITY RESPONSES TO THE LITTLEJOHN PETITION

Littlejohn's announcement aroused a good deal of community anger. Many written attacks on him were personal, ranging from his being called "LittleBrain," "Judas Littlejohn or Lazydick Arnold" in another letter to the editor of the *Bay Area Reporter*, the community's "traitor *extraordinaire*" by the *B.A.R.*'s editor himself,[55] and, in effect, the hemorrhoid on the asshole of the gay community by the owner of the Sutro Baths.[56] But Littlejohn seemed to maintain a steady confidence that a ban on bathhouse sex was for the community's greater good, and an awareness of his own good faith in proposing the ballot initiative.

Before he made his announcement, Littlejohn discussed his intentions with Shilts, Supervisor Britt, and with Carole Migden of the Milk Club, who all shared his view that the baths were more dangerous to the community than beneficial. Britt changed his position on the baths a number of times that year, and the reservations he sometimes did express were often very equivocal. Migden and Bill Kraus of the Milk Club became two of the community's most consistent advocates for the baths' closure. Kraus said it would be "increasingly difficult to tell straight politicians that there is a terrible crisis if we don't act like there is a crisis ourselves." Migden compared the baths to typhoid-infected swimming pools,[57] and said that since closure was now practically inevitable, community leaders should try to salvage control of the situation by calling for closure themselves. She also strongly opposed Littlejohn's initiative, saying it could "destroy all the political gains we've had" for the community.[58]

Littlejohn's announcement kicked off a frenetic series of meetings between dozens of members of community political, business, medical, legal, and activist organizations. Some people wanted Silverman to close the baths himself, and others were reluctant to assist in any DPH closure efforts. Michael Helquist and Rick Osmon wrote a clear, approximately 10,000-word summary of the next five days of community members' intense networking, brainstorming, resolutions, disagreements, retractions, and clarifications for the community paper *Coming Up!*[59]

The activity crystallized somewhat on the night of 29 March, when the president of the Stonewall Democratic Club and the activist owner of the Valencia Rose cabaret held a forum there on the looming possibility of the baths' closure. They invited Silverman and anyone who was interested to come and speak. Around a hundred people went, including "a large cross-section of the Lesbian/Gay leadership." Silverman was candid and forceful about the bind that he and the community were facing, saying that the ballot petition was "crazy," but that a recent rumor that AIDS incidence was dropping was "*bullshit.* It's going up everywhere." The meeting lasted over two hours, and speakers opposed to immediate closure outnumbered those in favor by about five to one.[60]

SILVERMAN'S FIRST PRESS CONFERENCE ON THE BATHS

Silverman had already called an 11 a.m. press conference for the next morning, 30 March; it was widely anticipated that he would close the baths. Over 200 people went to the conference, including a group of anti-closure demonstrators who smiled and wore towels around their waists. Different signs they carried read, "Today the Tubs, Tomorrow Your Bedroom," and "Out of the Baths and Into the Ovens?"[61] Another sign read, "Out of the Tubs and Into the Shrubs," expressing the belief that if the baths were closed, a number of men would keep meeting for sex in city parks and other places where condoms and AIDS-education materials were unavailable.

In a key, 1992-93 oral history conducted by Sally Smith Hughes, Silverman described a meeting he had that morning, before the press conference, with City Attorney George Agnost. Agnost told Silverman that the DPH needed far more information before a legally viable effort could be made to close the baths. Silverman had been open to the idea of closure before this talk, but now he decided against it. After consulting

Agnost, he met with Mayor Feinstein, Harry Britt, the chief of the SFPD, and a number of doctors and political activists. Silverman told them he had already made up his mind not to close the baths that day.

In the interview with Hughes, Silverman described how he said to everyone, "Just for the hell of it, how many of you now think I should close the bathhouses, and how many think I shouldn't?" The room was evenly divided. Silverman told Hughes, "The way it comes out in Shilts' book is as if that [question] was the determining factor. . . . One of the problems I had with Randy was his selective listening. His version is even going to be in the television movie that's coming out."[62] The biggest historical errors in the HBO film's portrayals of the bathhouse debates center on this event.

Silverman arrived at the auditorium almost an hour late.[63] A DPH official had received a telephone death threat for Silverman if he closed the baths, and he put on a bulletproof vest before he went in. When he was seated, Silverman simply announced, "I am not discussing the opening or closing of the bathhouses at this point." He said he was delaying his decision after considering various "facets of this issue, some of which had basically nothing to do with medicine and some of which do."[64] Years later, Silverman reread his own words to Hughes–"'and some of which do.' And I'm not sure what that 'some' would be. I may have thrown that in just to throw people off a little bit. But the real issue was the legal aspect" of the City Attorney's having told him, "You can't do it, because you don't have the necessary evidence to close them down."[65]

What Silverman called his "non-press conference" can still be seen as the first important City action on the baths that year: a public decision to postpone making a decision about regulation or closure. That day, Silverman announced that there was nothing to announce yet, apologized for keeping the crowded room waiting, said he'd try to issue a clear policy statement within a week or so, and left the room to the sustained applause of some audience members. Nevertheless, City Attorney Agnost hazarded a medical opinion for the *Chronicle* that day, that the "scientific basis is quite sound and quite convincing" to support a City move to close the baths.[66]

POSITIONS ON CLOSURE FROM ACTIVISTS AND THE MAYOR

Many letters about this controversy would be drafted in 1984 by coalitions of members of community organizations, delegates of single groups, and individuals. Gay author Frank Robinson had signed a tentative letter to Silverman favoring closure. He was concerned what would happen if AIDS "jump[ed] the fence," and began spreading widely among heterosexuals. He asked who would want to take bets on "whose lifestyle will be blamed? . . . What kind of defense could we offer as to having tried to contain the disease ourselves?"[67]

On 1 April, members of two of the community's Democratic clubs, bath-owners, and representatives of some AIDS service organizations held a meeting to draft a letter to Silverman opposing any "unilateral action by the city and to formulate alternatives" to closure. On 2 April, Bobbi Campbell, R.N., issued a response to the Littlejohn petition on behalf of the local chapter of People With AIDS (PWA). Campbell had been the first San Franciscan to come out publicly as having AIDS in 1981. He had been on the cover of *Newsweek* in August 1983,[68] and he would die in August 1984. His letter encapsulated many of the positions that other anti-closure groups took during the year.

Campbell said that PWA members believed that closing the baths "is not the real issue; rather, the issue is the education of gay men as to what *specific sexual practices*" carried risks for AIDS. He also suggested concrete changes for the baths. While he made risk behavior a more important issue than location, he wrote that the baths "should make structural and functional changes to encourage and facilitate low-risk, safe-sex practices," and discourage high-risk practices by turning up their lights, supplying educational materials and condoms, and closing orgy rooms–large, comfortable spaces for group sex.[69]

Campbell wrote that closing the baths could have "nationally detrimental effects on how gay men view ourselves and how we are viewed by society." He wrote that closure could give a green light to other city governments to close gay bars along with their baths, and that "increased discrimination against gay men in general and people with AIDS in particular" could follow. PWA doubted that other cities would understand that any San Francisco closure effort was only "a political shellgame to avert a more restrictive petition initiative" here. Campbell described the Littlejohn petition as "the worst possible approach to the AIDS crisis," and declared that PWA was now on the record opposing both the petition and any efforts to close the baths.[70]

Many community members shared Campbell's concerns that closure could have a city-by-city domino effect, leading to bath-closures in other places; and also what could be called a civil-liberties erosion effect on gay civil rights, in and beyond San Francisco. In an undated position statement, the National Gay and Lesbian Task Force (NGLTF) in

Washington also expressed its concerns that closure efforts could work towards "the reinstitution of sodomy statutes and other violations of the right to privacy," in American states where anti-sodomy laws had been revoked. In 1984 these laws were in force in half the states. The NGLTF affirmed a right to personal sexual decision-making that would recur in other community stances on the baths, emphasizing that "The regulatory powers of government . . . should not extend to the direct or indirect coercion of individuals regarding their private, consensual sexual activity."[71]

San Francisco's mayor, Dianne Feinstein, was the head of the AIDS Task Force of the U.S. Conference of Mayors and had organized an AIDS Awareness Week in 1983, inviting people with AIDS and their families to her office. Feinstein was widely known to feel real and deep concern for people with AIDS. However, her attitudes towards gay men's sexuality in general, and sexual creativity in particular, were less supportive.[72] Five days after Silverman's press conference, the mayor made her first on-the-record statement about the bathhouse controversy, saying, "My own opinion is that if this was a heterosexual problem, they would have been closed." She said, "The bottom-line question here is death. AIDS means one thing, and that is that you die. And therefore, if you want to avoid it, the message has to go out. Not in a namby-pamby way."[73]

SILVERMAN'S SECOND PRESS CONFERENCE ON THE BATHS

Five days later, on Monday, 9 April, Silverman announced that "all sexual activity between individuals [is to] be eliminated in public facilities in San Francisco where the transmission of AIDS is likely to occur." The ban was aimed at city "bathhouses, sex clubs and the back rooms of certain bookstores," as "Locations which particularly foster" meetings between gay and bisexual men who "indulge in multiple sexual encounters." In *And the Band Played On*, Shilts describes the order as "regulations to ban high-risk sexual activity";[74] this description is inaccurate. Silverman made no mention of risk levels, or distinctions between different sexual activities that were considered likely or unlikely to transmit AIDS.

Silverman announced his having met the week before with "a panel of national, state and local AIDS experts" to ask for recommendations for the baths. He said the ban represented "the unanimous position of this group," and had the support of both "AIDS experts and gay leaders."[75] He held this press conference seated at his desk at the DPH, flanked by a number of gay men he'd met with the day before, in a second consultation to discuss policies for the baths. He said, "Look at the group standing behind me," which included community activists and Drs. Don Abrams and Marcus Conant. "This is not a government-against-group thing."[76]

Unfortunately, Silverman's statements created the impression that it was the men standing around him as he announced his ban who had unanimously approved this new regulation policy, rather than the first group he'd convened on 3 April. The day before his announcement, 8 April, Silverman had neglected to tell this second group of local men about the earlier group's unanimity or any resolutions he'd come to, himself, to ban all sex in the baths. But Silverman now called "upon all members of the gay community to work with us as we move through these uncharted waters together."

A *San Francisco Examiner* sub-headline on the story read, "Gay leaders support policy, Silverman says."[77] But many of the people Silverman had met with the day before had disagreed and would disagree with this attempt to regulate the baths. Several of the people who literally stood behind Silverman as he made his statement were taken by surprise by his blanket ban on all sexual activity in the baths, regardless of condom use or fluid exchange, and withdrew their support.

For instance Tom Peretti, of the community's Concerned Republicans for Individual Rights, said that the Monday press conference Silverman had held "came off quite different than at the meeting" on Sunday. Peretti said, "I feel used, manipulated."[78] Psychiatrist Rick Andrews attended the 3 and 8 April meetings. When he was asked whether he supported Silverman's ban, Andrews said, "I support what I believe is his intent," but also confirmed that at the Sunday, 8 April meeting, Silverman "told us he was going to leave the area of 'safe sex' open."[79] Steven Richter of Bay Area Lawyers for Individual Freedom wrote in an open letter to Silverman that he was "more than annoyed" to hear that Silverman had implied that Richter supported the ban, when no vote had been taken on Sunday. Richter advised Silverman "that I intend to vigorously oppose the action you announced."[80] And Rev. James Sandmire of the Metropolitan Community Church (MCC) wrote, in an open letter to Silverman,

> I am disturbed by several statements you made at the news conference yesterday. I understand my concern is shared by others who

attended the meeting with you on Sunday. . . . it was my understanding that both bathhouses and other establishments would be allowed to develop creative programs that were erotic in nature and that sexual activity not involving the exchange of blood and semen would be encouraged. . . .

I want you to know I believe in your ethics and motives. Please clarify this issue for us. . . . We minister to [AIDS patients] and their families [at MCC] and we see them die. Accordingly, we will support any reasonable course to combat this disease.

However, some of us are among the early supporters of gay liberation. We will not support anything that diminishes our rights.[81]

FOLLOWING UP THE BAN, AND EIGHT LOCAL BATHS

Littlejohn announced he would drop his petition initiative, since Silverman's ban covered the petition's regulatory measures.[82] Silverman left the "legal fine points" of his ban's actual enforcement for the City Attorney's Office to draft in time. Silverman said he would ask for health inspectors to be empowered to make unannounced visits to bathhouses and report on any sexual activity, for which the owner's license could be revoked. Bathhouse patrons would not have been penalized.[83]

Silverman faced significant legal obstacles if he tried to enforce the ban, because bathhouse licenses were granted by the Police Department, not the DPH. And years later, Silverman described how "there was absolutely no regulation on sex clubs. None. We charged $300 to license a pretzel vendor, and yet sex clubs, which were making tons of money, were unlicensed."[84] Silverman did have the state-issued, emergency authority to quarantine any building whose premises were contaminated with a pathogen, but it was well understood by 1984 that AIDS was only directly spread by people, not rooms.

Silverman's ban may have contributed, along with very steep declines in business, to the self-closures of four local baths in the next two months, starting on 15 April with the Liberty Baths. In contrast to Shilts's description of the "cold, hard stares of the bathhouse attendants," a former patron described the place as having had a "wonderfully good-humored" staff, "thrilling" wall paintings, and the most intimate atmosphere of any local bathhouse.[85]

On 21 April the Catacombs, a club mainly known for fisting, held the last in its series of closing parties. Former patrons described the owners' providing condoms, gloves, showers, and surgical soap, and said, "They started educating their clientele from the start about safety."[86] Hal Slate, the owner of the Caldron, closed it in May; the club was especially known for watersports (sex play with urine), but had also hosted twice-weekly, masturbation-only nights, and had sponsored safe-sex education events in the previous year.[87]

The Sutro Baths was closed by its owner Bill Jones on 3 June.[88] The business had attained a good standard of accuracy with its 1983 AIDS slogan, "It's Not *Where* You Do It, It's *How* You Do It." In late April 1984, four other local bathhouses produced an ad that implied all sex on their premises would be inherently safe, whatever patrons did. The Club Baths at Eighth and Howard, the Club San Francisco bathhouse on Ritch Street, Animals, and the 21st Street Baths ran this ad along with three out-of-town baths. It was titled, "baths . . . not the problem but part of the solution!" It stated that "A full range of activities await your pleasure in our unique, clean environments," and "*You're invited* to be part of the solution. Redeem the coupon below and discover that sex can be safe and pleasurable." Above the coupon was the slogan, "your pass to safe sex."

A lower corner of the ad displayed a resolution by various baths' owners, in fine print, to "disseminate objective information about A.I.D.S." to their patrons.[89] But the ad itself contained no information about how AIDS could be either spread or contained. It ignored the links between AIDS risk and fluid-exchange sex, on or off the baths' premises–making no mention of condoms, risk levels of different sexual activities, or activities that the owners encouraged or discouraged at their businesses. This combination of invitations and omissions was as misleading as Harry Britt's and the mayor's previous implications that all sex at the baths automatically equaled risk and death.[90] The ad only made a simplistic negations of Britt's and Feinstein's equations of bath-attendance with AIDS risk, by implying that the baths, as places, were risk-free.

THE MAYOR AND THE SFPD

In a 27 March statement made on the day the Littlejohn petition was announced, Feinstein had acknowledged that "The closure and non-closure of the bathhouses is a public health issue not in the jurisdiction of the mayor," but said she had asked Silverman to make sure that AIDS-education materials were updated in the baths weekly. Feinstein had also said, "It is fair to say I am greatly concerned about the rapid spread of this deadly disease and I am watching the situation as closely as I can."[91]

A 31 May *Examiner* story revealed that the mayor's watch on the situation had been close enough to be considered municipal espionage by very angry community members. Within four days of Littlejohn's petition announcement, Feinstein had ordered on-duty, plainclothes San Francisco policemen to go into the baths, pose as patrons, and write a report for her on the sexual activities they saw. When the chief of the SFPD sent the mayor this report, he included another report of secret bath-surveillance made at an unspecified date, which the police had produced on their own initiative.[92]

The *Examiner* article marked the beginning of the SFPD's brief, open role in the bathhouse debates. When the police surveillance was revealed, Feinstein insisted that "the mayor has a right to get the facts about a situation," that her orders had been "entirely justified," and that "My concern with this has nothing to do with anything I may or may not think about morality. It has to do with life versus death."[93]

Feinstein refused to make the reports publicly available.[94] She claimed, "I cannot release them," though she had shown the second report to Silverman, who said, "It just described what goes on in bathhouses. It didn't tell me anything new."[95] Two unidentified city officials who also saw the report confided to Randy Shilts that it was "very explicit, very graphic," and said, "It definitely would get an X-rating."[96] The reports were never released to the public.

COMMUNITY RESPONSES, AND PAST INTERACTIONS WITH THE SFPD

A broad array of community members condemned the police surveillance. Harry Britt called the reports " 'unconscionable,' and expressed disbelief that the mayor would even order them." Sal Rosselli of the Alice B. Toklas Democratic Club said the mayor "should call a meeting with gay leaders and commit herself against ever doing this again." A political aide to one of the City Supervisors said Feinstein "did make the concession that she would never do it again using police." Rosselli said that in light of the "close relationships" between Feinstein and many community members, "we would expect her to come to us and ask for this information." The owner of Animals also said, "There are enough people in the gay community who frequent bathhouses who the mayor could just ask about what goes on there."[97]

The SFPD surveillance revelations provided the "immediate impetus" for two investigative articles by Helquist and Osmon on the baths' different environments and patrons' behavior in them, which ran a few months later in the community paper *Coming Up!* The journalists toured the baths as fellow patrons and openly gay men, for the sake of putting two community members' perspectives into the public record. They described individual men they met in different baths, covering the land-mined controversy in straightforward language. The articles are further described below, and are reprinted in this volume.

The community paper the *Bay Area Reporter* ran an editorial by publisher Bob Ross on the mayor's surveillance order, called "Big Sister's Watching." Protest letters to the editor in the paper were deeply critical of Feinstein. Most were reasonably polite, but two letters also ran without comment by editor Paul Lorch, saying, "One understands and accepts that there are probably as many pussy-whipped males under the dome of City Hall as there were eunuchs in the harem of the Ottoman Sultan," and calling Feinstein a "Jewish Princess."[98]

Dorothy Ehrlich, executive director of the Northern California chapter of the American Civil Liberties Union, wrote Feinstein "to express our profound objection" to the surveillance, which "unjustifiably invaded the privacy rights of the patrons of these establishments," who had gone "with a reasonable expectation that their activities will be free of government intrusion and that other patrons will be persons who share a common purpose." She wrote, "It is inconceivable" that patrons "would have expected that intimate and perfectly legal activities were being observed by an on-duty government agent and recorded for a police report."[99]

The SFPD had made advances against homophobia, but in 1984 many transgendered, lesbian, gay, and bisexual San Franciscans had experienced harassment, entrapment, extortion, arrest, mass arrests, announcements of their arrests at workplaces and in the media, or battery by local police in the previous years and decades, for their gender-expressions or sexuality alone.[100] From 1978 to 1979, many members of the SFPD had expressed sympathy for Supervisor Dan White in the months after he shot gay Supervisor Harvey Milk and the city's progressive Mayor George Moscone, whose death had automatically raised Feinstein from president of the Board of Supervisors to mayor.

A wave of police harassment of the community followed the murders, culminating after the White Night riot in May 1979, after White received the lightest possible verdict for the shootings–manslaughter. Five to ten thousand outraged community members rioted at City Hall, smashing windows and setting police cars on fire. Later that night police stormed a Castro bar, shouting "dirty cocksuckers" and "sick faggots," and indiscriminately battered patrons there and people on the street for two hours.[101]

Trust between the local police and the community had only been restored very gradually. In the fall of 1983, Feinstein had sent a letter to the U.S. Attorney General to say that because of the gravity of White's crimes and the lightness of his sentence, "talk of his impending parole has in my view rekindled the passions that erupted five [and four] years ago." Feinstein vigorously urged White's continuing punishment,[102] but 1984 had begun with White's release from jail.

On 6 January 1984, an afternoon protest rally at Union Square had drawn four thousand demonstrators, and a rally that night in the Castro drew nine thousand, to bear witness to the community's continuing grief and anger.[103] That summer, any use of police authority by the mayor to restrict the baths might have hit the community on very old bruises. Gay and bisexual men had turned to the baths for decades to celebrate their sexuality without fears of outside violence, except for the community's memories and awareness of sometimes brutal police raids on the baths.[104]

THE MAYOR, THE SFPD, THE CITY ATTORNEY, AND THE SUPERVISORS

On 11 June, less than two weeks after the police surveillance of the baths was revealed, the mayor canceled public, Police-Department hearings that had been scheduled for 27 June. City Attorney George Agnost criticized the mayor's decision, since it disrupted regulatory plans for the bathhouses that his office, the mayor, and the police had been preparing together.[105]

Agnost was the City's primary legal advisor and representative. The SFPD hearings would have been an effort to give legal teeth to Silverman's 9 April sex ban, via authority given in the San Francisco Civil Code to the SFPD, since bathhouse licenses were granted by the Police Department rather than the Health Department. At the hearings on 27 June, new regulations for bathhouses would have been proposed for construction details and sexual behavior. Each bathhouse would have had to meet these new standards to keep its license, but the Code amendments could only have passed after public hearings.[106]

The new plans included a few changes that were similar to Bobbi Campbell's suggestions for the baths, for instance proposals for brighter lighting. But the plans also included a system of in-house monitors; the prohibition of oral sex, anal sex, analingus or rimming, fisting, and scatology; and the elimination of all private rooms and gloryholes (a hole in a wall that allows the performance of fellatio through it).

Like Silverman's ban, these regulations failed to mention AIDS-risk levels or sex with condoms, and solo and mutual masturbation were neither prohibited nor explicitly permitted. If a bathhouse had violated these regulations, it could lose its license for 90 days or permanently, and patrons who had sex could have been expelled. Bathhouses would have been required to post these guidelines on their walls.[107] Unlike the SFAF's and BAPHR's AIDS-education literature, the regulations were couched in highly clinical, roundabout language. The *B.A.R.* reported it was Feinstein who insisted that the earlier word *penis* be substituted with "the copulatory organ" and its placing.[108]

Twelve days after the *Examiner* revealed the police surveillance from that March, the mayor canceled the hearings for the SFPD regulation proposals, and switched political directions. On 11 June she encouraged the Board of Supervisors, the city's legislature, to pass an ordinance rescinding the SFPD's authority to grant and revoke bathhouses' licenses, and transfer that authority directly to the DPH.

City Attorney Agnost's evaluation was that even if the licensing transfer were successful, any later DPH action taken against the baths would fail a judicial challenge. Agnost believed that "the sex ban regulations could be enacted immediately" if the mayor stuck with the SFPD proposals, which his office had finished drafting three days before, rather than turning to the Supervisors. But Feinstein "described this as a helpful move to give [the Supervisors] an opportunity to act first," and said, "the board is going to be acting on the issue soon."[109]

Four days later, the Supervisors announced a forty-five-day postponement of their decision on the licensing transfer. Supervisor Richard Hongisto, a former San Francisco sheriff who was a staunch supporter of the lesbian and gay community, "said he wanted more information on the legal and social ramifications" of the proposed transfer.[110] A good deal of anger would have greeted any decision regarding the city's baths, and the Board stayed out of the controversy. The mayor threatened to reconvene the SFPD hearings, but never did. The proposed

SFPD regulations and the licensing transfer proposal were dead ends in the struggles over the baths.

The Bay Area Physicians for Human Rights' June newsletter included a position statement on the baths in terms broad enough to include the Supervisors, SFPD, and DPH, asserting that past governmental "Attempts at legislating sexual behavior have only changed locations of that behavior, not curtailed it." BAPHR's statement began, "There is no definite evidence" that "closing bathhouses would reduce the risk or incidence of AIDS." They "strongly state, however, that multiple, anonymous sexual contacts, occurring in any location," increased AIDS and STD risks and should be avoided. BAPHR renewed their commitment to promote "safe sex practices in all areas, including bathhouses." They stated their continuing beliefs "that voluntary efforts by the gay community are the appropriate methods to achieve this goal," and "that government intervention in the sexual behavior of consenting adults should be avoided."[111]

The Consenting-Adults Bill had been successfully sponsored in the state legislature in 1976, after persistent efforts by Assemblyman Willie Brown to repeal California's anti-sodomy laws. In 1978, the San Francisco District Attorney applied this law to the baths, saying "There's no question this was a private place." The DA's establishing city bathhouses as private places quashed an SFPD raid and set of arrests at the Liberty Baths.[112]

The crux of later prosecution of the local baths was whether their entire, enclosed premises could be considered private, or were fair targets for government restrictions as commercial, public spaces. Since 1984, the question at the center of local debate over the baths has been whether they should be permitted to have private, closed rooms inside their premises.

THE DNC, THE SUPERVISORS, AND JOHN O'CONNELL

Nineteen eighty-four was a presidential election year, and the Democratic National Convention was held in San Francisco, beginning on 16 July.[113] Feinstein was a potential vice-presidential candidate, and there was a widespread assumption that she'd wanted the bathhouse debates to be concluded before the convention started, and the national media arrived.[114] In large part due to the work of Bill Kraus of the Milk Club, the Democrats' final platform included commitments to a search for the causes of AIDS and a cure, an end to the exclusion of lesbians and gays from immigration and from the military, and an end to homophobic violence.[115]

On 29 July, homophobia in the Bay Area led to murder. A San Franciscan named John O'Connell was walking on Polk Street, when four men from Vallejo attacked him and a friend, and kicked and beat them. O'Connell's head hit the curb when he fell, and he never regained consciousness, dying three days later. His attackers had called them "motherfucking faggot queers" and attacked two other men that night.

They attacked O'Connell a dozen blocks due north of City Hall, on the forty-fourth of the forty-five days that the Supervisors had set aside before announcing their SFPD/DPH bathhouse-licensing decision. On 10 August, the Board announced their refusal to make the transfer. Supervisor Hongisto mentioned the murder of O'Connell, and said news of the transfer could look like an encouraging triumph for homophobia in the area. Echoing Bobbi Campbell's concerns about the Littlejohn petition, Hongisto said the transfer might also encourage politicians in other states and cities to close their baths as well as their gay bars. Campbell died five days later, on 15 August 1984.[116]

THE DPH AND AVAILABLE EVIDENCE ON AIDS AND THE BATHS

Silverman had supported the licensing transfer attempt; his position on the baths had hardened through the summer and fall, moving beyond his April ban on sex between individuals, and far beyond his 1983 letters to Littlejohn and his speech in early March 1984. One of the Supervisors had said the Board had "not been given one bit of evidence showing a causal link between the outbreak and spread of AIDS and people's behavior" in the baths.[117] There was very little clear research that Silverman could cite, linking bath-attendance with AIDS risk.

Two studies of AIDS and San Francisco's baths were made available in 1984; the first was conducted by Leon McKusick, William Horstman, and Arthur Carfagni, who had released their results in February. As the year progressed, the authors disagreed completely about how their data should be interpreted or used to argue for or against closing the baths. On 3 April 1984, McKusick and a fourth man, Steve Morin, sent a memorandum to Silverman "in part to refute the notion that there are no data indicating that the closing of the baths would reduce the incidence of AIDS." McKusick and Morin believed that "closing or altering bathhouses could have a major impact on reducing high risk sexual behaviors and therefore the incidence of AIDS transmission." Carfagni dissented altogether in October, writing that "The conclusions and interpretations in [McKusick and Morin's] Memorandum . . . do not represent the conclusions of the original study [by McKusick, Horstman, and Carfagni], and I do not concur in them." Carfagni said that the three men's original "study does not indicate that bathhouse closure would be effective or appropriate and those conclusions should not be drawn from this study."[118]

More seriously, Dean Echenberg, Silverman's deputy for communicable diseases, had received a letter on 10 July from William Darrow, a senior research sociologist with the AIDS Activity Office at the Centers for Disease Control (the CDC). In the words of Ronald Bayer in *Private Acts, Social Consequences*, after analyzing data from a study conducted with men from San Francisco, Darrow questioned "the very foundation of the public health case for regulation or closure" of the baths.[119]

Darrow had looked for antibodies to LAV in frozen, stored blood samples that had been drawn from gay men in San Francisco in a 1978-80 study of hepatitis B. Some of the same men had been re-examined in 1984, with renewed questions about their sexual behaviors. In his letter to Echenberg, Darrow reported his conclusion that "Although numbers of partners and AIDS are significantly related, and men who go to bathhouses tend to have greater numbers of partners, bathhouse attendance [itself] is *not* significantly associated with AIDS" (Bayer's interpolation and Darrow's emphasis).

Citing a 1986 interview with Echenberg, Bayer writes that when Echenberg and Silverman received Darrow's letter, they "were furious and indeed would expend some effort to force a modification of the letter's conclusions by protesting to Darrow's superiors at the CDC. Ultimately, they were successful at wresting a new analysis, with conclusions that were more compatible with the effort to justify the regulation of the bathhouses. But that was not to be for three months," in October–exactly in time for the court case on the baths. In the meantime, Darrow had also sent his letter to another man in the city, and its contents became public. Bayer writes that over that summer, Silverman and Echenberg

> had to confront the inevitable political consequences of the new CDC findings as gay leaders seized upon the Darrow letter in an effort to force a retreat.
>
> Silverman resisted such pressure and continued to bridle under the bureaucratic restraints that had thwarted his plans to regulate the baths.[120]

In October, the Bay Area Physicians for Human Rights sent Silverman an open letter which was printed in the *B.A.R.*, announcing that they had obtained the Darrow information "which you, Dr. Silverman, have had since August." (This was a very late estimate of the letter's arrival time.) BAPHR warned that "Closure of bathhouses will harm the public health objective" of raising AIDS awareness, and that it would create "a dangerous precedent" for the DPH to order closure "without supporting data, without sufficient input, [and] in contradiction to existing medical information."[121]

THE HUMAN RIGHTS COMMISSION
AND COMMUNITY-BASED INVESTIGATIONS

In August the City's Human Rights Commission unanimously adopted a resolution opposing "any action by the City of San Francisco to . . . prohibit or regulate private consensual sexual activity in any bathhouse or sex establishment, absent a showing that it is a necessary and essential public health measure supported by clear and convincing medical and epidemiological evidence." The Commission noted that "health professionals cite types of sexual behavior, and not location, as the causative factors in the transmission of AIDS."[122]

That summer, journalists Helquist and Osmon completed their investigative tours of all the men's baths or regular sex parties in the city, and printed their findings in the July and September issues of *Coming Up!* In a 1995-96 interview with Sally Smith Hughes, Helquist said that the *Chronicle*'s and *Examiner*'s coverage of the baths had been "very lurid, but they didn't really tell you what it was that was going on" in them. Helquist said, "a lot of lesbians didn't have an idea" of what the baths were like. "A lot of gay men didn't have an idea. They were either scared, intimidated, or not interested." Helquist told Hughes, "The popular notion of, you go in the door and you walk into an orgy was far from true. A lot of people would point out, you can end up walking for hours up and down the hallways and it wasn't very interesting or exciting [laughter]."[123]

Helquist and Osmon described how they and their partners at the businesses negotiated sexual safety boundaries. They also described how well or how badly each business provided condoms and AIDS-education materials. Among their conclusions were that the businesses "have a long way to go before they can accurately claim that all efforts are being taken to encourage low risk activities," but that the City's actions "need not interfere with an individual's right to privacy and free choice." Silverman and the main doctors in the city who were involved in the bathhouse debates all received copies of these articles,[124] but ignored them in their subsequent portrayals of the baths as sites promoting high-risk sex.

PUBLIC OPINION, THE MAYOR, AND SILVERMAN

Two sources help illustrate the opposing pressures on Silverman at this time. First, the writer Frances Fitzgerald visited the city in 1984, and interviewed a number of San Franciscans. A pregnant journalist said that officials had given varying estimates of the risks that AIDS posed to the general population. She told Fitzgerald, "Look, the doctors and the health department people . . . told us not to worry about going to restaurants since AIDS isn't contagious" via social contact. But there were new reports that "saliva might transmit the virus. . . . Well, the one thing they do know is that AIDS can be sexually transmitted. And yet they won't close down the places where all the sex goes on. It's unbelievable."[125]

This journalist saw City delays in closure efforts as being medically incomprehensible, whereas local sociologists Stephen Murray and Kenneth Payne stated in 1988 that "Traditional moralism better explains" many AIDS policies, including restrictions on the baths, "than does existing scientific evidence." The local journalist saw Silverman as stalling and failing to protect the public, but Murray and Payne implied that "Verifiable medical facts were not necessarily of interest" to Silverman in the end, and dismissed him as proving himself, in time, to be more of a politician than a doctor. They attributed his eventual restrictions on the baths to political expediency, and criticized him for caving in under pressure from the mayor and others.[126]

Silverman believed that Feinstein's express concern for public health was only the "surface issue" of her involvement with the bathhouse debates. In his 1992-93 interviews with Hughes, Silverman said, "What I think is, she wanted me to clean up the city." He mentioned the SFPD bathhouse-surveillance report from March 1984, saying, "There were a number of things that obviously indicated high risk behavior. There were a lot of things in there which had nothing to do with high risk behavior, but that were abhorrent to her. The interactions that took place in these locations were basically abhorrent to the mayor. I think sex is an issue for her. And especially this kind of blatant, raw sex."[127]

FIGURE 4. "**Dr. Mervyn Silverman, San Francisco Public Health Director,**" **with Mayor Dianne Feinstein, 1984.** Photograph by Mick Hicks, © and reprinted by permission of the photographer; scan courtesy of the Gay, Lesbian, Bisexual, Transgender Historical Society of Northern California.

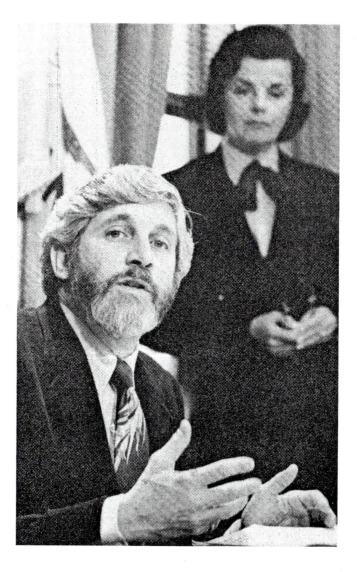

On 12 September 1984, the *Examiner* reported that the week before, Silverman had made a decision to close San Francisco's baths, and told the mayor so. Feinstein now said, "I am waiting for him to take the action he outlined to me," and said, "My feeling is that if you believe in what you're doing, do it. If your decision doesn't stand up in court, at least you've tried."[128]

The next day Silverman issued a statement, cautiously summarizing his current political planning. He acknowledged the "reduced patronage" at the baths, which had led to the closure of some of them. He also acknowledged that "To some extent, the community has begun to change as the result of alterations in individual behavior," and that individual behavior was the "major issue" for preventing the spread of AIDS.

However, he said that since "political considerations" had prevented the SFPD/DPH licensing transfer, there were two more options he was considering. He encouraged "the affected community to take action with regard to sex clubs, bathhouses, and other establishments which facilitate unsafe sexual behavior . . . to close *all* [these] remaining facilities." Otherwise, he himself might close "those facilities which encourage multiple anonymous sexual contacts. . . . Individual rights are an important consideration in this process. However, we consider health to be our uppermost priority." He said he would make no further statements on the issue until he had a decision to announce publicly–again demonstrating a readiness to wait, and let time pass before he declared any political commitments.[129] The statement of his plans and priorities was also a fair warning.

BATH OWNERS AND THE SFAF

Three days later, on 16 September, owners of area baths formed an Adult Entertainment Association. They committed themselves to certain kinds of self-regulation through closing orgy rooms, boarding up gloryholes, turning up the lights, distributing free condoms, and stepping up their AIDS-education efforts. Bob Owen, owner of the sex club the Academy, said he had passed out free condoms since April, and said, "As far as I know, all the orgy rooms in the City are closed."[130] A few days later, Helquist and Osmon let Owen know that the new wooden covers over the Academy's gloryholes were still easy to slide open, despite his claims to have seen to them. Owen initially threatened to eighty-six them from his club and from "every other place in the city," but later he apologized, and said he'd "freaked out, because those coverings were secured" as far as he knew.[131]

In late September, the AIDS Foundation announced that it had been consulting with community political clubs about how the community itself might promote low-risk sex at the baths. Together, the SFAF and club representatives reached a surprising consensus, across political-party and club-rivalry lines, about standards for the businesses. The standards would have included minimum lighting in the baths, prominent AIDS-awareness materials, SFAF representatives' in-house tabling, and periodic, P.A.-system announcements, reminding patrons of the dangers of the sexual transmission of AIDS and urging them to use condoms. SFAF executive director Jim Ferels hoped to bring the baths' owners into this coalition, and get them to agree to these guidelines. Baths that agreed to the guidelines would have been given signs for their doors to advertise their compliance. Baths that rejected the guidelines might have been picketed by members of the SFAF and political clubs.[132]

Modifying the baths hadn't been one of the possibilities Silverman had weighed in his last press statement. But Ferels said, "Silverman and I talk on the telephone almost daily," and he sent Silverman updates on the coalition's progress.[133] These talks and memoranda kept Silverman abreast of these community-based efforts to change and monitor the baths, as another apparent example of Silverman's efforts to gather input and work towards the broadest consensus that could be reached. He was famous in the city for preferring this kind of political networking, as the most stable groundwork for government action.

SILVERMAN AND THE PRIVATE INVESTIGATORS

On 27 September, the day the *Bay Area Reporter* ran the SFAF coalition story, Philip Ward and Daniel Collins of the City Attorney's Office wrote Silverman about how the DPH could gather information about unsafe sex in the baths, to prepare for a City prosecution of the businesses if they resisted a DPH closure order. Ward and Collins advised Silverman to "conceivably [utilize] private investigators to irregularly surveil [*sic*] the suspect establishments on five to ten separate occasions for purposes of determining if high risk behavior is taking place."

They cautioned that "Though it may be obvious to you that many bath houses and sex clubs are locations where such high risk behavior . . . takes place, it will be necessary to establish this as a matter of proof."[134]

High-risk sex was therefore still uppermost in the minds of City officials, despite Silverman's April ban on all sex between individuals in
the baths, regardless of an activity's AIDS risk; and despite the attor-
ney-drafted SFPD regulations that were scrapped in June, which would
have also ignored condoms and fluid exchange.

Silverman followed the City attorneys' advice, hiring four private investigators to go to different baths and write reports on sexual behavior
they saw between patrons. One of the investigators was an off-duty
Berkeley police officer. The mayor was informed of the decision to
send them into the baths.[135] The *B.A.R.* later stated that the owner of the
firm who employed the men was a friend and political supporter of the
mayor, though she hadn't been aware of the choice of his firm. The
DPH paid the owner $50,000, "without prior appropriation of funds."[136]
The *B.A.R.* said that an umbrella group for ten community organizations
investigated the expenses, and calculated that less than $10,000 of the
fee went to the private investigators. A DPH official denied this allega-
tion.[137] Fourteen businesses were investigated: six bathhouses, four sex
clubs, two adult bookstores,[138] and two adult theaters. The investigators
visited each business from two to four times, and their surveillance continued through 7 October.

In *And the Band Played On*, Shilts writes that "Even Silverman, who
was not naive about what went on in gay bathhouses, was shocked by
what the investigators found." According to Shilts, it was "when he read
the investigators' reports" that Silverman "had no doubt as to what
course of action he would take," since "Just about every type of unsafe
sex imaginable, and many variations that were unimaginable, were being practiced with carefree abandon at the facilities."[139]

The investigators wrote their reports with fewer claims to insight into
the patrons' feelings than Shilts makes and with less imagination, although one investigator estimated that a video lounge at the Ritch Street
bathhouse could seat twenty to thirty patrons, and declared that there
was "ample space for individuals to participate in almost any sexual act
desired, including anal intercourse," although he said only four or five
men were in the room at the time, and only two were engaged in a sexual
act–masturbation.[140] It was never stated whether any of the investigators were gay or bisexual; unlike Helquist and Osmon, all of them refused all offers by patrons to have sex.

The four men often noted the races of men at the businesses, including employees who weren't having sex. For example, "I observed a
white male of about thirty years of age orally copulating another white
male." "I saw two black males dressing who said that this area was great

because of the privacy." The "black male was having anal intercourse with this blonde white male." A "Latino-style male . . . masturbated and inserted a very large rubber penis-shaped object into his rectum." And "the oriental male then leaned over and took no. 5's penis into his mouth. The three relaxed and began to talk and I left the area."[141]

The investigators mentioned smelling poppers (amyl nitrite) several times, and smelling and being offered marijuana. They also gave two accounts of methamphetamine use, with one injection and an offer to share the needle, as Shilts writes in *And the Band Played On*. But Shilts's choice of the words "casually" and "cheerfully" to describe the IV drug use and offer are embellishments on the investigators' descriptions, which didn't convey a general atmosphere of light-hearted, willful perversity.[142] A typical statement in all four reports was, "At no time did I observe anyone who appeared to be an employee of the business attempt to control or stop the above described sexual activity." Sometimes there was none to describe–"There was no sexual activity seen on this floor. Men were watching Hill Street Blues on television."[143]

It's impossible to give a precise tally of the different kinds of sexual activities in the reports. The investigators were unable to name activities that they heard behind the closed doors of private rooms. They recorded many activities they did see without giving the numbers of men engaged in them, and wrote that they sometimes lost count of people, often because of dim lighting. They also mentioned sexual activities between men without saying how often an activity was performed, or between how many men. It was difficult to know if men swallowed semen during fellatio. Many of the reported activities were simultaneous or by the same man in one night, and none involved condoms. All the same, the investigators' mentions of anal sex were decidedly outweighed by lower-risk activities.[144]

In his description of Silverman's means and ends, Ronald Bayer sums up this surveillance in *Private Acts, Social Consequences* by writing that the four reports

> achieved the desired impact. Whatever the actual tabulation of safe, unsafe, and possibly safe sex acts observed might have revealed, the descriptions portrayed the existence of activity that would serve to shock the sensibilities of the conventional and disturb those concerned with the transmission of a deadly disease.
>
> With evidence in hand to buttress the decision he had already made, Silverman moved directly against fourteen sex establishments, declaring them public nuisances.[145]

SILVERMAN'S CLOSURE ORDER

On 9 October, Silverman ordered the closure of fourteen baths, writing that their space "encourages and facilitates multiple unsafe sexual contacts." (He allowed sixteen other investigated theaters, clubs, and other local adult businesses to stay open, as posing no AIDS risks.) In his closure order he asserted that "When activities are proven to be dangerous to the public and continue to take place in commercial settings, the Health Department has the duty to intercede and halt the operation of such establishments."[146] Bayer describes this assertion by writing,

> Thus did Silverman reject the claims of those who sought to protect the bathhouse by the invocation of the principles governing the state's relationship to private sexual behavior between consenting adults. . . . Gone were the concerns about privacy that had been so prominently featured in Silverman's responses to Larry Littlejohn. . . . Having obtained what he believed was the political support of important elements in the gay community for closure, he could discard the rhetoric of individual liberty.[147]

Silverman's order concluded, "Make no mistake about it. These fourteen businesses are not fostering gay liberation. They are fostering disease and death."[148] Laurie McBride, president of the Golden Gate Business Association, the community's unofficial chamber of commerce, said that "Rather than fostering health," Silverman's remarks were "fostering bigotry and hate."[149]

The SFAF issued a same-day press release on 9 October about the order. Jim Ferels was quoted as saying, "AIDS is not caused by places/establishments; all evidence indicates AIDS is primarily transmitted by specific behaviors which can take place anywhere." The general statement's last paragraph was, "We urge that our community not allow Dr. Silverman's action to distract gay men from their most important mission—individually protecting themselves and their partners from AIDS."[150]

Six of the businesses re-opened within a few hours on the advice of their attorneys, who considered that Silverman had no legal right to enforce his order.[151] All but two of the businesses reopened by the next night. The technical term was that the order was "to abate a public nuisance." The verb *abate* in this transitive sense means "to put a stop to," rather than the more usual intransitive sense, "to diminish gradually." But there were several indications that attendance levels and AIDS-risk activities in the baths had already been abating, in the second sense of the word, for months before Silverman's second order. These indications were five San Francisco baths' having gone out of business in the previous year, the conclusions that summer by Helquist and Osmon that most men they saw at the baths appeared "to have adopted the broader set of safe-sex guidelines" recommended by the SFAF and BAPHR,[152] and the community changes in sexual behavior and the dramatic reductions in business at the baths, which Silverman had acknowledged in his last press statement the month before.

In *And the Band Played On*, Shilts describes Silverman's 9 October closure order as "the final act of the San Francisco bathhouse drama." He says there was "little evidence that very many gays cared much about" it, because of a 300-member protest rally in the Harvey Milk Plaza.[153] The gathering was certainly small compared to the 6 January rallies over the release of Dan White, or the 1,000-strong August gathering to mourn Bobbi Campbell. But Shilts also acknowledges that only one community organization, the Milk Club, publicly supported Silverman's order. The Lesbian Rights Project and the board of directors of the California branch of the National Organization for Women (NOW) were among the organizations that opposed it.[154]

Other writers echo Shilts's descriptions–James Kinsella writes that when "Silverman finally closed the bathhouses, it was anticlimactic. There was little protest against a decision that had plagued Silverman for a year." Neil Miller states that "once Silverman made his decision, the bathhouse fight was essentially over. The baths never reopened. Eventually the issue just faded away."[155] These characterizations of the 9 October order as the culminating event of the local bathhouse controversy neglect the two months of intense legal fighting that immediately followed the order, the further 1986-89 rulings in the court case, and the fallout of the case in the 1990s.

PEOPLE OF THE STATE OF CALIFORNIA V. OWEN ET AL.: *THE PLAINTIFFS' CASE*

Bayer writes about the closure order that "Ultimately Silverman's decision transformed the political struggle . . . into a legal confrontation to be fought out in the courts," in "the adversarial system of justice."[156] In fact the City moved the next day, 10 October, with a 400-page complaint for the California Superior Court.[157] The City requested a temporary restraining order, a preliminary injunction, and a permanent injunction against the fourteen baths, with the case to be heard first by Judge William Mullins. The *Examiner* reported it was "the first time in history the San Francisco Health Department [had] to go to court in an attempt to have its mandate obeyed."[158]

The City declarations included eighty-five pages of the private investigators' surveillance reports. In his own declaration, Silverman wrote that the businesses' owners had ignored his repeated requests to prevent sexual behavior among patrons, and that they "foster, promote, harbor, encourage, and derive profit from multiple sexual encounters." Silverman wrote that when "sexual activity takes place in a commercial setting, this government has the prerogative and duty to intercede."

Dr. Marcus Conant described AIDS patients of his who told him they repeatedly went to the baths for unsafe sex, and saw no ethical problems in doing so. Drs. Donald Abrams and Paul Volberding both recounted a meeting that May at the AIDS Clinic at San Francisco General Hospital, when an unnamed bathhouse owner had said to them, "Let's face it–we both make money from these guys; we make money when they come to us, and you make money when they come to you." Volberding reported the statement as, "we make money from their sex, you make money when they're sick."[159]

COMMUNITY RESPONSES, JUDGE MULLINS' ORDER, AND THE COURT OF APPEALS

On 10 October, members of seven organizations released a statement that "Closing the baths is wrong and dangerous." They paraphrased Darrow's July opinion that "there is *no* correlation between the risk of acquiring the disease and bathhouses," and adapted Silverman's March 1984 claims that a closure effort "sends out the wrong message that government has finally done something effective and conclusive. It has not." The signers felt that Silverman's order also signaled to the general public that gays and lesbians were "worthy of censure," and concluded instead that it was the City's integrity that had been compromised, by the plaintiffs.[160] A flyer was also produced for a separate "Emergency Action Planning" meeting three days later, calling for suggestions for defending the baths, including a "call to oust" Silverman.[161]

Judge Mullins issued a temporary restraining order (TRO) on 15 October, finding for Silverman and the City attorneys, and ordering that the nine bathhouses and sex clubs remain closed for fifteen days. Mullins excepted the adult theaters and bookstores from the TRO on freedom-of-speech grounds.[162] He had denied the following organizations the right to submit friend-of-the-court briefs opposing closure: Bay Area Lawyers for Individual Freedom (BALIF), BAPHR, and the Northern California branch of the ACLU. Mullins said that when the TRO expired on 30 October, Superior Court Judge Roy Wonder, a Reagan appointee, would decide whether to grant the City's requests for preliminary and permanent injunctions.

On 18 October, attorneys representing the remaining defendants filed a petition in the State Court of Appeals to end the TRO. Two-to-one, the panel of appeals judges decided without prejudice not to vacate the TRO, leaving a way open for the defense attorneys to appeal their case again, if necessary, and leaving the next rulings to be made by Judge Wonder.[163] Defense attorney Thomas Steel requested that Wonder's review be delayed from 30 October to 8 November, so the defense could have more time to review the City's brief and seek declarations of support from medical experts in AIDS. The Appeals Court granted the delay, but the TRO was extended to 8 November as well.

The Court of Appeals' decision left the rulings to be made by a lower tier of the courts. Government officials' refusal to participate in the contentious regulation and closure efforts was therefore both vertical and horizontal–down levels of a single branch of government, as it also was in the Department of Health and Human Services' 1983 announcement to local health departments; and between different governmental branches and offices, as it was in the Board of Supervisors' decision not to make the SFPD/DPH licensing transfer.

THE DEFENDANTS' CASE, AND JUDGE WONDER'S FIRST RULING

The defense began gathering medical testimony from San Francisco and other cities. Shirley Fannin, the chief epidemiologist of Los Angeles, doubted that "closing the bathhouses would decrease the opportunities for high risk individuals" to meet for sex, "since the potential for transmission is carried with the individual wherever they choose to engage" in high-risk sex. Roger Enlow, director of New York City's AIDS Activity Office, declared for the defense that he had "become familiar with virtually all of the medical and epidemiological evidence" about AIDS transmission, and knew "of no evidence that definitely implicates the site of the intimate sexual contact, over and above individual sexual choices," as a determining factor for AIDS transmission.[164]

Outside the court, defense attorney Meriel Burtle pointed out to reporters that the sexual behavior of bathhouse patrons was, in itself, "completely legal and protected by state law." Burtle said, "I think the city is taking advantage of a certain distaste that some straight people have for gay sex," since "many straight people are tolerant of gays as long as they don't have to think about or read about what they do in bed."[165] But since the four investigators were unable to describe what happened in the baths' closed private rooms, most of the sex in their reports happened out of bed.

The progress of the case shifted on 9 November, when Judge Wonder allowed six patrons of the baths to file an intervening lawsuit in the proceedings, who claimed that their free-association rights had been infringed by the City's closure order. Among the group of new plaintiffs were two members of the Northern California ACLU's Gay Rights Chapter, and David Lourea, founder of the Bisexual Center and executive director of Bisexual Counseling Services. These plaintiffs' case was combined with the case of the City against the nine remaining businesses, with a single ruling to cover all complaints.[166] On 14 November, Wonder heard the arguments of the City, the defense attorneys, and the attorneys for the baths' patrons.

He issued his first preliminary injunction on 28 November, refusing to close the businesses as the City had requested. Wonder's three-page ruling focused instead on pragmatic ways to prohibit high-risk sex in the businesses. He ordered that they could legally operate as long as they contained no private rooms operated without a hotel license, and removed the doors from their rooms, booths, and video cubicles. The businesses were also to employ at least one monitor for an average of every twenty patrons, who would circulate every ten minutes, watching for "high-risk sexual behavior" as that phrase was defined by the AIDS Foundation, and expelling patrons who engaged in it.[167]

Wonder also ordered each business to "participate in the education of its patrons toward the prevention of high risk sexual activity including but not limited to that [education] suggested" by the SFAF, and post the injunction in each room and hallway. If the City became aware of violations of the injunction, it could write the business a complaint, which the business would have five days to correct. If the business ignored the complaint, the City could "proceed with all remedies allowed by law." The injunction was to remain in force until the public health director declared that the AIDS epidemic in San Francisco was over. This is the only authority that this ruling gave the director of the DPH over the defendant baths.[168]

RESPONSES FROM THE CITY, THE DEFENSE, AND OTHERS

The City had rebuffed previous defense offers to try to reach an out-of-court compromise. In a same-day statement, the mayor said that she was "very disappointed" with Judge Wonder's decision. She described the ruling as "vague and uncertain," creating "difficult problems of enforcement," and expressed concern that requiring the businesses to hire their own monitors "has the effect of setting up a spying system within bathhouses that must surely be repugnant to all–especially those who patronize the bathhouses."[169]

Silverman said years later that the mayor "was just about ballistic" when she heard Wonder had reopened the businesses.[170] On 3 December 1984, during a trip to New York City, Silverman said that if AIDS had been spreading in "a whorehouse" in San Francisco, he would have shut it down faster than the baths.[171] Silverman said he knew his closure effort "destroyed me politically in San Francisco, but I wouldn't have had it any other way." He said he was not "prohibiting sex. . . . If you can only get your rocks off in one building, you've got a problem. I don't." With some regional chauvinism, a *New York Native* reporter closed an article by writing that "With the baths closed, Silverman speculated that 'the guy' who otherwise could be 'laying on his stomach' there is prevented from having sex with as many partners as someone outside battling San Francisco's notorious wind and rain."[172]

Assistant City Attorney Philip Ward also expressed confusion over what he called the vagueness of the ruling. Defense attorney Thomas Steel replied that "The city attorney finds the order hard to understand because he doesn't want to understand it. Judge Wonder's ruling is completely clear. It reverses Dr. Silverman's order and sends a clear message to all that there is no legal basis to close the baths." Steel also called Wonder "more enlightened" than Silverman for making a clear distinction between high- and lower-risk sex, but he still described the injunction as "a serious violation of bathhouse patrons' privacy."[173]

Dennis Altman, an Australian, describes this ruling as the result of "an extremely American process. I can imagine no other country in which a Health Department order, based on claims about the transmission of an epidemic disease, could be overruled by a judge following a suit in which both the owners and patrons were represented."[174] Shilts ignores Wonder's second, December ruling in *And the Band Played On*, describing the bathhouse issue as "out of the way" after 28 November 1984, despite calling Silverman's 9 October closure order the final act of the drama of the baths.

Shilts also says the November ruling "put into effect the anti-sex regulations that Dr. Mervyn Silverman had proposed in mid-April"–implying that the November ruling and April ban were virtually identical.[175] But Wonder broke with Silverman's April ban on sex between individuals to make the first official distinction between impermissible high-risk and permissible lower-risk sexual activities in the businesses, as the SFAF then defined high-risk sex. The 28 November ruling was an authoritative order more in line with Silverman's statements in December 1983, when he'd urged local men who had sex with men to use condoms and not exchange body fluids.[176] Silverman neglected risk distinctions in both his 1984 orders for the baths.

SILVERMAN, THE CITY ATTORNEYS, AND JUDGE WONDER'S SECOND RULING

After Feinstein omitted Silverman from a task force whose job was to restructure the upper levels of the DPH, on 11 December he announced his resignation from the department, effective 15 January 1985, after seven years as its director. Silverman wrote the mayor an exit letter with genuine grace in it–wishing her well, and saying it had been a privilege to serve the City and County of San Francisco during very difficult years. A *Chronicle* reporter wrote that "His resignation was accepted promptly by Mayor Dianne Feinstein in a cool letter thanking him for his service but omitting any regret over his resignation."[177] Silverman went on to become a co-founder and executive director of the American Foundation for AIDS Research (AmFAR).

Also on 11 December, Deputy City Attorney Collins issued a subpoena for "any and all" documents held by the baths, including sign-in books and cards that recorded patrons' names and addresses. Thomas Steel announced his intention to ignore the subpoena and said the owners would risk jail before handing the lists over, which would force the City to apply for a court order. Collins said the City attorneys needed the records to calculate how many monitors each business would have to hire, at different times of the day and week. In the meantime, the owners had generally agreed to remain closed, pending a 19 December hearing in Judge Wonder's court which the City attorneys had requested. Only one club had reopened, posting the injunction and hiring monitors.[178]

On 20 December, Wonder issued a modified preliminary injunction, now granting the health director the right to define high-risk sexual behavior. The SFAF were to have some say in defining the term *high risk*, but in the event of any disagreements, the definitive authority would rest with the DPH's director.[179] From this decision through the last, 1989 reopening of the case, the guidelines Silverman drafted for the businesses remained static, applied only to sex between men, and took no account of condom use or fluid exchange in the assessment of the AIDS risk of oral or anal sex. Tom Steel pointed out that the new ruling contradicted "commonly accepted safe-sex standards that Silverman himself endorsed." He called it "pathetic" that "community-wide education" for AIDS had been compromised for "a measly advantage in a lawsuit."

Judge Wonder now allowed the businesses only one day, rather than five days, to correct their violations of the injunction in response to City complaints, and monitors were now expected to make weekly reports to the City attorneys of any violations that occurred. Collins dropped the effort to obtain the baths' records.[180] This was the final significant City decision made concerning the businesses in 1984, and the last significant decision made in this round of conflict over the baths.

SAN FRANCISCO'S BATHHOUSES AND SEX CLUBS AFTER 1984

Some events in the next few years lent weight to community members' fears that closing San Francisco's baths might have been the thin end of a wedge for further strikes at gay civil liberties. There was no national wave of bath or bar closures, but the Superior Court's rulings may have influenced other cities' and states' closure efforts for their baths. For instance in 1985, New York State's Public Health Council instituted local-discretion regulations for the state's baths. A number of baths were closed successfully in Manhattan, while a bathhouse in Buffalo was permitted to re-open by a New York county court, on the grounds that the business had been insufficiently investigated before its prosecution. In 1986, the governor of Georgia signed legislation outlawing businesses in the state that allowed oral or anal sex on their premises.[181]

In 1986, the U.S. Supreme Court upheld Georgia's anti-sodomy law with its *Bowers v. Hardwick* ruling, denying a national right to same-sex sexuality between consenting adults. Also, Proposition 64 was put on California's November 1986 ballot, to allow for the "discretionary quarantine by local health authorities" of HIV-positive people, and for discretionary bans on public funerals for people who died of AIDS. After an opposition campaign by community organizations and civil libertarians, California voters defeated Prop. 64 by 71%.[182]

As for San Francisco's baths, conflict over them was much more sporadic and less heated after 1984. But Judge Wonder's two rulings temporarily damped down and permanently transformed the controversy, rather than ending it. A few local baths remained open. One masturbation-only men's group has held parties at various San Francisco locations from 1983 to 2001.[183] Another masturbation-focused men's sex club remained open through 1984, was never prosecuted, and was torn down in the late 1990s to clear ground for the city's LGBT Community Center.

By the 1990s, local papers began making statements that were off base, to varying degrees, about when and how the city's bathhouses closed. A recent example is a 1999 *SF Weekly* article which began, "Officially, there have been no bathhouses in San Francisco since 1984, when health officials grappling with the AIDS crisis shut [them] down."[184] Four of the prosecuted baths did reopen in the months after Judge Wonder's second ruling, though all four closed within two years. A large bathhouse that had closed some years before also briefly reopened.[185] In 1986, Wonder revoked the hotel licenses of the Slot sex club and Animals bathhouse, on the grounds that their private "rooms are not being used for lodging . . . but for unsafe sexual activity." Both businesses closed afterwards, and also in 1986 the bathhouse at Eighth and Howard became a homeless shelter.[186]

The 21st Street Baths closed in 1987, after two of the same private investigators who made declarations in 1984 entered the business undercover, and made new reports for the ongoing *People v. Owen et al.* case. The owners agreed to close to avoid further prosecution. In 1989 a permanent injunction prohibited the business, technically San Francisco's last bathhouse, from ever reopening.[187] This was the only permanent injunction issued for the case, and its last ruling. Its rulings applied only to the defendants and not to other businesses in the city, but the case has continued to be influential.

New sex clubs were operating in the city by 1986, and continued opening as established businesses in the 1990s. The history of San Francisco's bathhouses and older sex clubs has often been blurred in coverage of these clubs. A *Chronicle* reporter wrote in 1993 that some gay people in the city favored closure of the new sex clubs, but "few city leaders are willing to speak out, lest they be branded homophobic. . . . When Dianne Feinstein was mayor, the bathhouses were closed. But . . .

Frank Jordan, The Nice Mayor, wouldn't want to hurt anyone's feelings." A doctor wrote to the *Chronicle*, in protest, that "closure of the bathhouses by Feinstein and Silverman in the early '80s was an error in public health"–making a similar, implied over-estimation of the mayor's and DPH director's independent spheres of authority. Two *Chronicle* columnists added to these mistakes in a 1996 article, by writing that sex clubs "are nothing new in San Francisco. They have, however, become increasingly popular since officials closed down the city's two dozen bathhouses." This sentence also glided too lightly over the word *closed*, and multiplied by four to get the number of bathhouses the City prosecuted twelve years earlier.[188]

Nineteen eighty-four was a watershed year for San Francisco's baths. A distinction that William Leap makes between the words *place* and *space* is useful for illustrating the changes that happened that year. Drawing on others' theories in his discussion of sexual spaces, Leap distinguishes place (an actual physical location) from space (various uses, meanings, perspectives, and practices that people impose on a place).[189] To use this distinction, in April 1984 the City tried to prevent all the baths in San Francisco from operating as sexual spaces, and that October it tried to eliminate certain baths entirely, as sexual, commercial places. By the 1990s, local baths' continued presence and operation became increasingly secure, and debate over the baths since then has focused on some San Franciscans' wishes to reintroduce visually private places to the premises of the city's baths.

Private rooms are still banned in local sex clubs. Despite the closing of the *People v. Owen et al.* case in 1989, the DPH has continued to claim the authority to ban private rooms, and require employee monitors in all sex clubs. The current DPH director stated in 1999 that bathhouses could also legally reopen in the city if they maintained the DPH's guidelines, although no bathhouses have opened, partly because saunas and pools are much more expensive investments than partitions.[190] Traditional men's bathhouses in Berkeley and San Jose, which respectively are about twenty- and sixty-minute drives from San Francisco, were open in 1984 and have remained open, and have continued to offer private rooms. None of San Francisco's current sex clubs have bathhouse licenses, private rooms, or the usual range of bathhouse amenities, although one club has steam and shower rooms and another has showers and a jacuzzi.

The 1984 debates over San Francisco's baths provide a necessary context for understanding the regulatory situation of the city's current sex clubs, but the clubs' story since the later 1980s is a separate phase of the baths' history. During the 1990s, the DPH relaxed its formal definitions of risk to permit sex with condoms in the clubs, achieving a better reconciliation of health priorities with both sexual liberties and generally received HIV-transmission guidelines. The current sex-club standards are therefore an unofficial blend of Judge Wonder's November and December 1984 rulings, with the same requirements for monitored, open rooms, but with much more rational DPH definitions of what constitutes lower-risk, permitted sex. Despite ongoing, municipally peculiar constraints, these San Francisco businesses continue to provide settings for consenting adults to meet for safer sex with latex supplies on hand, and affirm a value for sexuality itself.

ACKNOWLEDGMENTS

A number of people provided direct and indirect help with earlier drafts of this article. The author is especially grateful to several people who read it and made extremely constructive editorial and historical comments, many of which benefited the article, although remaining errors in it are the author's.

Terence Kissack took time from his dissertation to offer very useful writing suggestions. Michael Helquist loaned files of papers on the baths that he had kept from the mid-1980s, creating an initial, excellent starting base for understanding the topic. Both he and Rick Osmon provided supportive, detailed, and very helpful suggestions for the article.

Above all the author is indebted to William J. Woods for suggesting that a history article on the controversy over the baths would be a worthwhile project. His continuing encouragement has been invaluable.

NOTES

1. *And the Band Played On*, directed by Roger Spottiswoode with a screenplay by Arnold Schulman (New York: HBO Home Video, 1993), motion picture; and Randy Shilts, *And the Band Played On: Politics, People, and the AIDS Epidemic* (New York: Penguin Books, 1987). The HBO film includes an acknowledgement that some characters were invented, and "certain events were created or combined for dramatic purposes." I disagree with many of Shilts's written interpretations of events in San Francisco's mid-1980s bathhouse debates. I see him as having tended to embellish on people's actions and leap to assumptions about their motives, to sway public opinion against the baths with his news articles, and to infuse more drama into the narrative of *And the Band Played On*. Nevertheless, I admire the scale of the work he undertook in writing the book.

2. San Francisco has nonsexual bathhouses, but I've used the word "bathhouses" here to refer to businesses providing space for sex between patrons, as well as amenities like swimming pools, hot tubs, steam rooms, and private rooms. I've used the

phrase "sex clubs" for businesses providing private rooms and/or open spaces for sex between patrons, and used the phrase "the baths" for both these kinds of business, and sexually active back rooms in adult bookstores and theaters. The baths weren't brothels–patrons paid for the opportunity to meet other patrons for sex, not to have sex with employees. Some patrons at all-male baths had outside sex with women, and by the mid-1980s a few local baths had times when they welcomed people regardless of sex or gender.

3. I've used the word *City* with a capital *C* to refer to the government of the City and County of San Francisco, and *city* with a lower-case *c* to refer to San Francisco's population and land. I've also used the umbrella phrase "the community," rather than the usual contemporary phrases "the Gay community" or "the Lesbian/Gay community," to refer to San Franciscans who identified as bisexual and gay men, transgendered people, and bisexual and lesbian women. This community also extended across the Bay Area, although the evolving policies for the baths I describe applied specifically to San Francisco. Examples of this inclusive use of the term *community* appear in the minutes to meetings of the Lesbian/Gay Advisory Committee to the San Francisco Human Rights Commission, for instance on 15 May 1984, 2-3. Women in the community participated in local debates over the baths, especially Roberta Achtenberg and Carole Migden. Achtenberg was misidentified as a male attorney named Robert for two days running in the *San Francisco Examiner*, on 9 and 10 October 1984.

4. Charles C. Hardy, "Other AIDS cities unlikely to close gay sex clubs," *San Francisco Examiner*, 14 October 1984, preview edition, sec. B.

5. One measure of the year's importance is the *Annual Index to the San Francisco Chronicle*. In 1983, under the term BATHS, three AIDS-related articles were listed concerning San Francisco; in 1984 there were fifty-seven, in 1985 there were ten, and in 1986 there were four. In another brutal year, arsonists hit three local baths from 1977-78, causing a death at each. See Susan Stryker and Jim Van Buskirk, *Gay by the Bay* (San Francisco: Chronicle Books, 1996), 77-8.

6. R. King, "The Numbers Show . . . ," letter to the editor, *California Voice*, 19-25 April 1984. King managed the Liberty Baths, and said these figures could be "verified by numerical sequence registration cards" at the businesses.

7. Evelyn Hsu and Reginald Smith, "The Big Money in S.F. Gay Bathhouses," *San Francisco Chronicle*, 9 April 1984.

8. Armistead Maupin, *Tales of the City* (New York: HarperPerennial, 1978), 313. Maupin also positions three of the book's heterosexual characters in regard to another city bathhouse that welcomed women and men. Two women characters look at a magazine article on the Sutro Baths on pp. 6-7, and a male character goes there on pp. 127-32.

9. Maupin, *Babycakes* (New York: HarperPerennial, 1984), 253; cf. the 18 October 1983 *Chronicle* draft of the scene.

10. Frank Browning, *Paradox and Perversity in Gay Lives Today* (New York: Crown Publishers, 1993), 80-1.

11. Shilts, *And the Band Played On*, for instance pp. 23-4, 45-6, 57-9, and 89.

12. Gerre Goodman, George Lakey, Judy Lashof, and Erika Thorne, *No Turning Back: Lesbian and Gay Liberation for the '80s* (Philadelphia: New Society Publishers, 1983), 100-1.

13. Rick Osmon, electronic mail to author, Michael Helquist, and William J. Woods, 1 February 2002.

14. Allan Bérubé, "Prophesy, 1984," *Harvard Gay & Lesbian Review* 5, no. 2 (30 April 1998): 10.

15. See Stryker and Van Buskirk, 86-7, for descriptions of high STD rates among gay and bisexual men in San Francisco in the 1970s. See Gabriel Rotello, *Sexual Ecology: AIDS and the Destiny of Gay Men* (New York: Dutton, 1997), 58-64, for a description of how the baths provided very fertile initial ground for the spread of AIDS. For criticisms of Rotello's book see Mark Schoofs, "The Law of Desire," *Village Voice*, 15 April 1997; and Martin Duberman, "Epidemic Arguments," *The Nation*, 5 May 1997, 27-9. Schoofs calls *Sexual Ecology* "an ugly distortion of gay history and life" for tacitly "obliterat[ing] 15 years of HIV prevention accomplishments," and Duberman expresses doubts about Rotello's statements on historical patterns in anal sex between American men before the 1970s.

16. Michael Rumaker's narrator steps on a used condom in the orgy room in *A Night at the Baths* (Bolinas: Grey Fox Press, 1977), 61.

17. See three sources by Shilts: *And the Band Played On*, 90; "S.F. to Require Warnings on AIDS," *San Francisco Chronicle*, 1 June 1983; and "AIDS Continues to Spread–38 New Cases in S.F.," *San Francisco Chronicle*, 12 June 1984.

18. Michael Helquist, electronic mail to author, 13 February 2002. One example of a San Francisco official who fought AIDS with great dedication in the early 1980s is Dr. Selma Dritz of the Department of Public Health, a heterosexual woman honored in Shilts's *And the Band Played On* and played in the HBO film by Lily Tomlin.

19. Mervyn F. Silverman, MD, MPH, "Public Health Director: The Bathhouse Crisis, 1981-1984," an oral history conducted in 1992 and 1993 by Sally Smith Hughes, PhD, in *The AIDS Epidemic in San Francisco: The Medical Response, 1981-1984, Volume I*, Regional Oral History Office, the Bancroft Library, University of California, Berkeley, 1997, 146, 163. Quoted with permission.

20. Shilts, "Politics and Bathhouses: Local Complexities," *San Francisco Chronicle's This World*, 15 January 1984.

21. Mark Feldman, speech given at the Candlelight Memorial March: Fighting for Our Lives, San Francisco, 2 May 1983. My thanks to Michael Helquist for a copy of this speech.

22. Advisory committee, People With AIDS Coalition, "The Last Word: The Denver Principles," *The Body Positive*, July 2001. My thanks to Michael Helquist for this reference.

23. Silverman, "AIDS and the General Population," in *Cancer and AIDS, the 19th Annual San Francisco Cancer Symposium, San Francisco, 2-4 March 1984*, ed. Jerome M. Vaeth (Basel, NY: Karger, 1985), 168-70. My thanks to William J. Woods for this reference.

24. Helquist, "Journalist of the Early AIDS Epidemic in San Francisco," an oral history conducted in 1995 and 1996 by Sally Smith Hughes in *The AIDS Epidemic in San Francisco: The Response of the Nursing Profession, 1981-1984, Volume I*, Regional Oral History Office, The Bancroft Library, University of California, Berkeley, 1999, 16. Quoted with permission.

25. See Shilts, *And the Band Played On*, 448-51 for descriptions of the LAV and HTLV-III discovery statements by Centers for Disease Control and U.S. Cabinet representatives; and "Big step in isolating AIDS virus," *San Francisco Examiner*, 30 November 1984, morning edition, sec. A.

26. Brian Jones, "Silverman Says AIDS Experts 'Mixed' on Closing Baths; Health Director Explains Why He Changed His Mind," *Bay Area Reporter*, 29 November 1984.

27. Lawrence Mass, MD, "Cancer in the Gay Community," *New York Native*, 27 July-9 August 1981. Also see Edward Alwood, *Straight News: Gays, Lesbians, and the News Media* (New York: Columbia University Press, 1996), 220, for a description of Mass's promotion of the baths as sites for AIDS education.

28. For two very different examples of local, pro-closure views see Peter Collier and David Horowitz, "Whitewash," *California* magazine, July 1983; and Frank M. Robinson, "Not Just an Open and Shut Case: A Horror Story and a Challenge," *Coming Up!* April 1984.

29. Shilts, "An Evening at The Sutro Baths: How the AIDS era has affected patrons of the only coed bathhouse in S.F.," *San Francisco Chronicle*, 27 June 1983.

30. Clipping from the *Bay Area Reporter*, 1983, Ephemera Collection, the Gay, Lesbian, Bisexual, Transgender Historical Society of Northern California.

31. Shilts, "A Gay Bathhouse Closes Its Doors in S.F.," *San Francisco Chronicle*, 11 July 1983.

32. "S.F. Bills for AIDS Dumping," *California Voice Weekly*, 22-28 December 1983.

33. Bob Lynch, "Bathhouses, Sex Clubs Going 'Condom': Owners Reach Voluntary Agreement With City," *California Voice*, 2-8 February 1984.

34. San Francisco AIDS Foundation, "Can You Pass The Safe Sex Test?" June 1984. The chart was printed in a number of 1984-85 issues of the *Bay Area Reporter*, and as a stand-alone poster.

35. Richard F. Harris, "Saliva-AIDS link sparks fresh research assurances," *San Francisco Examiner*, 10 October 1984, East Bay edition, sec. A; and San Francisco AIDS Foundation, "Can AIDS Be Transmitted Through Kissing?" *Bay Area Reporter*, 28 February 1985.

36. Declaration of Robert K. Friedel, *People v. Owen et al.*, v. 3. See note 157 for a description of the case's full title.

37. Ronald Bayer, *Private Acts, Social Consequences: AIDS and the Politics of Public Health* (New Brunswick, NJ: Rutgers University Press, 1989). The first half of chapter 2, "Sex and the Bathhouses: The Politics of Privacy," pp. 31-53, is one of the best summaries of the debates over San Francisco's baths, with a very valuable account of Silverman's actions in 1984. I disagree with Bayer's evaluation of how moderate Silverman's policies were for the baths, but Bayer's account of the local bathhouse debates is notably balanced and evenhanded.

38. All the advertisements illustrating Bérubé's "The History of Gay Bathhouses" in the December 1984 issue of *Coming Up!*, the text of which is reprinted in this volume, were taken from issues of the organization's magazine, *Vector*. For a description of Littlejohn's activism in the 1970s see Bayer, *Homosexuality and American Psychiatry: The Politics of Diagnosis* (New York: Basic Books, 1981), 103-7.

39. Silverman, letter to Larry Littlejohn, 10 May 1983.

40. Silverman, letter to Littlejohn, 12 September 1983.

41. Bayer, *Private Acts, Social Consequences*, 33.

42. Alwood, 233.

43. Shilts, "Gay Bathhouses: S.F. to Require Warnings on AIDS," *San Francisco Chronicle*, 1 June 1983, sec. A.

44. Shilts, "AIDS Expert Says Bathhouses Should Close," *San Francisco Chronicle*, 3 February 1984, sec. A.

45. Stephen Kulieke and Nathan Fain, "CDC's Curran Says He Was Misrepresented On Bathhouse Closure," *The Advocate*, 20 March 1984.

46. Lynch, "Britt Embroiled in Bathhouse Controversy," *California Voice*, 9-15 February 1984.

47. Shilts, "AIDS Researchers Try To Stop Bathhouse Sex," *San Francisco Chronicle*, 4 February 1984, sec. A.

48. Kulieke and Fain, "Bathhouses: Scapegoat for AIDS Fears or Real Health Threat?" *The Advocate*, 20 March 1984.

49. Herb Caen, *San Francisco Chronicle*, 7 February 1984, sec. A.

50. Silverman, oral history conducted by Sally Smith Hughes, 120. Also see James Kinsella, *Covering the Plague: AIDS and the American Media* (New Brunswick: Rutgers University Press, 1989), 157-84 for descriptions of Shilts's private life, early career, and often "sensational–and wrong" stories (p. 159).

51. Collier and Horowitz, "Whitewash."

52. See W. E. Beardemphl, "Controlling the Queers," *San Francisco Sentinel*, 12 April 1984 for a description of the legal processes that would have followed a Yes vote, and been necessary to enact this new health policy for city bathhouses.

53. Dennis Altman, *AIDS in the Mind of America* (Garden City, NY: Anchor Press, 1986), 153. See pp. 147-55 for a short, excellent summary of San Francisco's bathhouse debates.

54. Silverman, "AIDS and the General Population," 171.

55. Scott O'Hara, "RE: LittleBrain," letter to the editor; Spinstar, "Traitor in Our Midst," letter to the editor; and Paul Lorch, "Killing the Movement," editor's Viewpoint feature, *Bay Area Reporter*, 5 April 1984. The *Bay Area Reporter* or *B.A.R.*'s editorial trend in 1984 was to oppose any effort to close the baths, sometimes with vitriolic personal attacks by Lorch. See Roger Streitmatter, *Unspeakable: The Rise of the Gay and Lesbian Press in America* (Boston: Faber and Faber, 1995), 251-9 and 274 for allegations of bias in the paper because of baths' advertisements in it. Streitmatter interviewed *B.A.R.* reporter George Mendenhall in 1993, and quotes him as saying that by 1983 the paper was "bleeding. Without the ads for the tubs, we weren't sure we'd survive. Our finances were in the toilet." The *B.A.R.* survived, and with a different tone is still the local LGBT community's main newspaper. See note 98.

56. Gary Schweikhart, "Littlejohn Agrees to Compromise at *Sentinel* Forum on Bathhouses," *San Francisco Sentinel*, 12 April 1984.

57. George Mendenhall, "Close the Baths? Community Voices Respond," *Bay Area Reporter*, 5 April 1984.

58. Helquist and Osmon, "The Bathhouse Controversy: A Time for Action: We Really Need to Think Carefully," *Coming Up!* April 1984. *Coming Up!* became the *San Francisco Bay Times* in 1989.

59. Ibid.

60. Ibid.

61. This slogan is an extreme example of the fear that closing the baths could begin an unraveling of legal protections for not only gay civil rights, but gay human rights. For contemporary conspiracy suspicions about the origins of AIDS, see for instance Paul Angara, "Homosexual Genocide!" letter to editor, *California Voice*, 29 March-4 April 1984; and Stryker and Van Buskirk, 112.

62. Silverman, oral history conducted by Sally Smith Hughes, 153.

63. Footage of his arrival appears in *After Stonewall: From the riots to the millennium*, produced and written by John Scagliotti (New York: First Run Home Video, 1999), documentary.

64. Shilts, "Silverman Delays on Gay Bathhouses," *San Francisco Chronicle*, 31 March 1984. Shilts was backtracking substantially from his previous day's headline–"S.F. Planning to Close Gay Baths."

65. Silverman, oral history conducted by Sally Smith Hughes, 154, 153.

66. Shilts, "Silverman Delays on Gay Bathhouses."

67. Frank M. Robinson, "Not Just an Open and Shut Case."

68. Helquist and Osmon, "The Bathhouse Controversy: A Time for Action"; and *Newsweek*, 8 August 1983, cover.

69. Bobbi Campbell, open letter from People With AIDS, 2 April 1984.

70. Ibid.

71. National Gay/Lesbian Task Force press statement, n.d., Ephemera Collection, the Gay, Lesbian, Bisexual, Transgender Historical Society of Northern California.

72. See Helquist, "The Sexual Politics of Dianne Feinstein," *Coming Up!* October 1984 for a history of Feinstein's sexuality-related political actions through 1984.

73. Larry Liebert and Hsu, "Feinstein Would Shut Bathhouses," *San Francisco Chronicle*, 5 April 1984.

74. Silverman, press statement, 9 April 1984; and Shilts, *And the Band Played On*, 446.

75. For a description of the 3 April meeting see Bayer, *Private Acts Social Consequences*, 38-9.

76. Cynthia Gorney, "San Francisco Banning Public Sex: City Health Director Trying to Halt AIDS," *Washington Post*, 10 April 1984, sec. A.

77. Seth Rosenfeld and Harris, "City bars sex at baths: Gay leaders support policy, Silverman says," *San Francisco Examiner*, 10 April 1984, morning edition, sec. A.

78. Lynch, "Silverman Dupes Gay Leaders, Bans All Sex," *California Voice*, 12-18 April 1984.

79. Ibid.; and Osmon and Helquist, "Physician Andrews Explains Baths Rationale," *California Voice*, 19-25 April 1984.

80. Steven A. Richter, "Proposed Bathhouse Regulations," open letter to Silverman with a letter to the editor, *Bay Area Reporter*, 7 June 1984.

81. James E. Sandmire, letter to the editor, *California Voice*, 19-25 April 1984.

82. Hsu, "S.F. Orders Ban on Sex in Bathhouses," *San Francisco Chronicle*, 10 April 1984.

83. Ray O'Loughlin, "S.F. Health Director Announces Ban on Sex In Baths, Sex Clubs," *Advocate*, 15 May 1984.

84. Silverman, oral history conducted by Sally Smith Hughes, 157.

85. Shilts, *And the Band Played On*, 89; and Bernard Spunberg, "A Retreat in the Sexual Revolution: Saying Goodbye to the Baths: Roar of the Saw is Deafening at the Liberty," *Bay Area Reporter*, 17 May 1984.

86. Fisting is the very careful and gradual engulfment of the fingers and then the heavily lubricated hand of a partner, by the rectum or vagina of a person with extensive experience of rectal or vaginal penetration and relaxation. See Osmon's sidebar on fisting and the Catacombs in *Coming Up!* July 1984.

87. Gayle Rubin, "Elegy for the Valley of the Kings: AIDS and the Leather Community in San Francisco, 1981-1996," in *In Changing Times: Gay Men and Lesbians Encounter HIV/AIDS*, eds. Martin Levine, Peter M. Nardi, and John H. Gagnon (Chicago: University of Chicago Press, 1997), 114-18. Rubin discusses the local baths' clo-

sures, Shilts's polemic writing on the issue, and safe-sex campaigns in the baths. She gives especially valuable insights into how the South of Market district, where many baths were concentrated, was destructively changed by AIDS.

88. Shilts, "A Farewell 'Orgy' at Sutro Baths: Casualty of AIDS Crisis Closes Doors," *San Francisco Chronicle*, 4 June 1984.

89. The ad ran on the back page of the *California Voice*, 26 April-2 May 1984.

90. See notes 43, 47, and 73 for Britt's and Feinstein's statements.

91. Shilts, "Gay Campaign to Ban Sex in Bathhouses," *San Francisco Chronicle*, 28 March 1984.

92. Dave Farrell, "Cops spy on bathhouses: Mayor ordered secret visits; report 'steamy,'" *San Francisco Examiner*, 31 May 1984, East Bay edition, sec. A.

93. Shilts, "Feinstein Defends Use of Bathhouse 'Spies,'" *San Francisco Chronicle*, 1 June 1984.

94. Osmon and Helquist, "Behind Feinstein's Police Surveillance Of Baths," *California Voice*, 7-13 June 1984.

95. Farrell, "Cops spy on bathhouses."

96. Shilts, "Feinstein Defends Use of Bathhouse 'Spies.'" Shilts wrote that the mayor ordered the operation in March and that it happened over a weekend. Littlejohn announced his petition drive on 27 March, so the police must have made their observations between Friday, 30 March and Sunday, 1 April.

97. Ibid.; and Brian Jones, "Cops Spy on Baths; Mayor Won't Apologize for Covert Mission," *Bay Area Reporter*, 7 June 1984.

98. Bob Ross, "Big Sister's Watching," publisher's Viewpoint feature, *Bay Area Reporter*, 7 June 1984; and letters to the editor by Martin F. Stow, "Dianne Cuts It," and Alan Grant, "More on Dianne's Spies," *Bay Area Reporter*, 14 June 1984. This was Lorch's last issue as the paper's editor; Brian Jones was its next news editor.

99. Printed in the *Bulletin of the Northern California Gay Rights Chapter of the American Civil Liberties Union* 1, no. 1 (1984): 2-3, Periodicals Collection, the Gay, Lesbian, Bisexual, Transgender Historical Society of Northern California.

100. For examples see John D'Emilio, "Gay Politics and Community in San Francisco Since World War II," in Martin Duberman, Martha Vicinus, and George Chauncey, Jr., eds., *Hidden from History: Reclaiming the Gay and Lesbian Past* (New York: Meridian, 1990), 456-73; Stryker and Van Buskirk, 73-81; and Helquist, "The Sexual Politics of Dianne Feinstein."

101. D'Emilio, 468-71.

102. "Mayor Urges U.S. Prosecution of Dan White," *California Voice*, 7 October 1983.

103. Dion B. Sanders, "SF Protests Mark White's LA Release," *Bay Area Reporter*, 12 January 1984.

104. For a description of police vandalism, assault, and battery in a series of concerted bathhouse raids in Toronto in February 1981, and a massive local-community protest of the raids, see Gerald Hannon, "Raids, rage and bawdyhouses," in *Flaunting It!: A decade of gay journalism* from The Body Politic, eds. Ed Jackson and Stan Persky (Vancouver: New Star Books, 1982) 91-4 (my thanks to William J. Woods for this reference); and Bérubé's "The History of Gay Bathhouses" in this volume.

105. "Agnost criticizes flipflop on AIDS," *San Francisco Examiner,* 14 June 1984.

106. San Francisco Civil Code, Article 26, sec. 2633.

107. "Regulations Proposed Pursuant to Municipal Police Code Section 2633 to Protect the Public Health by Preventing Activities Which Promote the Spread of Acquired Immune Deficiency Syndrome," 8 June 1984.

108. John E. Wahl, "The Fallacy in Closing the Bathhouses," guest editorial, *Bay Area Reporter*, 14 June 1984.

109. "Disgusting retreat on bathhouses," editorial, *San Francisco Examiner*, 17 June 1984, sec. B.

110. Smith, "Supervisors Postpone Bathhouse Decision: 45-Day Delay," *San Francisco Chronicle*, 15 June 1984.

111. "BAPHR's Official Statement on Bathhouses," *Bay Area Physicians for Human Rights Official Newsletter* 6, no. 6 (June 1984): 265, Periodicals Collection, the Gay, Lesbian, Bisexual, Transgender Historical Society of Northern California.

112. Bérubé, "The History of Gay Bathhouses."

113. See Dudley Clendinen and Adam Nagourney, *Out for Good: The Struggle to Build a Gay Rights Movement in America* (New York: Simon & Schuster, 1999), 499-508 for a discussion of Shilts, Silverman, Littlejohn, and the bathhouses in the contexts of American Democratic versus Republican politics in 1984, and the DNC specifically.

114. Bérubé stated three months earlier that "Traditionally before elections, conventions, Olympics and World's fairs, cities get cleaned up." See Gorney, "The Bathhouse War: San Francisco's Move to Fight AIDS Creates Rift Among Gays," *The Washington Post*, 19 April 1984, sec. D.

115. Shilts, *And the Band Played On*, 468.

116. Jones, "Supes Say 'No' to Sex Ban Rules," *Bay Area Reporter*, 16 August 1984; and Allen White, "Candles and Tears on Castro: 1,000 Mourn Bobbi Campbell," *Bay Area Reporter*, 23 August 1984.

117. Smith, "Supervisors Giving Up On Bathhouse Rules," *San Francisco Chronicle*, 9 August 1984.

118. Leon McKusick, William Horstman, and Arthur Carfagni, "Reactions to the AIDS Epidemic in Four Groups of San Francisco Gay Men," study conducted in November 1983; McKusick and Steve Morin, memorandum to Silverman, "Bathhouses and Public Policy," 3 April 1984; and Declaration of Carfagni, pp. 2-4, *People v. Owen et al.*, v. 4.

119. Bayer, *Private Acts, Social Consequences*, 43; see note 37.

120. Ibid.

121. Bay Area Physicians for Human Rights, open letter to Silverman, 8 October 1984, printed as "Gay Doctors Say Closure 'Not Medically Justified': Accuse Silverman of Withholding CDC Study Which Shows No AIDS-Bathhouse Link," *Bay Area Reporter*, 11 October 1984.

122. "Human Rights Commission Opposes Bathhouse 'Sex Ban,'" *Bay Area Reporter*, 30 August 1984.

123. Helquist and Osmon, "Sex & the Baths: A Not-So-Secret Report," and "Beyond the Baths: The Other Sex Businesses," *Coming Up!* July and September 1984, respectively; and Helquist, oral history conducted by Sally Smith Hughes, 17.

124. Helquist and Osmon, "Beyond the Baths"; and Helquist, electronic mail to author, 13 February 2002.

125. Frances Fitzgerald, *Cities on a Hill: A Journey Through Contemporary Cultures* (London: Picador, 1987), 96.

126. Stephen O. Murray and Kenneth W. Payne, "Medical Policy Without Scientific Evidence: The Promiscuity Paradigm and AIDS," *California Sociologist* 11, nos. 1-2 (Winter/Summer 1988): 13, 34-5, 30.

127. Silverman, oral history conducted by Sally Smith Hughes, 156-7. On p. 158, Hughes followed up Silverman's understanding of the mayor's motives by saying, "Well, it's an illustration of how personality enters into history," to which Silverman replied, "Absolutely."

128. Farrell, "Health chief told Feinstein last week," *San Francisco Examiner*, 12 September 1984, California edition, sec. A.

129. Silverman, press statement, 13 September 1984.

130. Farrell, "Clubs bow to City, ban risky sex acts," *San Francisco Examiner*, 19 September 1984.

131. Helquist and Osmon, "Getting Ready to Close the Baths," *Coming Up!* October 1984.

132. Jones, "Community Plan to Regulate Baths," *Bay Area Reporter*, 27 September 1984.

133. Jones, "Mayor Quizzes MDs On Closing Baths; Secret Meeting in City Hall; Is Silverman Odd Man Out?" *Bay Area Reporter*, 27 September 1984.

134. Philip S. Ward and Daniel E. Collins, "Closure of Bath Houses and Sex Clubs," memorandum to Silverman, 27 September 1984.

135. Silverman, deposition to defense attorney Thomas Steel, *People v. Owen et al.*, v. 6.

136. Human Rights Commission, "Resolution Opposing Government Surveillance of Consensual Sexual Conduct in Bathhouses and Sex Establishments in San Francisco," 10 January 1985, in *Minutes of the Human Rights Commission of San Francisco, 1985-6.*

137. Mendenhall, "Gays Block City's Attempt To Quietly Hire Sex Spies; Attempt to Rush Proposal Past Civil Service Board Fails; Delay Is Okayed," *Bay Area Reporter*, 31 January 1985.

138. In 1984 the Jaguar Adult Book Store had a bi-level sex club up- and downstairs.

139. Shilts, *And the Band Played On*, 481.

140. Declaration of James G. Campbell, pp. 15-16, *People v. Owen et al.*, v. 1.

141. Ibid., p. 3; Declaration of David Anderson, p. 6; and Declaration of Pierre Merkl, pp. 7, 22, and 21, from *People v. Owen et al.*, v. 1.

142. Shilts, *And the Band Played On*, 481. The description of the IV drug use is in the Declaration of Kevin Aiken, p. 4; and on p. 2 of his declaration Anderson describes being offered speed once and marijuana twice at one business (*People v. Owen et al.*, v. 1).

143. Aiken, pp. 15-16; and Anderson, p. 8, *People v. Owen et al.*, v. 1.

144. Having made these caveats, I tried to count only the discrete instances of sexual activities in the four reports. My own estimates are that they include the following, approximate, distinct instances of each activity: 142 instances of oral penetration, 80 of solo or mutual masturbation, 21 of anal penetration, 10 rimmings, 14 fistings or instances of anal penetration with one or more fingers, and 2 urine scenes.

145. Bayer, *Private Acts, Social Consequences*, 44-5.

146. Silverman, press release, 9 October 1984; and "Court fight ahead over bathhouses: Clubs still defy Silverman," *San Francisco Examiner*, 11 October 1984, East Bay edition sec. B.

147. Bayer, *Private Acts, Social Consequences*, 45.

148. Silverman, press statement, 9 October 1984.

149. Beth Hughes and Michael A. Robinson, "6 Sex clubs defy order: Bathhouses to sue to halt the shutdown," *San Francisco Examiner*, 10 October 1984, East Bay edition, sec. A. For an echo of Silverman's statement nine years later, see the conclusion of the cutting, sardonic article by Debra J. Saunders, "Tons of Safe Sex in the Nice City," *San Francisco Chronicle*, 2 July 1993, final edition, sec. A; also see note 188.

150. San Francisco AIDS Foundation, press release, 9 October 1984.

151. Carl Nolte and Shilts, "Gay Bathhouses Told to Close–6 Refuse," *San Francisco Chronicle*, 10 October 1984.

152. Helquist and Osmon, "Sex & the Baths."

153. Shilts, *And the Band Played On*, 490; also see Mendenhall, "300 Rally to Decry Baths Closure," *Bay Area Reporter*, 1 November 1984.

154. Bayer, *Private Acts, Social Consequences*, 45.

155. Kinsella, 178 (see note 50); and Neil Miller, *Out of the Past: Gay and Lesbian History from 1869 to the Present* (New York: Vintage Books, 1995), 446.

156. Bayer, *Private Acts, Social Consequences*, 46.

157. A partial title of the case is *People of the State of California v. Ima Jean Owen et al.*, or *People v. Owen et al.* The full, initial title included the names of three City plaintiffs (Agnost, another City attorney, and Silverman) versus over forty individual defendants owning fourteen businesses. The carton of case records contains eight substantial files, referred to here as v. 1-8.

158. Hardy, "S.F. to ask judge for bathhouse ban," *San Francisco Examiner*, 11 October 1984, Peninsula edition, sec. B.

159. Declarations of Silverman, Tab A; Marcus H. Conant, MD, Tab D; Donald Ira Abrams, MD, Tab C, p. 13; and Paul A. Volberding, MD, Tab E, p. 8, *People v. Owen et al.*, v. 2. Cf. Shilts, *And the Band Played On*, 421-2.

160. The signers were Roberta Achtenberg (who was later an attorney for patrons of the baths) of Bay Area Lawyers for Individual Freedom, Thomas Steel (who was later an attorney for baths' owners) of the Northern California Bathhouse Association, and members of Bay Area Physicians for Human Rights, the American Civil Liberties Union of Northern California, the Golden Gate Business Association, People With AIDS, and the American Association for Personal Privacy (a group of civil-rights scholars who worked to maintain sexual civil liberties).

161. "Safe-Sex Solidarity Against the Scapegoat Scam" flyer, Ephemera Collection, the Gay, Lesbian, Bisexual, Transgender Historical Society of Northern California.

162. Dennis J. Opatrny, "9 defiant gay sex clubs close down," *San Francisco Examiner*, 24 October 1984, sec. A. Jaguar Books was among the bookstores excepted; Mullins ordered the stores and theaters to exclude sexual facilities from their premises.

163. Michael A. Robinson, "Appeal court lets bathhouses and sex clubs remain closed," *San Francisco Examiner*, 24 October 1984, sec. B.

164. Helquist and Osmon, "The City vs. the Sex Businesses," *Coming Up!* November 1984.

165. Ibid.

166. Helquist, "Court Allows Patrons And BALIF to Join Suit," *Coming Up!* December 1984.

167. Judge Roy Wonder, Preliminary Injunction, 28 November 1984, *People v. Owen et al.*

168. Ibid.

169. Dianne Feinstein, press statement, 28 November 1984.

170. Silverman, oral history conducted by Sally Smith Hughes, 160.

171. Mitchell Halberstadt, "San Francisco Health Director in New York for Forum on Bathhouse Closure," *Connection*, 14 December 1984.

172. Steven C. Arvanette, "San Francisco Health Director Addresses New York Physicians' Group: Dr. Mervyn Silverman Talks About Baths Closure at Gay Community Center," *New York Native*, 17 December 1984.

173. O'Loughlin, "Judge Allows San Francisco Baths to Reopen: Sexual Activities to be Monitored," *New York Native*, 17 December 1984.

174. Altman, *AIDS and the New Puritanism*, 151.

175. Shilts, *And the Band Played On*, 498-9.

176. See note 32.

177. Maitland Zane, "Feinstein Left Silverman Off Her Health Team," *San Francisco Chronicle*, 10 November 1984; Silverman, letter to Feinstein, 10 December 1984; and Nolte, "Silverman Steps Down As S.F. Health Director," *San Francisco Chronicle*, 12 December 1984.

178. Opatrny, "Bathhouses to fight The City's subpoena for business records," *San Francisco Examiner*, 12 December 1984; and Jones, "City Demands Lists of Baths Customers: Subpoena Issued as Part of Nov. 28 Court Order; Clubs Will Challenge; Attorneys Express Outrage," *Bay Area Reporter*, 13 December 1984.

179. Wonder, Modified Preliminary Injunction, 21 December 1984, *People v. Owen et al.*

180. Jones, "Most Sex Banned At Gay Bathhouses: Judge Toughens Order, Gives Power to Silverman; Clubs Stay Closed," *Bay Area Reporter*, 27 December 1984.

181. See Bayer, *Private Acts, Social Consequences*, 53-71; and Dave Walter, "Georgia Bans Gay Bathhouses," *Advocate*, 27 May 1986.

182. Bayer, "AIDS, Public Health, and Civil Liberties: Consensus and Conflict in Policy," in *AIDS & Ethics*, ed. Frederic G. Reamer (New York: Columbia University Press, 1991), 33-6.

183. Jerry Zientara, co-organizer of SF Jacks, interview by author, 11 April 2002.

184. Joel P. Engardio, "Private Places—Gay activists push for return of traditional bathhouses," *SF Weekly*, 28 April-4 May 1999.

185. See four *Bay Area Reporter* sources: Mendenhall, "Baths Appeal Court Order; May Reopen Next Week," 24 January 1985; 25 April and 13 June 1985 advertisements for the Bulldog Baths; and Jones, "Plan to Close 'Baths' Seen as Ineffective," 14 November 1985.

186. Perry Long, "Crackdown on 2 Gay Clubs," *San Francisco Chronicle*, 26 March 1986, sec. A; and Mark Sandalow, "South-of-Market Foes Lose Bid to Stop Shelter," *San Francisco Chronicle*, 15 August 1986.

187. Charles Linebarger, "Owners, Facing Jail Term, Close 21st St. Bathhouse: Out-of-Court Settlement With City Attorney Allows Operators to Avoid Stiff Penalties," *Bay Area Reporter*, 7 May 1987. Also see *People v. Owen et al.*, v. 8 for the two private investigators' declarations, Judge Wonder's 16 April 1987 modified preliminary injunction, and Judge Ollie Marie-Victoire's 25 October 1989 permanent injunction against the business.

188. Saunders, "Tons of Safe Sex in the Nice City"; W. L. Warner, MD, "Know-Nothing," letter to the editor, *San Francisco Chronicle*, 8 July 1993, final edition, sec. A; and Philip Matier and Andrew Ross, "Plan in Works to License S.F. Sex Clubs: City would be first in nation with regulations," *San Francisco Chronicle*, 18 October 1996.

189. William Leap, editor's introduction to *Public Sex/Gay Space (Between Men–Between Women)* (NY: Columbia University Press, 1999), 7.

190. For the current City guidelines for sex clubs, see the DPH AIDS Office's undated "Minimum Standards for Operation of Sex Clubs and Parties." For an explanation of the need the DPH director perceives for these standards see Mitchell H. Katz, letter to San Francisco's HIV Prevention Planning Council, 20 May 1999, 4-5; and for a statement of the sources of the DPH director's authority to set the standards see Jean S. Fraser, Deputy City Attorney, and Louise H. Renne, City Attorney, letter to Health Commission President Lee Ann Monfredini and the DPH Health Commission, "Re: Authority of Director of Public Health To Issue Standards Relating to Sex Clubs," 15 June 1999.

Legal Aspects of Regulating Bathhouses: Cases from 1984 to 1995

Scott Burris

Temple Law School

SUMMARY. Public health measures regulating or closing bathhouses and other businesses facilitating consensual sexual activity among strangers have generally been upheld by courts. Using standard legal research methods, this study sought (1) suits brought by government authorities to close a sex-facilitating business (SFB) based at least in part on health concerns, and (2) suits filed by SFBs to invalidate state laws or local ordinances banning closed booths or other architectural features that facilitate sexual activity. The research yielded eight published and unpublished trial or appellate opinions between 1984 and 1995 in which local health or other officials filed a law suit to close or otherwise interfere with sex at a bathhouse or other SFB. In seven of the eight cases, the state prevailed entirely or in large part in securing the relief it sued for. Factors influencing these results include the traditional deference of courts to public health officials, stigma, and limited legal recognition of a right to public sexual activity. Major questions include the extent to which coercive health measures increase stigma or social hostility towards gay men, whether closure actions "educate" at risk-individuals about the danger of

Correspondence may be addressed: Temple Law School, 1719 N. Broad Street, Philadelphia, PA 19122.

[Haworth co-indexing entry note]: "Legal Aspects of Regulating Bathhouses: Cases from 1984 to 1995." Burris, Scott. Co-published simultaneously in *Journal of Homosexuality* (Harrington Park Press, an imprint of The Haworth Press, Inc.) Vol. 44, No. 3/4, 2003, pp. 131-151; and: *Gay Bathhouses and Public Health Policy* (ed: William J. Woods, and Diane Binson) Harrington Park Press, an imprint of The Haworth Press, Inc., 2003, pp. 131-151. Single or multiple copies of this article are available for a fee from The Haworth Document Delivery Service [1-800-HAWORTH, 9:00 a.m. - 5:00 p.m. (EST). E-mail address: docdelivery@haworthpress.com].

10.1300/J082v44n34_06

anonymous unprotected sex, and what effect legal action has on the frequency of unsafe behavior. *[Article copies available for a fee from The Haworth Document Delivery Service: 1-800-HAWORTH. E-mail address: <docdelivery@ haworthpress.com> Website: <http://www.HaworthPress.com> © 2003 by The Haworth Press, Inc. All rights reserved.]*

KEYWORDS. Bathhouses, public policy, legal issues, public health law

INTRODUCTION

Health officials struggle over the question of how best to reduce the transmission of HIV in bathhouses, sex clubs and other businesses that facilitate a high volume of anonymous sex. Caution is prudent. The value of closing or significantly limiting activity in these businesses depends on empirical questions like who has what sort of sex in these venues, whether sex prevented in these venues would simply occur elsewhere, whether educational interventions at sites of congregate sex reduce transmission more than closure, and whether the symbolic force intervention is helpful or harmful to the effort to change behavior–all questions which remain largely unanswered (Binson et al., 2001). Measures against sex-facilitating businesses (SFBs) must also be considered cautiously given the long and unsuccessful history of sex regulation in America (Brandt, 1987).

Some objections to interfering with SFBs are phrased in legal terms. The right of privacy, incorporating a freedom to make intimate personal choices, and the right of free association in the First Amendment, powerfully express a view that government ought not to interfere in the sexual behavior of consenting adults. In his account of the first bathhouse closure cases, Ron Bayer saw the discourse of privacy as central to the policy debate, and a major limitation on the discretion of health officials (Bayer, 1989). As we consider the future of public health regulation of SFBs, it is important to revisit the role of the law. In this paper, I want to take two steps towards a better understanding of law's role.

First, I want to show that legal doctrine does not generally stand as a serious impediment to a health official resolved to curtail sexual activity in bathhouses, theaters, bars, arcades, or any other place of business. The authority of state and local government to regulate sexual activity in public places is capacious, with or without the threat of HIV. Over the past ten years, courts in virtually every case have upheld closures and other restrictions in the face of sometimes intense and creative legal opposition. While health officials have sometimes provided extensive direct evidence of specific unsafe sexual acts, the burden of proof has generally been no heavier than a good soufflé. In many instances, rank hearsay or traces of dried semen have sufficed to establish the prevalence of unsafe activity, and in no case has the government been forced to offer any solid evidence that closure or other restrictions would, in fact, reduce the overall level of unsafe activity, much less the transmission of HIV. I will demonstrate these propositions by a review of the cases involving the regulation of SFBs.

Second, I want to suggest that law, as a formal limitation on health action, is only part of the story. Law and law-talk play other roles in this controversy, roles that are important and may often be overlooked when litigation seizes the focus. Law is a rhetoric of political action. Law expresses the values of the dominant culture, but also may give voice to the competing claims of less powerful subcultures. Law validates the exercise of power. It educates. It tends often to define the prerogatives and options of health authorities. In thinking about how to address the risks posed by SFBs in the future, a broader view of law raises important questions for discussion and research.

A SURVEY OF CASES INVOLVING
THE REGULATION OF SFBS

Background

There are no comprehensive data on the measures local health officials have taken to control sexual behavior in business establishments. This review is based on cases identified through standard legal research methods. The search was limited to cases involving businesses, open to the public, whose premises were designed in a way that facilitates voluntary, uncompensated sexual contact between strangers, and which were subject to regulation based at least in part on concerns of disease transmission. The scope of the research for this review did not include massage parlors, brothels or other sites of prostitution, nor short-stay motels or bars without special accommodations for sex, but it does include cases that do not mention HIV.

While published cases are the appropriate source of information about legal doctrine, they have serious limitations when used for other purposes. Efficient regulation depends upon voluntary compliance. Coercive authority is most useful when it does not have to be actually deployed to compel obedience (Tyler, 1990). We can assume that in at least some places, if not in many, health officials have secured compliance with an HIV prevention effort through persuasion and negotiation with operators and users of SFBs (Ayres & Braithwaite, 1992). In addition to saving resources, this use of regulatory authority will tend to be less divisive and stigmatizing, and may foster goodwill that can be transferred to the management of other issues. Health strategies that successfully avoid controversy, however, do not appear in a review based on litigation.

Nor are published cases necessarily representative of all litigation. As a general matter, most cases that are filed are settled or otherwise disposed of without a trial-court opinion or an appeal, and so would not appear in a sample based on such opinions. While there have almost certainly been more actions taken against SFBs than are reflected in this survey, these cases are unlikely to have had different outcomes than the ones that resulted in written, published opinions. The most likely reason for a case being disposed of before a judicial ruling or without an appeal of an unwritten trial-court judgment is acquiescence by the SFB operator. The government, having brought the action, would be very unlikely to make major concessions, or to forego appealing an adverse ruling by a trial judge. It is possible, nonetheless, that there are instances of public health officials being prevented by courts from acting, or of being deterred from taking action by the possibility of a court defeat. These cases would not be discovered by the research methods used here.

Results in Summary

The bulk of the case law can be divided into (1) suits brought by government authorities to close an SFB based at least in part on health concerns, and (2) suits filed by SFBs to invalidate state laws or local ordinances banning closed booths or other architectural features that facilitate sexual activity.

The research yielded eight published and unpublished trial or appellate opinions since 1984 in which local health or other officials filed a law suit to close or otherwise interfere with sex at a bathhouse or other SFB (see Table 1). In seven of the eight cases, the state prevailed entirely or in large part in securing the relief it sued for. In the cases in which the state was not completely successful, it appears from other sources that the SFB was eventually put out of business. Half of these

TABLE 1. Cases Involving Closure of an SFB, 1984-1995

Case and year of Initial Action	Type of Facility		Remedy	
	Bath or sex club	Bookstore, arcade or theater	Sought	Granted
City of New York v. Dana, 627 N.Y.S.2d 273 (1995)		X	Closure	Closure
Commonwealth of Pa. v. Danny's Bookstore, 625 A.2d 119 (1993)		X	Closure; ban on video booths and "California Couch Dancing"	Preliminary injunction banning booths and "California Couch Dancing"[1]
City of Ramsey v. Amusement Center, 498 N.W.2d 25 (1993)		X	Closure [2]	Closure
City of Lincoln v. ABC Books, 470 N.W. 2d 760 (1991)		X	Closure	Closure
California v. Three 3 MCS, unpublished (1988)	X		Closure	Closure
City of New York v. St. Marks Baths, 130 Misc. 2d 911 (1985)	X		Closure	Closure
City of New York v. Big Apple Spa, 497 N.Y.S. 2d 988 (1986)	X		Closure	None[3]
California ex rel Agnost v. Owen, unpublished (1984)	X		Closure	Ban on booths and unsafe sex; patron education

1. The Commonwealth's petition to close the entire premises of the bookstores as nuisances was put off for a trial. The case reported only the operators' appeal of the preliminary injunction. The Commonwealth eventually decided not to pursue closure.
2. Pending compliance with open-booth ordinance only.
3. Closure sought based on prostitution. The court ruled that the evidence was insufficient to justify a preliminary injunction.

cases involved bathhouses or sex clubs. The remaining four concerned adult-oriented businesses featuring closed booths where unsafe sex was alleged to take place. Customers intervened in only two of the eight cases–the early San Francisco and New York bathhouse cases–to raise privacy and free association claims that were not available to the operators in their own right. Only in the Los Angeles case did a civil liberties group (Lambda Legal) participate.

The second group of cases consisted of challenges, brought by operators of SFBs, to local ordinances (and one state law) banning closed booths and other dark nooks and crannies in adult-oriented businesses. (Two other cases, *Martinez v. Texas*, 1987, and *Rahmani v. Texas*,

1988, were unsuccessful appeals of criminal convictions for violating an open-booth ordinance.) This group consists of at least fifteen cases, all of which focused on First Amendment claims. These "open-booth" cases are a subset of a far larger group of over five hundred reported cases concerning the regulation of adult-oriented businesses generally, primarily through zoning restrictions and licensing schemes. The discussion here is limited to those cases in which the primary or substantial focus of the decision was on the validity of open-booth laws as a means of preventing public sex, and so it does not include decisions like *City of Colorado Springs v. 2354 Inc.* (1995) where booth rules were upheld with little or no discussion in the course of a decision involving other, more controversial forms of regulation.

The issue of how far a state or local government may go in using zoning, licensing and other regulatory devices to restrict businesses that trade in sexually-oriented books, movies or performances is much disputed, and many such regulations have been struck down as unconstitutional (*FW/PBS, Inc. v. City of Dallas*, 1990). The narrower question of structural limitations on businesses, including primarily lighting and open-booth rules, has been easier for courts: in all fifteen of the cases reviewed here, the open-booth requirement was upheld. (There are cases in which an ordinance that included an open-booth requirement was found partially or completely invalid on other grounds (*FW/PBS Inc. v. City of Dallas*, 1990; *Ellwest Stereo Theater, Inc. v. Bonner*, 1989).)

The cases for the most part deal with the operator's interest in purveying books, movies and performances without undue interference. In only one case have patrons been parties to raise personal claims, though in some cases courts have put aside the question of standing and allowed operators to argue claims based on the customers' rights (see, e.g., *City News and Novelty, Inc. v. City of Waukesha* (1992); *Suburban Video, Inc. v. City of Delafield* (1988)). No civil rights organization participated as a party or friend of the court in any of the cases.

Only two states–Delaware (1994) and Tennessee (1995)–have passed statewide open-booth rules. North Carolina has a statute prohibiting more than one person from occupying a booth (N.C. Gen Stat. § 14-202.11 (1995). It is not known how many towns, cities and counties have such ordinances, but as discussed below, virtually every local government that has zoning authority has the authority to pass one. While the misdemeanor penalties contained in these ordinances are typically fines of less than $1,000, violation sets the stage for closure of the business as a nuisance, or pending compliance with the law.

Legal Bases of Regulation

As a general matter, regulation of SFBs is based on the "police power," the great reservoir of authority conferred on the state to take action necessary to preserve the health, welfare and morals of the community. Nuisance law, the primary vehicle for closing an SFB, is a traditional tool of the police power (Gostin, 2000). A nuisance is commonly defined as "whatever is dangerous to human life or detrimental to health" (New York City Administrative Code, 1994). A condition may be categorized as a nuisance in several ways. The legislature may do so; New York law, for example, declares any place that harbors prostitutes to be a nuisance (New York Consolidated Laws Public Health, 1994). Judges may do so on a case by case basis. Administrative agencies may do so. The New York closure cases are based on a resolution of the State Public Health Council, subsequently made a permanent part of the state Sanitary Code, defining as a nuisance an establishment that makes "facilities available for the purpose of sexual activities in which facilities high-risk sexual activity takes place" (New York State Sanitary Code, 1994). This was later changed to be more specific, and currently reads: "No establishment shall make facilities available for the purpose of sexual activities where anal intercourse, vaginal intercourse or fellatio take place. Such facilities shall constitute a threat to the public health" (New York State Sanitary Code, 2001). The police power is also the basis for the open-booth rules. The authority to regulate for health and safety is inherent in the state, and is routinely delegated by the state to local governments (Connecticut, 1989; Gostin, 2000; Miller, 1997).

Why Does the State Always Win? The Dance of Facts, Rights and Values

While the pattern of case outcomes is simple, that of cause is a thick tangle of strands ranging from the social status of the parties to the Byzantine tautologies of contemporary constitutional doctrine. A thorough analysis of the determinants of case outcomes is well beyond the scope of this paper. For present purposes, it must suffice to note briefly the leading factors.

The Play of Status: Pornographers and Promiscuous Pederasts versus the Public Health

Litigation over bathhouses takes place on the same field of social ambivalence about sex and sexual orientation as any other HIV case, only perhaps more so because the issues of homosexual behavior, and its role in the construction of modern gay identity, are explicit. Litigation over open-booth ordinances adds the spice of the pornography debate. Any dispute about HIV regulation reflects prevailing understanding of the disease itself, as a plague, a chronic disease, or some combination of both (Fee & Krieger, 1993). A rich body of research has traced the roots, expression and impact of stigma in the HIV epidemic (Herek and Cogan, 1995; Herek & Capitano, 1999; Burris, 2002).

Stigma also affects court decisions. Musheno and colleagues have found that, consistent with earlier sociolegal research, the social status of parties, and the degree to which their claims run counter to established norms or authorities, do influence the outcome of litigation across doctrinal lines. Their qualitative quantitative analysis of early HIV cases found that "the courts show a strong tendency to legitimate the standing of dominant parties . . . In so doing, the court lent support to restrictive claims, showed a great reluctance to give equal standing to stigmatized parties, employed divisive AIDS metaphors to rationalize their decisions, relied on traditional legal presuppositions to justify rulings, and used the language of rights while selectively applying right to manage AIDS contestations" (Musheno, Gregward & Drass, 1991; Aiken & Musheno, 1994). There is thus support beyond common sense for the proposition that gay men and the operators of sex clubs and dirty bookstores will tend to be losers in fights over sex regulations brought by the government in the name of public health.

The closure cases have been notable for a relative avoidance of dramatic characterizations of the epidemic or moral criticism of bathhouse patrons. Yet the very posture of litigation imposed by the law is stigmatizing. To justify closure of an SFB, health officials must in essence establish that gay sex is a nuisance–like gambling, prostitution, or crack dealing or crowding too many people into an unsanitary tenement. This dishonorific depends in turn upon a showing that gay sex is a danger to public health and safety. Anal and oral sex are anatomized as acts allowing the introduction of semen into cavities studded with cuts and sores. The patrons of SFBs are at once victims and villains, and in both roles are equal threats to the public health. The value of gay sex, the distinctive if problematic role of sex in gay culture, the richness of gay identity beyond sex are all invisible in the complaint brought by the state, or the findings of a city council passing an open-booth ordinance.

The problem of sex itself figures largely in cases–often by omission. There is a widespread though not universal tendency on the part of courts in the open-booth cases to ignore the fact that these cases are about preventing people from masturbating or having sex while watching sexually explicit programs. Upholding open-booth laws as "content-neutral" time, place and manner restrictions, courts have noted that they are only coincidentally being applied to sexually explicit material: these laws, we are told in *Berg v. Health & Hospital Corp of Marion County* (1989), "would apply to a showing of *Rebecca of Sunnybrook Farm* as well as any other form of performance" (p. 802). This kind of abstraction renders the practical stakes of the case largely invisible, which, one senses, many of the judges believe it ought to be.

The Limits of Judicial Fact-Finding

To the extent that the question of SFB regulation comes down to the set of factual questions I raised in the introduction to this paper, courts are not helping illuminate the best course. (See Table 2.)

The main factual predicate for intervention is the occurrence of sexual activity per se. The closure cases usually, but not always, included evidence of actual activity witnessed by undercover investigators. All the bathhouse cases have had such evidence. Indeed, the main reason for the denial of closure in the Big Apple Spa ("Plato's retreat") case was the investigator's inability to find sufficient evidence of unsafe sex or prostitution. This is consistent with the rules of nuisance law, which place a burden on the government to establish that a dangerous condition actually exists. The open-booth cases, which are for the most part challenges to laws that have yet to be applied, have had less decisive proof of sex. Cases tend to rely on the general legislative findings of the body which enacted the law, even if these findings are based on nothing more than the legal research of counsel drafting the ordinance. In several of the cases, the presence of dried semen or masturbation is sufficient.

The harder questions get shorter shrift. Courts have had nothing of substance to say about the important distinction between safer and unsafe sex. In at least two open-booth cases, judges based their rulings in part on the finding that HIV might be transmitted by contact with semen left on the floors and walls of booths. In one case, the judge wrote that the operator's medical expert "testified that there is only a *slight* possibility that AIDS and other diseases could be spread by masturbation or by ejaculated semen left exposed on the interior of the booths. This court finds this testimony to be credible but notes that even Dr. Travis admits that it is a *possibility*, however slight, of such transmission and that the medical field does not use the word 'impossible' when making

TABLE 2. Challenges to Open-Booth Ordinances

Case	Plaintiff	Type of Law	Evidence Presented that Business Presented a Risk to Health
Mitchell v. Commission on Adult Entertainment Establishments, 10 F.3d 123 (3rd Cir. 1993)	Owner	State statute	None
Libra Books, Inc. c. City of Milwaukee, 818 F. Supp. 263 (E.D. Wis. 1993)	Owner	Local ordinance	None
City News and Novelty, Inc. v. City of Waukesha, 487 N.W.2d 316 (1992)	Owner	Local ordinance	None
Bamon Corp. v. City of Dayton, 923 F.2d 470 (6th Cir. 1991)	Owner	Local ordinance	None
Doe v. City of Minneapolis, 898 F.2d 612 (8th Cir. 1990)	Owner & 2 patrons	Local ordinance	Police testimony of unsafe sex; general evidence of disease risk from public health authorities
Adult Entertainment Centers, Inc. v. Pierce County, 788 P.2d 1102 (1990)	Owner	Local ordinance	Police and citizen testimony of unsafe sex, general evidence of disease risk from public health authorities
Berg v. Health & Hospital Corp of Marion County, 865 F.2d 797 (7th Cir. 1989)	Owner	Local ordinance	Hearing record with testimony of unsafe sex, general evidence of disease risk from public health authorities
Grunberg v. Town of East Hartford, Connecticut, 736 F. Supp. 430 (D. Conn. 1989)	Owner	Local ordinance	Parties agreed there was no evidence of unsafe sex in plaintiff's facilities
Movie & Video World v. Board of Commissioners of Palm Beach County, 723 F. Supp. 695 (S.D. Fla. 1989)	Owner	Local ordinance	Evidence of masturbation and that transmission of HIV via masturbation was not "impossible"
FW/PBS, Inc. v. City of Dallas, 837 F.2d 1298 (5th Cir. 1988)	Owner	Local ordinance	None
Suburban Video, Inc. v. City of Delafield, 694 F. Supp. 585 (E.D. Wis. 1988)	Owner	Local ordinance	None
Wall Distrib. v. City of Newport News, 782 F.2d 1165 (4th Cir. 1986)	Owner	Local ordinance	Some evidence of masturbation
Broadway Books, Inc. v. Roberts, 642 F. Supp. 486 (E.D. Tenn. 1986)	Owner	Local ordinance	Sex crime arrests; presence of semen, blood and feces; "glory holes" allowing inter-booth sex
Ellwest Stereo Theater v. Wenner, 681 F.2d 1243 (9th Cir. 1982)	Owner	Local ordinance	No health evidence or justification; ordinance based on sex crimes
Postscript Enter. v. City of Bridgeton, 905 F.2d 223 (8th Cir. 1990)	Owner	Local ordinance	None

predictions based on scientific testing and data" (*Movie & Video World v. Board of Commissioners of Palm Beach County*, 1989). The decision in *Broadway Books, Inc. v. Roberts* (1986) relied on "expert" witnesses and the medically questionable "findings" of the city commission:

> One of the Commission's paramount concerns was the health hazard created by these establishments and the increased incidence of Acquired Immune Deficiency Syndrome (AIDS) which have been reported in the Chattanooga area. Dr. Katherine Hankins of the Hamilton County Health Department testified that exposure to the blood and semen in these booths could transmit the HTLV-III virus that carries AIDS, not to mention the exposure which could be generated by sex acts conducted through the "glory holes." (*Broadway Books, Inc. v. Roberts* (1986), p. 491)

Even in some of the bathhouse cases, the distinction between fellatio and anal sex–of great significance to gay men and public health authorities–is glossed over. Nor do the decisions closely consider whether intervention will actually reduce the rate of disease transmission, or whether there are alternatives that would be more effective and less restrictive.

This reflects various practical and doctrinal limitations on the role of courts. Courts do not do independent fact-finding. They depend on what the parties provide, and the data that would allow reasonable decisions about the value of bathhouse closures or open-booth laws were largely lacking at the time of the litigation. In the early bathhouse cases, the evidence consisted primarily of battling conclusions drawn by experts, based largely on experience and intuition. The judicial process did not fill the lacunae, although sometimes the rhetorical needs of the opinion writer, or his limited grasp of the medical issues, would lead to a decision making the health stakes sound much higher than they were.

The most apparent reason for the weak fact finding in the cases reviewed here, however, is the formal legal doctrine. Courts, and the law, recognize that the regulation of SFBs is largely a political question, to which there is not really a "correct" answer. The role of courts in such matters is, in theory, only to prevent serious mistakes–excessive or pointless infringements on individual rights. Thus public health actions and legislation like open-booth ordinances are presumed to be legal, and any factual disputes are dispatched as they were in the St. Mark's case:

To be sure, defendants and the intervening patrons challenge the soundness of the scientific judgments upon which the Health Council regulation [declaring baths a nuisance] is based, citing, *inter alia*, the observation of the City's former Commissioner of health . . . that "closure of bathhouses will contribute little if anything to the control of AIDS." . . . Defendants particularly assail the regulation's inclusion of fellatio as a high-risk sexual activity and argue that enforced use of prophylactic sheaths would be a more appropriate regulatory response. They go further and argue that facilities such as St. Mark's, which attempts to educate its patrons with written materials, signed pledges, and posted notices as to the advisability of safe sexual practices, provide a positive force in combating AIDS, and a valuable communications link between public health authorities and the homosexual community. While these arguments and proposals may have varying degrees of merit, they overlook a fundamental principal of applicable law: "It is not for the courts to determine which scientific view is correct in ruling upon whether the police power has been properly exercised. 'The judicial function is exhausted with the discovery that the relation between means and end is not wholly vain and fanciful, an illusory pretense.'"(*City of New York v. New St. Mark's Baths* (1986), p. 917)

Similarly, in assessing a time, place and manner restriction such as an open-booth rule, the Supreme Court has instructed lower courts not to engage in independent collection and evaluation of the evidence supporting a law, but to defer to the law-making branch as long as it can show that the evidence it relied on "is reasonably believed to be relevant to the problem that the city addresses (*Renton v. Playtime Theaters, Inc.*, 1986; *Broadway Books v. Roberts*, 1986). As one court summarized the law, the city" was not obligated to conduct independent research on the link between AIDS and anonymous sex. . . . Members of the . . . Common Council were entitled to rely on the experiences of the other cities and counties cited in the introduction to its ordinance" (*Suburban Video Inc. v. City of Delafield*, 1988).

Public Sex in Legal Doctrine

The "black letter" law is the easiest part of the explanation of case outcomes. The police power gives the government the authority to act in furtherance of public health, safety and morals. Actions taken are presumed to be proper, and will only be countermanded by courts if they infringe upon a fundamental right. The core question in the cases, then, has been whether restrictions on sex do violate any rights. Several have been proposed in the cases. Opponents of closure or open-booth ordinances have argued that these measures interfere with sex between consenting adults, and that this violates their general right of privacy (which has a variety of proposed sources in the Constitution) or their right to free association guaranteed by the First Amendment. In cases involving bookstores and theaters, patrons (or operators trying to argue on their behalf) have argued that closings or booth restrictions interfere with their right of access to ideas, protected by the first amendment. None of these have fared well in litigation.

The notion that there is a right to have the sex of one's choice in a public place has been rejected root and branch. The early *Ellwest* case is unusually frank:

> The essence of the argument is that the customers have a constitutional right to fondle themselves; therefore, argues *Ellwest*, the City may not constitutionally require that the theater open the booths and thus chill the patrons' exercise of the right to masturbate. We assume with a fair degree of confidence that the activities *Ellwest* seeks to protect may be enjoyed without governmental interference in the sanctity of the customers' homes. *Ellwest* must establish, however, that there is a constitutional right to engage in such activities in a public place. That issue has been decided against *Ellwest* in *Paris Adult Theatre I v. Slayton*, 413 U.S. 49, 65-67, 93 S. Ct. 2628, 2639-40, 37 L. Ed. 2 446 (1973). The Court there held that the constitutionally protected right to watch obscene movies in the privacy of one's own home did not import a similar right to watch the same movies in a public place. The court reasoned that while viewing obscene movies in one's home, *Stanley v. Georgia*, 394 U.S. 557, 568, 89 S. Ct. 1243, 1249, 22 L. Ed. 2d 542 (1969), and engaging in sexual intercourse in the marital bedroom, *Griswold v. Connecticut*, 381 U.S. 479, 485-86, 85 S. Ct. 1678, 1682, 14 L. Ed. 2d 510 (1965), are both protected by the constitutional right to privacy, that protection ceases when the locus of the conduct shifts to a place of public accommodation such as a theater. The Court "declined to equate the privacy of the home relied on in Stanley with a 'zone' of 'privacy' that follows a distributor or a consumer . . . wherever he goes. The idea of a 'privacy' right and a place of public accommodation are, in this

context, mutually exclusive." *Paris Adult Theatre*, supra, 413 U.S. at 66, 93 S. Ct. at 2639 (citations omitted). In defining the limits of the constitutional right to privacy, the Court invoked Justice Cardozo: "(o)ur prior decisions recognizing a right to privacy guaranteed by the Fourteenth Amendment included 'only personal rights that can be deemed "fundamental" or "implicit in the concept of ordered liberty." ' " Id. at 65, 93 S. Ct. at 2639, quoting, inter alia, *Palko v. Connecticut*, 302 U.S. 319, 325, 58 S. Ct. 149, 151, 82 L. Ed. 288 (1937). While we certainly agree with *Ellwest* that its customers have a constitutional right to view its films, we cannot agree that the interest in simultaneously engaging in sexual activity is similarly protected. We decline to hold that the "right" to unobserved masturbation in a public theater is "fundamental" or "implicit in the concept of ordered liberty." (*Ellwest Stereo Theatres, Inc. v. Wenner* (1982), p. 1248)

Since these words were written, the case for a right of sexual privacy has only gotten weaker, particularly for gay men. A right to sexual privacy in public would seem to depend on a right of sexual privacy anywhere. In *Bowers v. Hardwick* (1986) decision, however, the Supreme Court upheld Georgia's sodomy statute against the challenge of a gay man who had been arrested for having sex with another man in his own bedroom. The majority opinion, relying on the long history of criminalization of homosexuality, concluded that "to claim that a right to engage in such conduct is 'deeply rooted in this Nation's history and tradition' or 'implicit in the concept of ordered liberty' is, at best, facetious."

The First Amendment claims raised in bookstore and theater cases have fared no better. Sex, according to the courts, does not become protected just because it happens near or because of or during the use of a protected video or book. "First Amendment values," as the Supreme Court dismissively put it, "may not be invoked merely by linking the words 'sex' and 'books'" (*Arcara v. Cloud Books Inc.* (1986)). Thus courts have rejected the claim that the first amendment right of privacy or the first amendment confer on peep show customers the right to watch movies in seclusion. "[T]he [customers] do not have a privacy right to watch the material conveyed in the viewing booths in seclusion. The right to view public entertainment in the seclusion of a closed booth simply falls outside the ambit of the personal intimacies of the home, family, marriage, parenthood, procreation, and child rearing" (*Doe v. City of Minneapolis* (1990), p. 615-16 n. 11).

In the first closure case, in San Francisco, the several bookstores and theaters initially targeted along with the bathhouses were quickly allowed to reopen because of First Amendment concerns. Ten years later, in the recent *Dana* case in New York, these claims were of no avail to the operator. The change reflects the emergence of a clear rule from the Supreme Court that "the First Amendment is not implicated by the enforcement of a public health regulation of general application against . . . physical premises in which [business people] happen to sell books" (*Arcara v. Cloud Books Inc.* (1986), p. 707). Strictly speaking, the *Dana* case did not involve federal law, but even more protective state law in New York. In a challenge to the closure of a bookstore as a nuisance (based on prostitution), the Court disparaged "the fallacy of seeking to use the First Amendment as a cloak for obviously unlawful sexual conduct by the diaphanous device of attributing protected expressive attributes to the conduct" (*Arcara v. Cloud Books Inc.* (1986)). Closure imposed a "dubious" burden on the operators, who were free to move their business to a new location.

Gostin and other commentators on public health law have stressed the importance of the concept of the least restrictive means in the rational formation of policy (Gostin, 1995). The least restrictive means analysis, which essentially requires the state to show that its coercive measures reflect a reasonable weighing of alternatives and the avoidance of unnecessary infringements of individual rights, is a feature (albeit in an attenuated form) of the First Amendment analysis used in the open-booth cases. Under the so-called O'Brien test, measures that have a goal unrelated to speech, but which have an effect on speech, must be "narrowly tailored" to their purpose so that "they leave open ample alternative channels for communication of information" (*Ward v. Rock Against Racism* (1989), p. 791 (quoting *Clark v. Community for Creative Non-Violence* (1984), p. 293)). Operators have frequently argued that partial doors, occupancy restrictions or patrols would be as effective as open-booth requirements without the same negative impact on patrons' enjoyment. This passage is typical of the courts' response:

> Adult Books' argument that there are better means to deter sexual contact in the booths without inhibiting freedom of expression is rejected. . . . The choice of one among several legitimate statutory means to obtain a legitimate end is a matter for the legislature not the judiciary. Moreover, it does not appear that use of partial doors open only at the bottom, booths spaced further apart, or booths with the bottom two feet of the door removed would adequately

accomplish the legislative goal of deterring promiscuous sexual contacts that can spread deadly disease. Doors of this kind would not inhibit sexual activity between two individuals in adjacent booths through the use of holes in the common dividing partitions, or inhibit masturbation within the partially enclosed booths. Therefore, we reject Adult Books' contention that the legislative purpose of preventing unprotected sexual activity arguably could be served by spacing the booths one foot apart as well as its suggestion that this spacing, combined with partial doors, would reduce undesirable sexual conduct within the booths with less impairment of the privacy that encourages persons using the booths to engage in the kind of expressive activity Adult Books seeks to promote. Moreover, Delaware did not have to adopt the means. Adult Books preferred to regulate the undesirable health effect of the marginally protected speech and expression it purveys. The state must be allowed a reasonable opportunity to experiment with solutions to problems, *Renton*, 475 U.S. at 52 (quoting Young, 427 U.S. at 71), and the regulation "need not be the least-restrictive or least-intrusive means of doing so." *Ward*, 109 S. Ct. at 2757-58 (footnote omitted); see also *Bamon Corp.*, 923 F.2d at 473-74. But see *Berg*, 865 F.2d at 803-04 (requiring least restrictive means analysis but concluding it was easily met with open-booth ordinance). "So long as the means chosen are not substantially broader than necessary to achieve the government's interest . . . the regulation will not be invalid simply because a court concludes that the government's interest could be adequately served by some less-speech-restrictive alternative (*Ward v. Rock Against Racism* (1989), p. 2758)." (*Mitchell v. Commission on Adult Entertainment Establishments* (1993), p. 143)

WHAT WE DO NOT KNOW

The main burden of this paper so far has been that law—in the form of legal rules applied by courts in litigation—is not a barrier to action against SFBs. In some places, like New York, we see a high level of professional competence being brought to bear by health and legal authorities in creating regulations governing SFBs, developing a record of unsafe sex, and making a thorough case to the court. Another notable instance was *Ellwest*, in which the local health director had accumulated data about STDs traceable to the establishments affected by the open-booth ordinance. In other places, open-booth regulations were adopted with little serious fact-finding, based largely on moral concerns about public sex generally (e.g., *Bamon Corp. v. City of Dayton* (1991); *Movie & Video World v. Board of Commissioners of Palm Beach County* (1989)). Either way, the government wins and the regulations are upheld. Yet the law applied by courts in litigation is not all the law there is, and law is not all that matters. In the remaining pages of this paper, I will present a series of questions whose answers would be of considerable value in assessing the use of law to regulate SFBs in the cause of public health. There are many gaps in the empirical foundation for action.

Law and Politics

Law provides a vocabulary for political struggle over gay sexuality. The use of law in this sense is largely unconnected to the constitutional doctrine of courts. Indeed, the gay claim to a fundamental right to live gay without government harassment is made more, rather than less, urgent by the fact that courts do not recognize it. The claim of government to regulate gay sex is reasonably seen by many gay people as having more to do with scoring points against homosexuality than protecting public health (Dangerous Bedfellows, 1996). Precisely because they entail the exercise of power, coercive health measures can be unsettling to their target communities even when the measure itself is recognized as reasonable (Burris, 2000). Likewise, measures focus on the behavior of individuals at risk without considering the social drivers of the behavior can be perceived as assigning blame (Marks et al., 1999). How is the language of legal rights being used in the political debate over regulating SFBs? What can health officials learn from this language about the nature and intensity of concern about sex regulation? In such an environment, how can public health officials exercise their authority in ways that draw upon and build support within the gay community?

Public Knowledge, Attitudes and Beliefs About SFB Regulation

It is often said that coercive measures drive people with HIV underground, but there is little evidence to support this claim in its broadest forms (Burris, 1998). Affluent urban gay men have tended to make rights claims during the HIV epidemic, but we should not assume that they or any other segment of the gay community are actually very conscious of health laws or court decisions, much less of the details of doctrinal interpretation. If we abandon this assumption, it is clear that we must speak cautiously about the impact of law on gay men, or the society as a whole. How do those who are regulated–gay men in particular–perceive the law as expressed in court decisions? How does this affect their views of public health officials? To what extent are people aware of this body of law? Do they regard these decisions as legitimate/fair? Does SFB regulation add to the anger/stigma/fear felt by gay men and others with or at risk of HIV?

Law as Education

If people with or at risk of HIV are aware of court decisions, we should be concerned about what the outcomes, legal reasoning and factual findings are telling the audience about HIV and its control. Men who have sex with men themselves are a key audience for this message, particularly if one believes that attitudes towards or norms about sexual behavior are important community-level influences on individual men's behavior (Rotello, 1997). How do court decisions (mis)educate the public and those at risk about HIV? How and what do people learn about court decisions? Do decisions convey accurate information about HIV transmission? Do decisions upholding coercive measures add to stigma? Do they tend to suggest HIV is a disease of the promiscuous other? Does failure to act undermine the legitimacy of public health policy among other important constituents?

Law as an Effective Regulatory Tool

Legal health measures, like nonlegal ones, are often not validated. We should be concerned about how well various approaches to regulating SFBs are working. Are closure, open-booth rules and other limits on sex reducing the rate of HIV transmission, or shifting its location? Is this the right measure of success? Are there others? What works better to close bathhouses, local market pressure, negotiation or coercion? Has the capacity to use coercion been useful in securing voluntary compliance with health guidelines or programs? How has market pressure affected sex clubs over the years? Do sex clubs cause or reflect patterns of unsafe sex? How important are local cultural and political factors? Have closed booth ordinances stopped sexual activity in adult businesses? Are they being obeyed? Have operators found new ways to facilitate sex among patrons? Are there other strategies that will work better? Are the enumerated powers of health departments appropriate to this task?

CONCLUSION

Despite its role of dispute-resolver-of-last-resort, the judicial system tends to mirror rather than solve significant social dilemmas. Ten years of legal experience with HIV shows that health officials have great power to regulate sex in public places, but sheds little light on whether it is a good idea to do so. Arguments about rights such as privacy have their place in assessing the regulation of SFBs, but decision-making and rights debate would alike be enriched by empirical answers to basic questions about law's operation and effects in this area. With evidence of a resurgence in risky sexual behavior in San Francisco and potentially other epicenters of homosexually transmitted HIV, the legal issues may once again become urgent.

ACKNOWLEDGMENTS

This paper was prepared for a Kaiser Family Foundation meeting on "Public Policy Aspects of Regulating Bathhouses and Sex Clubs," co-sponsored by the Center for AIDS Prevention Studies, in New York, in December 1995. It was revised for publication without updated research in 2001. The author is grateful for the research assistance and editorial advice of Jennifer Ward, a JD candidate at Temple Law School.

REFERENCES

Aiken, J.H., & Musheno, M. (1994). Why have-nots win in the HIV litigation arena: Socio-legal dynamics of extreme cases. *Law & Policy*, 16, 267-297.

Arcara v. Cloud Books Inc., 478 U.S. 697, 705 (1986).

Ayres, I., & Braithwaite, J. (1992). *Responsive regulation: Transcending the deregulation debate*. Oxford University Press.

Bayer, R. (1989). *Private acts, social consequences: AIDS and the politics of public health*. New York: Free Press.

Binson, D., Woods, W. J., Pollack, L., Paul, J., Stall, R., & Catania, J.A. (2001). Differential HIV risk in bathhouses and public cruising areas. *American Journal of Public Health*, 91, 1482-1486.

Bowers v. Hardwick, 478 U.S. 186, 190-91 (1986).

Brandt, A.M. (1987). *No magic bullet: A social history of venereal disease in the United States since 1880*. New York, N.Y.: Oxford University Press.

Broadway Books, Inc. v. Roberts, 642 F. Supp. 486 (E.D. Tenn. 1986).

Burris, S. (2002). Disease stigma in public health law and research. *J. Law, Medicine & Ethics,* 30(2), 179-190.

Burris, S. (2000). Surveillance, social risk and symbolism: Framing the analysis for research and policy. *Journal of Acquired Immune Deficiency Syndromes*, 25 (Suppl. 2), S120-S127.

Burris, S. (1998). Law and the social risk of health care: Lessons from HIV testing. *Albany Law Review*, 61, 831-895.

City of Colorado Springs v. 2354 Inc., 896 P.2d 272 (1995).

City News and Novelty, Inc. v. City of Waukesha, 487 N.W.2d 316 (Wis. App. 1992).

City of New York v. New St. Mark's Baths, 130 Misc. 2d 911(1986).

Clark v. Community for Creative Non-Violence, 468 U.S. 288 (1984).

Dangerous Bedfellows (eds.) (1996). *Policing public sex: Queer politics and the future of AIDS activism*. Boston: South End Press.

Delaware, 24 Del. Code § 1631 (1994).

Ellwest Stereo Theater, Inc. v. Bonner, 681 F.2d 1243 (M.D. Tenn. 1989).

Fee, E., & Krieger, N. (1993). Thinking and rethinking AIDS implications for health policy. *International Journal of Health Services*, 23, 323-346.

FW/PBS, Inc. v. City of Dallas, 493 U.S. 215 (1990).

Gostin, L. (2000). *Public health law: Power, duty, restraint*. Berkeley: University of California Press.

Gostin, L. (1995). The resurgent tuberculosis epidemic in the era of AIDS: Reflections on public health, law and society. *Maryland Law Review* 54, 1-131.

Grunberg v. Town of East Hartford, Connecticut, 736 F. Supp. 430 (D. Conn. 1989), aff'd 901 F.2d 297 (2d Cir. 1990) (per curiam).

Herek, G.M., & Capitano, J.P. (1999). AIDS stigma and sexual prejudice. *Am. Behav. Scientist*, 42:1126-1143.

Herek, G., & Cogan, J. (1995). *AIDS and stigma, a review of the literature*. Public Media Center.

Marks, G., Burris, S., & Peterman, T. (1999). Reducing sexual transmission of HIV from those who know they are infected: The need for personal and collective responsibility. *AIDS* 13, 297- 306.

Martinez v. Texas, 744 S.W.2d 224 (App. 1987).

Miller, C.A., Gilbert, B., Warren, D.G., Brooks, E.F., DeFriese, G.H., Jain, S.C., & Kavaler, F. (1977). Statutory authorization of the work of local health departments. *American Journal of Public Health*, 67, 940-945.

Mitchell v. Commission on Adult Entertainment Establishments of State of Del., 10 F.3d 123 (Del. 1993).

Movie & Video World v. Board of Commissioners of Palm Beach County, 723 F. Supp. 695 (S.D. Fla. 1989).

Musheno, M., Gregware, P., & Drass, K. (1991). Court management of AIDS disputes: A sociolegal analysis. *Law and Social Inquiry*, 16, 737-774.

New York Administrative Code (1994). N.Y.C. Administrative Code § 564-15.0.

N.Y. Cons. Laws Public Health § 2320 (1994).

New York Sanitary Code (1994). N.Y. Compilation Codes Rules & Regulations tit. 10 § 24-2.2.

New York Sanitary Code (2001). N.Y. Compilation Codes Rules & Regulations tit. 10 § 24-2.2.

N.C. Gen. Stat. § 14-202.11 (1995).

Rahmani v. Texas, 748 S.W. 2d 618 (App. 1988).

Regan v. Time, Inc., 468 U.S. 64 (1984).

Renton v. Playtime Theaters, Inc., 475 US __ (1986).

Rotello, G. (1997). *Sexual Ecology: AIDS and the Destiny of Gay Men.* New York: Penguin Putnam.

Suburban Video, Inc. v. City of Delafield, 694 F. Supp. 585 (E.D. Wis. 1988).

Tenn. Code Ann. §§ 7-51-1401 to -1406 (1995).

Tyler, T.R. (1990). *Why people obey the law.* New Haven, CT: Yale University Press.

United States v. Albertini, 472 U.S. 675 (1985).

Ward v. Rock Against Racism, 491 U.S. 78 (1989).

Sex and the Baths:
A Not-So-Secret Report

Michael Helquist
Rick Osmon

SUMMARY. During the 1984 debate about closing the baths in San Francisco the mayor directed the police to investigate sexual behavior in the bathhouses and write a report for her. The directive had been a secret, but when the community learned of the report, its response was quick and furious. The mayor squelched the report and no one but the report's authors, the mayor, and probably a handful of intermediaries ever saw the written report. In response to this investigation, two local journalists conducted a more open investigation that resulted in a newspaper article for *Coming Up!*, a lesbian and gay community newspaper published monthly in San Francisco (California). This article is reprinted here in large part because of its scientific rather than journalistic or historical value. These investigators approached their work systematically (certainly much more so than many other scientists, journalists or police professionals at the time), and as a result, their article provides a much more thorough description of what was happening in the baths at that point in the AIDS epidemic. Interestingly, many public policy options considered today were already part of the discussion then and, at times, already in place in the San Francisco bathhouses. Of note, at the time, orgy rooms were con-

This paper reprinted here by permission of the San Francisco *Bay Times*.
Correspondence may be addressed to Michael Helquist, 2088 Golden Gate Avenue, San Francisco, CA 94115 (E-mail: HelquistSF@aol.com).

[Haworth co-indexing entry note]: "Sex and the Baths: A Not-So-Secret Report." Helquist, Michael, and Rick Osmon. Co-published simultaneously in *Journal of Homosexuality* (Harrington Park Press, an imprint of The Haworth Press, Inc.) Vol. 44, No. 3/4, 2003, pp. 153-175; and: *Gay Bathhouses and Public Health Policy* (ed: William J. Woods, and Diane Binson) Harrington Park Press, an imprint of The Haworth Press, Inc., 2003, pp. 153-175.

sidered likely to be contributing to transmission, thus the authors gave particular attention to its presence/absence and use. The original paper was published in the July 1984 edition (pp. 17-22). As with all the reprinted papers in this volume, no editorial changes were made to the paper and only minor typographical errors were corrected. The editor of *Coming Up!* included a preface to the article in the original publication, and that preface is also reprinted here.

KEYWORDS. AIDS, HIV prevention, gay bathhouses, history

Coming Up! *has authorized and supported the research and writing of this bathhouse report. The debate over what action our community should take regarding the status of the bathhouses has sharply divided us. Discussion often takes place in the arena of personal prejudices, political agendas, and uninformed speculations. Factual information about the sexual activity that takes place in the baths and the possible risks that gay men are exposing themselves to has been virtually non-existent.*

The immediate impetus for this report was the disclosure of the bathhouse report prepared by the San Francisco Police Department at the request of Mayor Feinstein. That report remains confidential, and has only publicly been described as "steamy." Coming Up! *has not been secret with our report. The Northern California Bathhouse Association was notified in advance, and they welcomed the opportunity for a factual reporting on bathhouse activity.*

Reporters Michael Helquist and Rick Osmon centered their research on the six gay bathhouses in the city; sex clubs are not included in the report. Their visits to the bathhouses occurred over an eight-day period in mid-June. They spent a minimum of three hours at each facility. Frequently they told bathhouse patrons that they were writing about the baths; sometimes they simply said they had come to see what was happening.

Helquist and Osmon describe their experiences in graphic language. Sexual institutions need to be talked about in sexual terms. Clinical descriptions used by doctors and politicians ignore the erotic nature of the baths. Civil rights advocates often defend the baths on grounds of rights to privacy, while sidestepping the reality of the sexual activities.

The terrible sweep of AIDS through San Francisco will only claim a greater toll if decisions about education and prevention for gay men are not based on frank discussions and acknowledgments of the actual means of transmission.

In order to understand what was happening at the baths, it was necessary for Helquist and Osmon to enter the private rooms. They write, "We decided to have sex ourselves in the bathhouses and felt our activities would provide greater insight into the nature of current bathhouse behavior, high-risk and safe sex. We also decided that our sexual experiences could illustrate such activity in the baths.

"We saw our challenge clearly: to recreate an actual environment for our readers' greater understanding. We had already established our individual standards for appropriate risk reduction in our own sexual behavior. We maintained our standards throughout these visits. We suggest only to others that they seriously consider and adopt standards of risk reduction based on guidelines provided by the San Francisco AIDS Foundation."

By printing this report, Coming Up! *neither encourages nor discourages the use of bathhouses by gay and bisexual men. Additionally, since the report does not address the sex clubs, porno movie theatres and bookstores, there is still no factual accounting of the situations there. Could those institutions also stand the test of the spotlight? The information on the bathhouses is presented here to assist each individual in making his own decision about appropriate and safe behavior.*

–Kim Corsaro, Editor

AN EROTIC ENVIRONMENT

We observed from 15 to 60 men at the individual facilities during our visit to the six baths. Clearly a great majority of gay and bisexual men no longer go to the baths; many never did. Others–gay and nongay–may find them unappealing, impersonal, and unsatisfying. For those men who continue to frequent the baths, the major attraction is the erotic stimulation found there.

Our descriptions here result from an appreciation of the sexual energy found in bathhouses. A nongay observer may only see long, lurid hallways with rooms on either side, doors opening and closing, men entering and leaving, and a seemingly endless walking around routine with apparently little sex. But gay and bisexual men who are "into it" often experience a sense of intrigue and anticipation, an overall sense of sensual arousal, an appreciation of gay male sexual identity, and sometimes an obsessive compulsion. Stimulation can occur without any sexual activity at all. The dynamics of all these elements can be volatile;

not uncommon are periods of boredom, a sense of wasting time, a frustration over lack of sexual contacts, and an uneasiness over compulsive feelings. The experience involves a very complex set of emotions, expressed by many of the men with whom we spoke.

There's an immediate sense of relief upon entering the baths. The attendant buzzes you through the door into a warm, controlled environment where the worst thing likely to happen is boredom. The facility is relaxing, removed from the alcohol and smoke of the bars, from the judgmental eyes of society, from the insanity and random violence of the streets, and from the pressure to be either politically correct or socially correct for the benefit of others. Other amenities often take the edge off the sexual energy. There's usually plenty to do without having sex at all, including exercise classes, gyms, feature movies, reading, parties, sunbathing. Fantasies can easily be realized without fear of offending lovers, friends, wives or family. The nonthreatening aspect of the baths, a place where men acknowledge their common sexuality, sometimes without a word spoken, establishes them as an erotic environment.

It was late; I was getting tired and feeling less motivated to initiate any more "bathhouse behavior" conversations. I stood in the video porno room watching the scenes of one very hot man getting fucked by another. The actors didn't seem to be very passionate, or maybe it was just my growing fatigue. As I turned to leave the room, a tall muscular man walked by. He was naked, with a towel wrapped around him. His body was firm, with one of those washboard stomachs and a well-developed chest. And he had a large cock—all in all a good enough reason to walk around naked.

We exchanged eye contact as he passed me; I paused and then followed him down the hallway. I turned down the aisle to my room, unlocked the door, and stood in the doorway, excited that he might be interested and circle back to my room. And there he was at the end of the hallway. We watched each other, quickly oblivious to others walking by. He began to rub his hands over his body. I retreated into my room, dimmed the light a bit, left the door open, and reclined on the bed, awaiting his arrival.

In moments he stood outside my door, leaning against the opposite wall. His gaze was intense and serious. He pulled on his cock; it was now in full erection. I did the same. Finally he came into the room. I leaned around him and closed the door.

We found that several men were drawn to the baths especially for this erotic excitement. Sometimes the men with whom we spoke were in long-term relationships and would come to the baths with their lovers to spark flickering sexual desires in each other.

I paid the one-time charge, got my towel and complimentary rubber, along with a key to a locker. I decided against wearing just a towel as I would usually do. Instead, I just took off my shirt. On the third floor, in one of the many rooms along the hallway, I saw a man lying on a double bed on his stomach. He was wearing only a black leather vest. Neatly laid out on the bed beside him were a condom, a jar of lubricant, a butt plug, and five flesh-colored latex dildoes, all shaped like erect cocks, of increasing size from the standard 8 inches to the largest, which was nearly the size of a forearm.

I was a little impressed, intrigued, and intimidated. The man looked over his shoulder at me and smiled. He was handsome with a trim body. After a few trips past his door—each time he smiled, sometimes he raised his butt some—I decided to enter.

"How are you?"

He smiled and said, "Sit down."

He asked how my evening was going; then we talked for awhile about the baths. He remained lying on his stomach, and I put my hand on his thigh, caressed his leg, and gradually moved to his ass, which was firm and inviting.

"You have a really nice ass," I told him.

He encouraged me, "Why don't you play with it."

So I rubbed his ass, massaged it, and moved around to sit more comfortably on his bed. Meanwhile, he reached beside him and flipped a narrow black leather collar over his ass, an unmistakable invitation. I felt hesitant; I had decided earlier not to fuck around tonight, and I didn't want to be a tease.

But the invitation was almost irresistible, and I slapped his butt a few times with the leather strap. He was enjoying it, gasping a bit with each slap. It was more fantasy than pain, because I wasn't using that much strength.

I stopped and explained, "I'm not going to do more right now; I don't want to lead you on."

"Fine," he said, "but just let me lie across your lap so you can spank me a few times."

I liked that idea, and thought to myself, "If this isn't having sex, what is?" So he positioned himself over my lap. During the next few minutes, his excitement mounted. He was hot to the touch, beginning to sweat. I stopped the spanking and helped him take off his vest. Then I continued a few more times. Finally, we stopped, sat up, smiled at each other, and began to talk, first exchanging names. His was Steven.

I told Steven that this was my first visit here, and that I was curious to see what was happening at the baths these days. He said that this has become his regular place, since the Hothouse closed last year. The bathhouse we were in is known as a place for fisting.

"I come here every few months, sometimes alone, sometimes with my lover. We usually get together with one or two others whom we know well. One man—who I only see here—I've had sex with for the last year. That's not anonymous sex in my mind. In fact, the main reason I came here tonight was to get the phone numbers of these other regulars so I can meet them if the baths close down."

"What will you do if they are closed?" I asked.

"I'll go somewhere else; I'll make arrangements with my regular sex partners so we'll have a place to go. Perhaps my home, but I come here because of the atmosphere. All the basics are taken care of: the music's always playing, someone else does the laundry, the rooms have slings in them."

Steven was very up-to-date with the news about AIDS, the medical research, the science behind the discovery of HTLV-3, the possible AIDS virus. I was impressed with how much he did know—from the recent behavior change symposium held in the city to the politics of AIDS that he felt ran rampant at City Hall.

"I think a few of the gay doctors are advocating outright celibacy," Steven declared. "These doctors are letting themselves be used by the politicians."

"Do you know of anyone with AIDS? Have you seen the physical damage AIDS can cause?" I asked.

"Who among us anymore doesn't know someone who has died of AIDS? Someone I liked a lot and used to work with—I also tricked with him several years ago—died a year ago last June. I was very upset, and in some ways I still am. There have been others; their deaths have affected me deeply."

Steven added, "You know, a lot of what my lover and I have learned about reducing risks with sex we found out at the baths."

"What's it like coming here with your lover?"

"We've been together for over four years now. After that amount of time together, our sexual interest in each other comes and goes in cycles. One of the ways we rekindle the interest is to come to the baths together. Here we can fantasize in our sex play, using these rooms, sometimes letting others watch us."

Steven continued, "What I find so ironic about all this bathhouse business is that these people encourage gay men to couple up for sex, and they tell us to use fantasies for safe sex. That's what my lover and I do at the baths, and now they're trying to close them!"

We were in a room that came equipped with a sling—black leather straps hung from the ceiling with chains allowing someone to lie on his back suspended comfortably with his legs supported. I asked about the safety of his preference for getting fisted.

He replied, "My doctor has given me the same advice now about fisting that he did years before AIDS appeared. 'Do it with someone you trust and with someone who knows how to do it safely.'"

We continued to talk some more, stroking each other a little.

"Can I include some of what you told me in my writing?" I asked him.

"Sure. You can use all of it."

As our conversation stalled, he put on a jock strap and said he was going to go to the john. We hugged and said good-night.

AIDS AWARENESS

It's difficult to realize, at least in the gay and lesbian community of San Francisco, that in May of 1983, the city noted "AIDS Awareness Week." Now, only 14 months later, AIDS awareness frequently seems so high that a little relief from awareness would be welcome. Still, the relentless epidemic remains and increases with new diagnoses and deaths nearly every day in this city.

During the past two years health activists have committed themselves to informing the general public and high-risk groups about AIDS, believing information on prevention to be the necessary first step towards slowing the epidemic. In the midst of the bathhouse controversy, basic questions gained spotlight attention: Do gay and bisexual men know about AIDS and how to prevent it? And do these men alter their sexual behavior at the baths to protect their lives and the lives of their sexual partners?

Signs about hygiene and risk reduction are everywhere in most of the baths. They recommend "Use A Condom When You Play" and "Take A Shower Before And After Sex," or some other helpful hint. An erotic AIDS poster exhorts patrons to "Have Fun And Be Safe, Too." The messages are brief and to the point. Almost all of the facilities provided brochures that include safe sex guidelines. Some of the baths had the popular "Can We Talk?" brochure developed by the Harvey Milk Lesbian and Gay Democratic Club, others offered the "Risk Reduction Guidelines" (see Figure 1) written by the Bay Area Physicians for Human Rights. A few bathhouses had both. The signs and brochures have been provided to the bathhouse owners free of charge by the San Francisco Department of Public Health. Owners have displayed the signs prominently–at the top of stairways, the end of hallways, near the showers–so they cannot be missed or ignored. The continual visual reinforcement makes it easier to mention safety and health concerns to prospective partners.

I had been going to the baths nearly every night for a week, and it was all beginning to catch up with me. If the halls I had walked down were put in a straight line, I'd have been halfway to L.A. In my conversations, I was starting to take on the persona of Miss Manners of Safe Sex.

I was sitting quietly in my room with the door halfway open when this redhead walked in.

"Hi, my name's Eric. What's yours?"

This direct, non-sexual approach immediately put me at ease, so I told him my name and invited him to have a seat. Eric is a professional who works with a number of gay organizations. We talked about theatre and books, business and cooking.

Then he initiated a short discussion on the importance of safe sex. Both of us felt relaxed and comfortable. It seemed much easier to rub and touch each other after our pleasant getting-acquainted session. His concerns for safety made him all the more attractive to me. The mood grew increasingly erotic while we took turns giving massage, chewing or nibbling on ears, necks, and fingers.

"I want to fuck that ass of yours," he whispered in my ear.

"Oh yeah?" I said.

"Yeah, but first let's clean up together in the shower and find a condom. I want us to feel good about this."

"Even with the condom on, I'd rather you not come inside me. Is that OK with you?" I asked.

"That's fine. Now, let's go wash."

The signs and brochures, the distribution of the condoms–these contributed to the awareness of taking safety precautions while having sex. While this was one kind of AIDS awareness, we wondered how much people actually knew about what AIDS does to someone. A few men readily mentioned knowing someone diagnosed with AIDS. And yet they still went to the baths.

FIGURE 1. Inset from Page 20 of the Original *Coming Up!* Article

Risk Reduction Guidelines

The most up-to-date brochure of risk reduction guidelines, "Play With It Safe," was developed by the Bay Area Physicians for Human Rights and distributed by the San Francisco AIDS Foundation. The varieties of sexual activities are arranged in three categories: Safe, Possibly Safe, and Unsafe.

Each category lists the following activities:

SAFE:	hugging, massage, jerking off, fucking between the thighs.
POSSIBLY SAFE:	fucking with a condom, sucking to near climax, french kissing, water sports (on, not in).
UNSAFE:	rimming, taking cum or piss in the mouth, fisting, fucking without a condom, blood contact, sharing sex toys.

"I come to the baths because I can relax here; it's an enclosed environment, and I enjoy looking at attractive male bodies."

That was one patron's response to my questions about his regular visits, perhaps once every other week, for the last few years. His name is Jack; I've known him for a few years, but we haven't been in contact for some time. We met in the shower room, and began talking as we were drying off.

Jack appeared to be somewhat troubled, with a pervasive sadness behind his smile, shadowing his eyes. He referred to my writing about AIDS and said he appreciated the sharing of feelings. And he revealed his own difficulties adjusting to the toll of the disease.

"None of my immediate family or friends has been diagnosed, but one of my clients died of AIDS last week. And now I'm seeing a pair of lovers, one who is near death with AIDS." Jack has been a therapist for several years.

He continued, "I'm very upset and very sad about this. I have trouble dealing with the helplessness and the frustration."

Jack spoke freely of his feelings; he knew I understood and that I had experienced them as well.

"I still come to the baths," Jack explained. "It's a pleasant part of my routine. It helps me relax and unwind and reduce the tension I've been feeling. I don't rely on the baths for much of my sex, but sometimes I have sex here."

AIDS PREVENTION

However well informed any person may be about the need for adopting more healthful behaviors, the real question remains as to whether people have actually changed their behavior. Everyone is familiar with the difficulty of quitting smoking, continuing a diet, or maintaining a regular schedule of exercise, despite advice from their doctors. Doctors themselves, of course, face the same struggles with behavior change. Such difficulties were frequently mentioned by bathhouse patrons who spoke of their efforts to adopt safe sex practices.

GROUP SEX/PUBLIC SEX

We have both been to the baths many times. Over the last several years, public and group sex were not unusual in the orgy rooms at most of the baths. On Lesbian/Gay Freedom Day in 1982 we remember going to the baths and seeing bodies of every description crowded together in the orgy room. It was dark enough to make discrimination practically impossible. Men were fucking, sucking, and exchanging partners frequently. Not all the bathhouse patrons were in the orgy room–some preferred more one-on-one contact–but those that were, eagerly observed or participated in the group activities.

Have things changed at the baths since then? Are the orgy rooms still busy? We chose busy nights with specials (e.g., "buddy night" and "$2 night") and the weekends to see what was happening now. We were surprised to find activity in the orgy rooms an extremely rare event; in fact, we only noticed one occasion during the eleven visits to baths that we undertook. Two baths still have open orgy rooms with beds (see Figure 2). But another has removed the mattresses. We frequently walked by the rooms, but they were always empty. We thought that perhaps there would be a spontaneous group jack-off, but there weren't any during the busy late evening hours.

During one visit, however, a single couple was in the orgy room. The room was well lit enough to see clearly. A man in his 40s was giving a massage to a younger man who was lying on his back on one of the lower bunk beds. It was probably more "erotic touching" than massage. The younger man had an erection. Checking back on the same scene 20 minutes later, the couple was still there. This time the older man was bending over and sucking on the young man's cock. There were four other men in the room, standing some distance apart. Virtually all of the sex in the room was solitary masturbation, very little activity "between individuals"–to use the phrase of Dr. Mervyn Silverman of the Department of Public Health. Things very seldom even made it to the "footsie" stage.

FIGURE 2. Matrix of Prevention Education by Bathhouse

BATHHOUSE	CONDOMS	SAFE SEX CARDS	SAFE SEX SIGNS AND BROCHURES	ORGY ROOMS	GLORY HOLES	AMENITIES
CLUB SAN FRANCISCO (ALSO KNOW AS RITCH STREET BATHS)	Not distributed upon registering, but available free for the taking from an open container located on the main counter inside the facility.	Not distributed, not available.	Prominent sign suggesting condom use plus brochures ("Can We Talk?") available outside at registration area, signs located throughout facility in prominent location (e.g.: top of stairways, end of hallway, and near shower rooms).	Open but well-lit bunk beds with mattresses; room seldom used.	Glory hole cubicles gone. Area now an open room without beds or anything else.	Full gym with Dyna-Cam equipment and free weights; gym instructor aerobic classes three evenings a week, feature movie one night each week, full snack bar, large screen TV room, large jacuzzi, sauna, steam room, large sun deck, video porno room, social area available for reading and talking, tasteful fresh flower arrangements, lockers and rooms, shower on two floors, disco music throughout.
CLUB BATHS (AKA 8TH AND HOWARD)	Not distributed at registration but one found in each room and allegedly in each locker. Extras available upon request; no difficulty encountered when receiving another.	Not distributed, not available.	Signs posted on each floor in noticeable areas and near showers. Brochures available near registration area.	Open with some beds but without any mattresses, dimly lit but not dark; not used by patrons.	Areas blocked off, no longer accessible.	Large hot pool in wood paneled room, large maze-like steam room, large porn video room, sex toy store, vending machines, large screen TV and viewing area, small sun deck, generally loud disco music, lockers and room.
ANIMALS	Given upon registration: extras available in open container at front counter.	Not distributed, not available.	"Play Safe" posters mounted throughout facility, with risk reduction brochures nearby in noticeable areas. Metal signs "Use Condoms," "Shower After Sex" posted.	Downstairs, bottom floor has open space with beds which might be used for sexual encounters, but none noticed during our visits.	No special area provided. Note: Animals is known primarily as a bathhouse for "fisting."	Steam room, video porno room with seating on mattresses, reading area on main floor, disk jockey, friendly and helpful owner working at registration desk, vending machines, lockers and room, several areas for sitting, along hallways floors need to be cleaned (indoor-outdoor carpeting that should have been put outdoors long ago).
THE SLOT	Not distributed upon registration but available upon request.	Not distributed, not available.	Poster displayed at top of stairs and on main floor, brochures available, metal signs "Use Condoms," "Shower After Sex" posted.	Two rooms at end of hallways on upper floors, each more darkly lit than hallways: each with beds and mattresses, patrons visited room frequently with some sexual activity ensuing.	No area provided. Note: The Slot serves those men who are especially interested in "fisting and bondage."	Reading/social area, porn video room, roof-top area (undeveloped) but with good view of city, vending machines, rooms and lockers, sign up blackboard for patrons to list their specialties and room numbers, (e.g., "fit play room 231," "vanilla sex - blank"); floors, walls, door handles need to be cleaned (sometimes cruising resembled sliding).

163

FIGURE 2 (continued)

BATHHOUSE	CONDOMS	SAFE SEX CARDS	SAFE SEX SIGNS AND BROCHURES	ORGY ROOMS	GLORY HOLES	AMENITIES
JACK'S	Not distributed at registration, but available upon request. However, the staff had to search to find them.	None available.	Poster prominently displayed, risk reduction brochures available.	None	None	Small sauna, small steam room, vending machines, room only (no lockers) wrap around sheet distributed as well as towel.
SAN FRANCISCO HEALTH CLUB (AKA THE "ELLIS BATHS")	None distributed; condoms must be purchased from vending machine inside facility for .35 cents each.	None available.	"You Can Have Fun and Be Safe Too" poster mounted on wall near entrance. One risk reduction brochure taped to wall, brochures not available for distribution.	None	None	Huge tiled sauna with comfortable chairs, steam room, small swimming pool but large enough for laps, regular size TV screen and viewing rooms, gym with Universal-type equipment, reading room, sun deck, rooms only (no lockers), wrap around sheet distributed as well as a towel.
TWENTY-FIRST STREET BATHS	One distributed at front door upon registering, others available upon request.	None available.	Poster prominently displayed just inside the entry door along with risk-reduction brochures. Metal signs "Use Condoms." "Shower After Sex" posted.	Former orgy room on main floor closed; upstairs open room now a porno video viewing area; lower level area near jacuzzi has several bunk beds with mattresses allowing for some sleeping and resting but with no sexual activity observed.	None available now, nor were there any in recent years.	Sun deck, steam room (very darkly lit) jacuzzi pool, video porn viewing room, lockers and rooms, social reading room (resembling a doctor's office waiting room).

AIDS Information and Risk Reduction: A Bathhouse Comparison

This is a comparison related to the encouragement of safe sexual practices at the gay bathhouses in San Francisco. The San Francisco AIDS Foundation staff have consulted with bathhouse owners for the last several months suggesting specific changes. The Foundation has also offered free of charge a number of education materials for each bathhouse facility. These include posters ("You Can Have Fun. ... And Be Safe, Too"), metal signs ("Shower Before and After Sex," "Use a Condom When You Play"), brochures ("Can We Talk?", "Risk Reduction Guidelines"), and wallet-size cards that list safe sex guidelines. The six measures used to compare each facility are the following:

(1) **Condoms:** distribution and availability of condoms. *
(2) **Safe Sex Cards:** availability and distribution of wallet-size cards with risk reduction guidelines.

(3) **Safe Sex Signs and Brochures:** whether signs and brochures are available, where the signs are posted.
(4) **Orgy Rooms:** whether a facility provides an orgy room, generally an open, dimly-lit area with or without beds where multiple contact, anonymous sex of varying degrees of risk might occur.
(5) **Glory Holes:** whether glory hole cubicles for generally anonymous cocksucking are available.
(6) **Amenities:** description of what other features or services--sexual and non-sexual--that a facility offers its patrons.

*All condoms distributed at all of the baths surveyed are Trojans in the orange packet.

The video rooms can be very erotic, with men jerking off while watching hot men on the screen fucking, sucking, whatever. Sometimes viewers will watch each other tantalizing each other with their hard cocks, beating off to a more immediate audience.

At times there was mutual masturbation. Once we noticed a man bold enough to sidle over to the man beside him and tentatively go down on his cock.

Men would come in and go out, sometimes to sit and take a break from walking the hallways, sometimes to cruise those in the room. When someone left the video room, he might be followed by another, hopeful for a contact.

A note about the video features themselves: Some bathhouse owners have suggested that they offer "safe sex" videos. A long-time tradition, certainly pre-dating AIDS, requires video sex partners to "cum outside" for the benefit of the viewing audiences. Because of this, there is frequently no exchange of bodily fluids, the mainstay recommendation for safe sex practices. But the same films may also feature higher risk activities, such as rimming, multiple partners without benefit of showering in between, and sometimes fisting.

Whatever the group sex scene in the baths may have been six or nine months, one or two years ago, we found that the baths have now become facilities almost exclusively devoted to individual or couple sexual activities.

INDIVIDUAL SEX/PRIVATE SEX

Sam was a cute redhead, about 5'6". I watched him go to his room, lean over to pull the key on its elastic cord away from his calf and over his foot, open the door, and enter. Soon the light in his room dimmed a bit, and I walked past his door. He was lying on his bed, propped against a pillow and looking out into the hallway. His towel was draped over one thigh and just covered his crotch. He said "hello" as I entered his room.

Sam and I talked a little before, and more after, some very energetic safe sex, mutual jerking off. Sam came to the baths "just to do something different," he said. His lover of five years had left earlier in the day for the Russian River.

Sam smiled and said, "Joseph's spending the weekend with his new boyfriend—an affair on the side."

"Did Joseph know that you were coming to the baths?" I inquired.

"Oh, yeah, I told him. He just said, 'Take condoms and be careful.' "
Sam and Joseph are new to the city, I learned. Until last July, they had lived in Houston.

"AIDS hadn't hit Houston very hard then. Since coming to San Francisco, we've been more careful. We don't have any more wild evenings of three-ways and we don't have risky sex. Now we both use rubbers when we have sex together. We also use them when we have sex with our boyfriends." [Sam has been seeing someone else as well.]

Bathhouse patrons are not necessarily regular customers. One man, Peter, said this was his first visit to any bathhouse in 5 ½ years and only his second visit in a total of 8 years. He also said he hadn't *any* sexually transmitted diseases for 11 years. So why was he at the baths this particular evening? Peter explained, "With all the controversy about the baths, it got me thinking about going to one. But most of all, I've got back problems and I wanted to use the jacuzzi here–this place has got the best one in town."

Whether patrons are regular visitors to the baths or not, almost every gay man we met and spoke with had developed his own standards for behavior. For example, one man was willing to suck a man's cock and to let his partner fuck him without using a condom. When questioned about the safety of this practice, he responded, "I said I'd let someone fuck me; I wouldn't let him cum inside me. I figure if I've decided a cock is clean enough to put in my mouth, it's clean enough to put up my ass." An observer judging his decision might question the wisdom of trusting a new partner's ability and willingness to fuck without cumming. He simply believed he was enough in control of the situation to be safe.

Another man, Charles, said he "loved to get screwed" but he wouldn't allow his partner to do so without wearing a rubber.

Both "safe sex" and higher risk sex occur in the baths. We noticed, however, a much higher proportion of safe sex. The standard precautions were mentioned over and over–no fucking without a condom, sucking but without cumming, no rimming. Our experience was that approximately 90% of the men with whom we talked had adopted these guidelines and observed them fairly consistently. Higher risk activities do occur, however. These include rimming, swallowing cum, fucking and being fucked without benefit of condoms, sharing lubricants. A few men had not established personal limits to risk. And some couples had not dealt with how AIDS affected their relationship.

I made a brief tour of the place and discovered only a few men. Coming around a corner, an attractive blond stepped into my path. I had seen him earlier in another corridor and had caught a flash from his soft, blue eyes. He put his hand boldly on my crotch, setting a stern gaze on my face. Before the scene developed any further, I invited him back to my room.

"What's your name?" I asked.

"Stan, and I'll bet you're just a little teddy bear." A small bead of sweat slid down his forehead. He was still flushed from a hot shower a few minutes before. We sat somewhat shyly together on the bed and looked at each other. Stan appeared to be healthy as well as clean, and I didn't object when he turned the light down a little.

We kissed, hugged, and massaged affectionately for about ten minutes before Stan started sucking my cock. My eyes were closed, but I felt his tongue move in ever-wider circles until he was under my balls and my legs were in the air. I flinched. "Can we have a break?"

"Why? You look OK to me," Stan said.

"Well, I'd just like to talk for a while."

"Not now!" Stan seemed kind of sad and reckless. He asked if I would fuck him.

"Do you have a condom?" I inquired.

"No, that's OK. I don't care with you. Besides I haven't been fucked in several months anyway. Be careful going in."

I stroked his anxious ass. "Do you want me to come inside you too?"

"Baby, you can do anything you want."

"Then let's just jack-off," I suggested.

Stan looked a bit confused, but the situation was still pretty hot and we found our erotic adventure underway in this new direction in no time. I gasped for breath in the last seconds before I came. Within moments, Stan's cock exploded on my leg and we collapsed into the bed. As we relaxed afterward and chatted, Stan's sadness became more apparent.

"You're very warm and open physically, maybe a little too much so," I said. "But I think you're holding back on some other level. Something's really bothering you, isn't it?"

He sat up to answer, and those clear blue eyes turned very thoughtful. "Yeah, well, I had a fight with my boyfriend. We haven't had sex for weeks."

For twenty minutes or so we talked about Stan's boyfriend, then the discussion went back to sex.

I wanted to know why he had been willing to rim me a short while before. "You know how dangerous it is. For you and your boyfriend."

"Yeah, but you look clean," he replied.

"That's bullshit. Haven't you read anything about safe sex?"

Stan said he'd read "Can We Talk" and the "Risk Reduction Guidelines" and that he kept up with the gay papers. "But I don't go out much anymore, not like I used to. And I don't go to the dangerous places you read about in the papers."

"What does your boyfriend think about what's OK?" I asked.

Stan replied, "We don't discuss sex outside the relationship. He'd never abide by what I say anyway."

"But if you're going out because the two of you aren't having sex together, then maybe he's going out too."

"You don't understand," Stan insisted. "My boyfriend would never admit it and doesn't want to know that I go out either."

I felt I was missing some crucial link in his logic, so I repeated what I thought I had been hearing.

"Because your boyfriend doesn't want to talk about sex outside the relationship, you can't set standards for yourself?"

Stan nodded and explained, "He just wouldn't listen."

I thought to myself, "We're talking about some serious denial." But, I responded, "For your own sake, at least set some standards for yourself and by all means find out what your boyfriend is doing. You could really be exposing yourself to a lot."

Stan said he would think about it.

Nonverbal communication plays a role in sexual interactions. A sensitive man can read the physical responses of another and will reassure a concerned partner about his intentions without making him feel self-conscious and without altering the sexual mood that has developed. Such assertiveness and responsiveness allows both men to relax and enjoy the moment.

Dominic presented a sight that I would tuck away in my memory for some time. I felt I was having sex just by looking at him.

He looked healthy, and all my senses told me he was clean. And his cock was erect. I teased myself by first nuzzling at his inner thighs and then sucking on his balls before filling my mouth with just part of his cock.

Dominic slid his hand between my legs, probing with an insistence that clearly indicated his desires. The potential for rimming was there and had to be resisted. I sensed that I had to be the one to set the limits

There was something uncertain about him; he was larger and stronger than me and had a dominant edge to him. I knew he could be force-

ful. Without sufficient rapport between us for me to feel comfortable, I told him, "I don't want to get fucked tonight."

Although disappointed, Dominic made it clear that he wanted to stay. He rolled me over on my stomach; I felt some steely inner tension, "Was I going to have to be forceful in my resistance?" I looked over my shoulder at him. He read the question on my face.

"It's OK. I just want to see your ass and lay on top of you."

In those few seconds, Dominic had departed from his own erotic image to connect with me. After that, I relaxed and felt OK. The limits were set; I could enjoy everything else that I realized was about to happen.

Alcohol and drug use may alter one's steadfastness in maintaining resolutions, certainly in adhering to safe sexual practices. We did not observe any illegal drug use during our several visits to the gay baths. Three patrons did say they were pretty "high." One mentioned marijuana; another, cocaine; and the third, "crystal," an amphetamine. No one indicated whether their drug use occurred inside the facility or outside previous to entry. A few men displayed and sometimes used bottles of "poppers" (nitrite inhalants). Poppers–which are legally available on the general market–were also sold in many of the bathhouses. Those facilities that did sell poppers also posted the city-mandated warning about nitrite use.

With only three examples of illicit drug use, there really isn't any conclusion for us to draw about effects on sexual behavior. Two of the three men maintained safe sexual behavior while the other was willing to participate in high-risk sexual activities.

There was no doubt in our minds at the conclusion of our visits that patrons of bathhouses had implemented limitations on their sexual behaviors. Self-esteem and caring friends were mentioned frequently as important elements for accepting personal standards. Those few who denied some of the responsibility for sexual conduct inevitably mentioned some other related problem areas in their lives.

It was quite apparent to us that sex remained a very important element in the lives of bathhouse patrons, one that they would not relinquish to external restrictions.

AMENITIES

While the bathhouses provide a place for sex for gay and bisexual men, other needs are met as well. One man told us, for example, that he and his lover of four years go to the baths three times a week for aerobic classes. "I also like to use the gym equipment there. The mirrors and just the whole atmosphere allow an erotic exercise program, too." He admitted, "Sometimes I'll go upstairs to look around and maybe have sex with someone; but if I don't, that's OK, too."

Another man in his 30s, Charles, goes to one bathhouse maybe once a month, but usually only if he doesn't have a boyfriend. "Sometimes I just want to be around other men and have a chance to touch and be touched. Those times when I'm feeling lonely and want to be affectionate . . . often I don't have sex at all." Charles explained further, "I was never one to go into the orgy rooms. I've always wanted to see who I was about to have sex with. I want to do it with someone I'm attracted to."

The evening I spoke with Charles, he said he had come to the baths "out of defiance . . . I'm angry that they're trying to close them. I thought I should come and *support* the business, a bit." Charles hadn't always felt so supportive of the baths. Several months ago he was busy with his graphic design work and had a boyfriend. "Then I didn't care as much about the baths. I wasn't even thinking of them," he remembered. When his relationship ended, however, the baths became an option for meeting other men, sometimes for having sex.

Randy has studied dancing for most of his life. A year ago he injured his knees in a fall and has undergone extensive therapy since. The accident was severe enough to prevent him from ever dancing again. He joked, "Well, this sounds like a standard line, but in my case it's true. The main reason I came here tonight was to use the jacuzzi. It really helps my knees, and I can relax here." Asked if he expected to have sex also, he replied, "Oh sure. Well, maybe, I'll have to wait and see who is here."

Since the baths have a rather timeless quality about them, I checked on the wall: it was 8 p.m. The 20 men in the aerobics class had just finished their final movements; several of them stepped into the gym and talked with a few of the five or six men there. A few joked about "checking out the upstairs," while others headed for the showers. The rest just visited, lingering awhile, as if in transition, coming off the exercise.

I continued to sit in the jacuzzi, trading a few glances with a middle-aged couple having a bite to eat in the restaurant area. I wondered what my roving colleague was doing across town in the baths that he was visiting. Later that evening he told me of one of his conversations in the facility's sauna:

"The temperature in the sauna was very hot. I saw a man reclining, reading the paper."

"May I have a section?" I asked.

"Sure, take what you want," he replied.

"This place is clean, the people seem friendly, and I love this sauna."

"Yeah, I've been coming here for twenty years," he said proudly. "It's the best place in the city. Quiet and relaxed. I like to get away from all the mess out on the street, so I bring myself here twice a week as a treat to myself. I can't afford to join one of those big fancy gyms."

"Well, I haven't been going to the baths much lately," I told him. "AIDS has made me a little nervous. But after the cops went in, I thought I'd come see for myself what's going on and maybe write about it."

The man frowned. "This AIDS is really a tragedy. I read about it all the time in the bar rags."

"How are the men responding to it? Are they aware of safe sex guidelines?"

"How could they not be? It's all over the gay papers."

He continued, "I don't have sex when I come here; oh, maybe, once every couple of months. But I like to look at the pretty boys. I got mugged about two months ago on my way home. That's what's really dangerous. And friends of mine drink themselves to death worrying. Sex—you have to decide for yourself what you can live with. I come here to be nice to myself."

PERSONAL CONCLUSIONS AND RECOMMENDATIONS

Our observations result from a combined total of some 45 hours spent in the six gay bathhouses in San Francisco. The activities and general environments we witnessed led us to draw several personal conclusions and recommendations.

Personal Conclusions

- For all the added amenities in several of the bathhouses–movies, TV, exercise classes, gyms–gay and bisexual men in San Francisco go to the baths primarily for sex and affection, or at least to be a participant in an erotic environment charged with male sexual energy. We found that bathhouse patrons participated in a broad range of sexual experiences, not all of which involved sexual acts.

- Most men do not limit their sexual activities to the current guidelines outlined by Dr. Mervyn Silverman, Director of Department of Public Health. (He has proposed a ban on sex "between individuals.") Most bathhouse patrons we talked with appear to have adopted the broader set of safe sex guidelines supported by the Bay Area Physicians for Human Rights and the San Francisco AIDS Foundation [see inset].
- Awareness of risk reduction guidelines, health concerns, and of AIDS was very high among bathgoers. It's difficult to imagine how the majority of men we talked with could be more informed about the basics, AIDS 101. The path to safe sex will be longer for some than for others, but every person with whom we spoke has taken at least the first tentative steps. Most have come a great distance already. The facts that a few could be better informed and that there are always visitors and newcomers to the city support the notion that AIDS education efforts should continue with the basic information while a newer focus about behavior change develops.
- While the bathhouse owners have no power to control private sexual activities, they can discourage high-risk behavior. Many have done so already. Some facilities no longer provide glory holes for anonymous cocksucking. Mattresses have been removed from beds in what was formerly the "orgy room" in one of the major bathhouses. We would suggest that the general consensus among gay men to reduce high-risk sex has as much to do with the disuse of orgy rooms as the removal of mattresses does.
- The fear that someone diagnosed with AIDS may go to the baths leads to easy scapegoating. Indeed, the person not yet diagnosed with AIDS may be a carrier of the AIDS agent; people who may never develop AIDS may be carriers; and for that matter, there is no medical evidence one way or the other as to whether people with AIDS can transmit the disease. That means everyone should recognize their own responsibility to themselves and to others. There is no reason, in our opinion, to restrict persons with AIDS from going to the baths as long as they share only in safe sexual activities. At the same time, someone with AIDS may be reluctant to put himself in some of the facilities that pursue hygiene less strenuously than others. If anyone has a compromised immune system,

he may wisely hesitate to expose himself to such things as possible fungal infections.

- Many have said that if only a gay man witnessed the physical effects that can be wrought by AIDS, then he would no longer go to the baths, or have high-risk sex, or have any sex; seeing the tragic effects of AIDS is a numbing and sobering experience that likely would lead to the curtailment or elimination of high-risk sex. But there's little reason to expect that a man would thereafter avoid gay sexual activities at the baths or anywhere else.

- Good health requires that we recognize and safely nurture our sexuality. Analogies of sexual activity to alcohol intake, cigarette smoking, or drug use are limited in their usefulness. Addiction to substances is not instinctual and is therefore clearly a matter of choice. The bathhouse patrons appeared not only to acknowledge but also affirm their needs for affection and sex.

Personal Recommendations

- Each bathhouse patron should recognize his responsibility for his own actions at all times. It is not safe to assume another's good health by mere visual observation over a brief period of time and thus discard any standards of conduct. A consistent set of personal standards makes it easier to enjoy yourself if you choose to go to the baths.

- In some cities in the country, for example Los Angeles, the local health departments conduct testing and treatment for STDs (Sexually Transmitted Diseases) on a regular basis at the bathhouses. San Francisco bathhouse owners should cooperate to bring these services to bathhouse patrons.

- Easy access to condoms should be encouraged at all facilities. The bathhouse with a container of rubbers on the registration counter–free for the taking without even having to ask for one–offered the best approach. Condoms should also be given directly to each patron upon registration. They might also be placed in the rooms and lockers.

- "Safe sex" cards should be distributed at registration. They serve as introductory reminders of safe behavior to the patrons. "Play Safe," "Shower Before and After Sex," and "Use Condoms" signs should be posted on all floors of buildings and should be placed near restroom and shower facilities.

- Bathhouse owners should supply one-time use lubricants–a small tube perhaps–to each patron at the door upon registration. Additional supplies should be available, like condoms, on a counter top. An individual's open jar of lubricant–used during several encounters and perhaps dipped into by both partners–can provide a good medium for germs to grow and spread.
- To specifically address the adoption of safe sexual practices, special behavior guidance counseling with profiles of personal health status should be available at the baths on a regular basis. This service is already provided at health centers in the community with the coordination of the San Francisco AIDS Health Project. An effective undertaking at the bathhouses will require the cooperation and commitment of the bath owners and staff as well as that of city health officials.
- Education efforts should acknowledge the needs and interests of gay couples. Some couples can rekindle mutual sexual interest by visiting erotic environments such as the baths, and "sex talk" about this should be encouraged. Other couples may need support to deal realistically with the possibility for sex outside a relationship. This can be a very threatening issue for the couples. The need exists for counseling on frank and constructive communication within relationships to arrive at mutually agreed-upon standards for outside sexual behavior.
- Education efforts should emphasize talking about sex and the details of sexual activities in explicit language understood by specific high-risk target groups. The taboo against discussing sex contributes not only to a diminished enjoyment of sex, but also to misunderstandings between partners, to a hesitancy to set safe practice limits, and to much self-deprecating guilt about one's natural desires and interests.
- The practice of fisting should be re-evaluated in light of the AIDS epidemic. [See sidebar.] Lesbians and gay men have a responsibility, in our opinion, to prevent any segment of our community–including those who engage in fisting–from becoming outcasts.
- Gay and lesbian businesses–especially the bars–should be more involved in efforts to educate the community about AIDS and STDs and to promote prevention methods. Bars could also distribute free condoms, one-time use lubricants, and safe sex wallet-size cards to their customers. Bar owners could use posters to advise their customers of the possible links between drinking alcohol and wavering commitments to safe sex behaviors.

Special AIDS prevention campaigns could be sponsored by the Golden Gate Business Association, the Tavern Guild, and individual businesses. In our opinion, it's time for business leaders to establish committees to develop specific plans for the full and active participation of every business that makes its money from the lesbian and gay community.

- The public discussion of the gay bathhouses, in our opinion, needs to be more frank and honest. The bathhouses are first and foremost sexual institutions, and sexuality needs to be recognized as the central issue of the debate.

Beyond the Baths:
The Other Sex Businesses

Michael Helquist
Rick Osmon

SUMMARY. After their successful review of the local bathhouses, Helquist and Osmon conducted another investigation, this time of other sex businesses in San Francisco, including sex clubs. Once again, these investigators approached their work systematically. Their article provides a thorough description of what was happening in the sex clubs and other sex businesses at that point in the AIDS epidemic. The original paper was published in the September 1984 edition of *Coming Up!* (pp. 19-24). As with all the reprinted papers in this volume, no editorial changes were made to the paper and only minor typographical errors were corrected.

KEYWORDS. AIDS, HIV prevention, sex clubs, sex businesses, history

"Sex and the Baths: A Not So-Secret Report" appeared in the July issue of *Coming Up!* and provided the first gay-identified look at the San Francisco bathhouses, and the changes they have undergone to cope with the AIDS crisis. This report focuses on the other gay sexual institutions in San Francisco. We hope to inform the public about the sexual activities that occur in these facilities, to reflect upon the role of these

This paper reprinted here by permission of the San Francisco *Bay Times*.

Correspondence may be addressed to Michael Helquist, 2088 Golden Gate Avenue, San Francisco, CA 94115 (E-mail: HelquistSF@aol.com).

[Haworth co-indexing entry note]: "Beyond the Baths: The Other Sex Businesses." Helquist, Michael, and Rick Osmon. Co-published simultaneously in *Journal of Homosexuality* (Harrington Park Press, an imprint of The Haworth Press, Inc.) Vol. 44, No. 3/4, 2003, pp. 177-201; and: *Gay Bathhouses and Public Health Policy* (ed: William J. Woods, and Diane Binson) Harrington Park Press, an imprint of The Haworth Press, Inc., 2003, pp. 177-201.

10.1300/J082v44n34_08

sexual institutions in the lives of gay and bisexual men, and to report on efforts taken by sex businesses to promote low-risk sex play among their customers.

In early August we visited eleven sex bookstores, four sex theaters, six clubs, and two safe sex social groups. Our research took us to the Tenderloin, Polk Street, South of Market, and the Castro. Most visits occurred during the evenings, but the all-day popularity of some businesses required daytime visits as well. Conversations with customers in bookstores and theaters were infrequent. Talking is not the rule in such facilities and we chose not to be intrusive.

As in the earlier article, "Beyond the Baths" includes graphic language, in the belief that sex institutions need to be talked about in sexual terms. We have again tried to capture the erotic aspect of these places without resorting to sensationalism. We decided to have sex ourselves in these sex facilities and felt our activities would provide greater insight into the nature of current behavior. We had already established our own individual standards for minimum risk in our sexual behavior.

We do not encourage or discourage men about their frequenting of these businesses and social groups. We do advise gay and bisexual men to inform themselves and adopt standards of risk reduction based on guidelines provided by the San Francisco AIDS Foundation.

AVERTED GLANCES

Located in a few of this city's neighborhoods—the Tenderloin, Polk Gulch, and South of Market mostly—are what might be considered the mainstays in the world of sexual businesses. They're known simply as "adult bookstores," but might better be called "sexual emporiums." In these storefronts are racks along the walls which often feature hundreds of gay and non-gay magazines and paperbacks. Titles as well as photos and stories are variations upon predictable themes of sexual enticement and sexual acts. Many of the gay magazines are glossy reproductions with very attractive, well built, often well-hung men engaged in various sex acts: jacking off alone or with others, sucking, fucking, rimming, or S&M adventures.

In display cases is a potpourri of what were once known as "marital aids" but are now directly called "sex toys." These include dildos of all shapes and sizes, cock rings, tit clamps, leather halters and restraints, inflatable dolls for sex play, condoms of all textures, lubricants, and "sensual lotions." Many bookstores now also carry the hottest commercial item, videocassette packs.

These businesses have managed to survive the years and years of police raids, political attacks from elected officials, crusades by church groups, and charges of sexism by many anti-pornography feminists. Although the cultural merits of the bookstores are frequently debated, the historical significance for many gay men has been considerable.

I hadn't been to one of these bookstores for years. My pursuits for sexual contacts had long since focused on the baths, the bars, sometimes the clubs, and most frequently in relationships, those lasting from several months to several years. I immediately remembered my first tentative forays into the "adult bookstores" of my hometown. They were located in the older downtown district areas that would be called "sleazy." For me at the time they were the true embodiment of dens of iniquities, and I was interested.

I never entered the bookstores of my youth for real sexual contacts. Just to be in there looking at magazines of nude muscle men posing in jock straps and less seemed a pretty bold sexual assertion on my part. I would be nervous, hoping to appear simply intent. I would leaf through one magazine and then another, always nonchalantly perusing the non-gay porn before "happening upon" the gay section. I was curious about the apparatus in the display cases. The dildos seemed self-explanatory, but my inexperience left me wondering about the other devices.

I would never look at anyone directly; most of the customers were much older men. I saw men go into the back room and I understood that movies in little booths were shown there. I also understood that I wasn't ready for that world of exploration. After a respectable time–or what I thought was allowable without getting accusations of loitering–I left the bookstore, nervously wondering if my parents just might be driving by outside.

Now many years later I was standing in a very similar bookstore again. This time I had walked directly to the gay section of the pornography. I realized how crucial a role these storefront operations had played in my initial "coming out"–not so much as a gay man, but mostly as a sexual person.

Most bookstores offer more than glossy magazines and sex toys. (See Figure 1.) Usually a back room features a video arcade with individual booths and screens for viewing selections of sex films. These, of course,

FIGURE 1. Matrix of Prevention Education by Eleven Bookstores

	FFA BOOKSTORE	FOLSOM STREET	ADONIS BOOKSTORE	TURK STREET NEWS	LOCKER ROOM BOOKSTORE	DISCOUNT BOOKS
CONDOMS AND LUBRICANTS	Various brands of condoms (mostly as novelty items) and lubricants for sale.	Various brands of condoms (mostly as novelty items) and lubricants for sale.	Various brands of condoms and lubricants for sale.	Various brands of condoms and lubricants for sale.	Available for sale at counter.	Condoms for sale mostly as novelty items. Lubricants for sale.
SAFESEX CARDS	None available or distributed.	None available or distributed.	None available or distributed.	None available or distributed.	Sometimes available on counter at entryway.	None.
SAFESEX SIGNS AND BROCHURES	None posted or available. One sign posted about the alleged danger implicit in recently proposed ballot measure to close the baths. One BAPHR poster advising on the adoption of safe sex practices.	None posted. "Can We Talk?" and Department of Public Health brochures at video arcade entrance.	None posted nor available.	None posted nor available.	Risk reduction brochures, including "Can We Talk?" available on counter. No "safe sex" signs of any kind posted in magazine and none in video arcade area	None.
ORGY ROOMS	None provided.	None provided.	None provided.	None provided.	None provided.	None.
GLORY HOLES	None. Video booth for individual use only.	Active area, with holes at various heights in back room. Video booths in back room. Holes large enough for sex and for viewing.	Active area, with holes at various heights between video booths in back of arcade. Very busy just after 5 pm on weekdays.	Active area with holes at various heights between video booths in back of arcade. Very busy just after end of workdays.	None provided.	Active area in video arcade.
AMENITIES	Discreet display of sex toys. Specific effort not to sell anti-woman sexual material. Very extensive library of videocassettes catalogued. Many gay and non-gay magazines and paper back books and also poppers for sale. Helpful friendly staff. Classical music played. Customers observed in friendly banter with man behind desk. A mutual respect communicated.	Many gay and non-gay magazines and paperbacks for sale; sex toys and poppers for sale. Can for donations to San Francisco AIDS Foundation on counter.	Many gay and non-gay magazines and paperback books for sale, video games. Sex toys and poppers for sale.	Many gay and non-gay magazines and paperback books for sale; sex toys, and poppers for sale. Video games.	Several hundred gay and non-gay magazines and paperbacks; large selection of video films to purchase; also available for sale are sex toys, inflatable "sex" dolls, dildos, lubricants.	Video games. Magazines, videocassette packs, and books for sale. Also poppers and sex toys.
GENERAL HYGIENE	Clean but well worn. No toilet or sinks available.	Floor in video booths dirty. Toilet and sink available with key from the front desk.	Smell of poppers in large video arcade area. Floor in video booths dirty. No toilet or sinks available.	Smell of poppers in large video arcade area. Floors in video booths dirty. No toilet or sinks available.	Magazine area brightly lit and clean. Video booths area generally clean. Bathroom very dirty; toilet, no sink.	Smell of urine in video arcade. Floor in booths dirty. No toilet or sinks available.

180

	GOLDEN GATE BOOKS	SPRINGMEADOW BOOKS	CITY BOOKS	PLEASURE PALACE	BEN-HER BOOKSTORE
CONDOMS AND LUBRICANTS	Condoms for sale, mostly as novelties. Lubricants for sale.	For sale.	Condoms for sale, mostly as novelty items. Lubricants for sale.	Condoms for sale, mostly as novelty items. Lubricants for sale.	Prominent display of various brands of condoms for sale.
SAFESEX CARDS	None.	Not available.	None available.	None available.	None available or distributed.
SAFESEX SIGNS AND BROCHURES	None.	None.	None.	None.	"Enjoy Sex" and "Play Safe" posters near entrance.
ORGY ROOMS	None.	None.	None.	None.	None provided.
GLORY HOLES	Video arcade area under construction.	Booths designed for individual use. Little sharing observed. One glory hole set up in back room that gave little privacy.	Between some of the video arcade booths. Active area. Blue haze lighting in arcade.	Between some of the video arcade booths. Active area. Blue haze lighting in arcade.	None provided.
AMENITIES	Many gay and non-gay magazines, videos, books, sex toys, poppers for sale. San Francisco AIDS Foundation donation can at counter.	Used magazines for sale, inexpensive. Many titles, videos, books, sex toys, poppers for sale. Chosen for these reporters' "Best Name" award.	Many gay and non-gay magazines, books and videos for sale. Sex toys and poppers for sale. Video games.	Many gay and non-gay magazines, books and videos for sale. Sex toys and poppers for sale. Video games.	Several 100 gay and non-gay magazines and paperback books for sale; stacks of dildos of all sizes and shapes for sale. Videocassette packs for sale.
GENERAL HYGIENE	Books and magazine areas clean; the rest under construction.	Relatively clean bathroom. No paper towels. Video booths remarkably clean.	Toilet and sink available. No paper towels. Not a particularly clean place. Sink very dirty.	Toilet and sink available. No paper towels. Not a particularly clean place. Sink very dirty.	Staff seemed indifferent to customers, but "regulars" elicited a friendlier response. Bookstore public area clean and brightly lit. Backroom area of video booths generally clean. Generally clean toilet available, no sinks provided.

These charts aren't meant to be a consumer's guide with observations about best sexual ambience or best quality video pornography. Instead they are a comparison related to the encouragement of safe sexual practices at some of the sexual facilities for gay and bisexual men in San Francisco.

The six measures used to compare each facility are the following:
1) CONDOMS AND LUBRICANTS: distribution and availability of condoms and lubricants. 2) SAFE SEX CARDS: availability and distribution of wallet-size cards with risk reduction guidelines. 3) SAFE SEX SIGNS AND BROCHURES: whether signs and brochures are available, where the signs are posted. 4) ORGY ROOMS: whether a facility provides an orgy room, generally an open, dimly-lit area with or without beds where multiple contact, anonymous sex or varying degrees of risk might occur. 5) GLORY HOLES: whether glory hole cubicles for generally anonymous cocksucking are available. 6) AMENITIES: description of what other features or services--sexual and non-sexual--that a facility offers its patrons. 7) GENERAL HYGIENE: the appearance and apparent cleanliness of the facility.

are available at a price, usually 25 cents. One arcade has a posting of rules for customers. These state that customers must keep moving at all times, stopping only to consider the films advertised on the door of any given booth. Once a customer enters a booth and closes the door, he must keep feeding the slot machine that regulates the movie clips. Management also warns customers against any "lewd behavior." What the rules advise and what many patrons seek are often two different things.

I step from the sidewalk and into the storefront, where I am met by a turnstile. There is no free admission. At the counter to my left, I give the clerk a dollar in exchange for four brass tokens. There are no words exchanged; he appears indifferent at best. One token to pass through the turnstile, and I look beyond the display cabinets with the stacks of dildos and beyond the magazine racks with the familiar titles, beyond these to the back room. At the entrance of the video booth area is a poster on the wall: "You Can Have Fun (And Be Safe, Too.)" That, I realize, is the only acknowledgement by the management that there's an epidemic in our midst.

It's darker in the back room, but my eyes readily adjust. Two dozen booths are lined up next to each other following the contour of the room. Two rows of booths form a corridor. Each booth has a TV size video screen with a slot for the tokens. The newer machines have a six-button selector for choosing which video clips you want to watch: man with man, two women with one man, man with woman, etc.

A dozen men walk about. This is a small space and there's a continual shifting of positions from walking a few steps to the end of the corridor, leaning against the wall, walking to a booth, and standing. The presence of most of the men outside the booths belie any thought that men come here just to watch the video clips and jack off alone. There's an avoidance of glances, and eye contact is uneasy. Connections are infrequent, but if a glance has been met and held, the next step will usually be for one man to walk into a booth, leaving the door open as an invitation.

I had been standing and walking about for a half hour. A short blond man wearing a tight navy blue sweatshirt and 501s stepped back into a booth—waiting. I was leaning against the wall across from him. We had exchanged glances earlier; now he nodded at me. I walked over and stepped into the booth. It was so small that we had to position ourselves in the corner to swing the door closed. It was then almost completely dark.

We stood close to each other. There was that familiar sexual charge of two men about to have sex. He felt for my crotch rubbing against my Levi's. He reached for my shirt buttons, undid them, and pulled aside my plaid shirt. He rubbed his palms against my chest as I began to massage his cock through his Levi's. He reached to the top button of my Levi's, loosened it and all the others to free my erect cock. He held it in his hand and began to jerk on it.

By now he had unbuttoned his Levi's as well and had pushed them to his ankles. Now I could reach and feel his ass as it contracted with the attention paid to his cock. He wanted to suck my cock and began to bend down. I caught his chin and interrupted his descent. He seemed a little surprised, but I touched his head gently and started jerking on his cock, now moist with pre-cum. He leaned back against the door and breathed heavily as I continued. He came with several moans, and then he kept my hand away from his cock; it had become so sensitive.

We relaxed and leaned against each other. He pulled up his Levi's. I re-buttoned my shirt. We hugged briefly, and he spoke the only two words that had passed between us, "Thank you."

For a great many men the bookstores continue to be an opportunity to explore their desires for sex with men; this is especially true for those who do not identify themselves as gay men. Wherever they are located in the city, nearly every bookstore provides both gay and non-gay magazines and books. Whatever the commercial reasons for this combination, it means that a man could frequent the bookstores without a challenge from others about his sexual orientation. With the gay and non-gay video clips in the backrooms, the same could be said about a man who is seen in the video arcades. For married men and for others who choose not to be open about their homosexuality, the bookstores provide a real outlet.

However busy the action outside the booths, there were some men who would go into a private booth alone (one without a gloryhole into the adjoining booth), close and lock the door, and watch several video clips by themselves. After perhaps ten or fifteen minutes the door would open and the man would walk out of the arcade area and out of the store. Some men do use the bookstores for solo masturbation with the stimulation of video pornography. For some men we suspect this is a convenience and a preference; for others there appears to be a likely issue of economics. Some customers clearly cannot afford to own an expensive video home recorder for their private viewing of video porn. Instead they can see some of the same features for a dollar at the bookstores or a few more dollars at the sex theatre. Bookstores are generally located in poorer areas of the city, and their customers are presumed to be less affluent men. The sexual activities at the bookstores are no different from those that occur elsewhere in town, yet public attitudes about lower economic status seem to prejudice notions about the quality of sex.

Before city officials, supervisors, medical doctors, and gay leaders rush to close sexual institutions, some thought might be given to the needs of that group of men who find that the bookstores, the theaters, and sometimes the baths provide their only opportunity to be in a sexual environment with other men. Due to the dictates of a culture clearly focused on youthful attractiveness, men who are older and who are less attractive frequently find themselves coping with very few sexual opportunities. Orgasm may not be their ultimate pursuit. Watching other men have sex, touching other men, and being even minimally affectionate can maintain and affirm one's own sexuality and positive self-image.

I paced the arcade. Around the corner several men loitered, keeping an eye on the moves of the others. Some were very attractive and others were not. I walked through a group of them and into a booth, shut the door and dropped a token in the slot. Al Parker started his sexual acrobatics on the screen. Doors on both sides of me opened and closed. I saw an older man through the viewing hole on my right and a corpulent man dressed like a banker on the left. Both peered through other holes to see what I was doing. Fingers appeared in the glory hole. I put my cock in the hand. In another second lips had encased it. I withdrew quickly. Not a safe gamesman, I thought. Soon his cock came through the hole. I grasped it lightly, stroking it as he stood next to porn star Casey Donovan on the screen in his booth. He came in a quick, strong climax, all the while the older man watched. I heard him gasp as he moved away from the peep hole, jerking himself off quietly next door. Video, fantasy, and voyeurism had created an intense erotic energy between us.

In short order the two men rearranged their disheveled clothes. The doors opened sharply, and they returned to the arcade lights. Both were satisfied and none the worse for wear.

AT THE MOVIES

What characterizes a sex business as a bookstore, a theater, or a club? The distinctions often blur. The Jaguar Bookstore, for example, is known as much for its two floors geared to sex play as it is for the selection of gay magazines for sale. The Circle J Club resembles a theater of sorts, with two small video screens. Savages offers a maze of glory holes, orgy rooms, full-screen films, and live performances: Granting the confusion over the categories, there are nevertheless a few businesses that do provide full length sexual features.

Generally the theaters provide a relatively sedate environment for customers to view sex films. The videos or films may play for 45 to 60 minutes each, with actors–mostly men in their 20s and 30s, usually white but sometimes Black or Hispanic–engaged in the usual repertoire of sex acts. During a visit to one of the largest theaters, twenty men sat apart from each other throughout the seating area. Some men cruised those nearby. Some jerked off during the screening of the "fuck films." The more restless and sexually ambitious men stood in the back of the theater cruising each other and members of the audience while keeping an eye on the screen. Eye contact would sometimes prompt one man to leave the theater area for more private space to await his prospective sex partner.

Patrons were of all ages, from early 20s through late 60s, and of all races. A number of men sat and watched the films and then left the building after they had seen enough. Restrictions against sexual activity would be irrelevant to these customers. Closure of the facility would effectively prevent them from watching films in the presence of other men, an activity that hasn't appeared on the risk reduction lists.

Many customers do engage in sexual activities at the theaters. All the facilities provide glory holes and orgy rooms. The owners and managers provide minimal, if any, educational messages about AIDS or risk reductions. Free condoms are provided by only a few businesses. The number of AIDS diagnoses in San Francisco continues to increase at an alarming rate, but for several sex business operators, promotion of AIDS prevention remains at ground zero. (See Figure 2.)

Some men do go to the theaters and get what they want: a sexual adventure, sometimes in the company of other men directly, sometimes from the feature film. In a few theaters eager audiences await the scheduled live entertainment: erotic male dancers.

I couldn't wait for the hot dancer I had heard about. It sounded like a different sexual experience. The theater had a crowd of about 30 men. The film showed the tedious acts of an amazingly un-friendly group of men. Behind the screen I discovered a hallway with glory hole booths on either side and a dark space at one end. Nothing was posted about hygiene or safe sex. Before I could explore any further, I heard the music begin for the dancer, and I rushed eagerly to find a seat.

The front row filled up first. The man on stage was nothing short of beautiful, with bronzed, smooth skin, and well-developed muscles. At first he wore a pair of gym shorts and a tank top. He began dancing to some Bolero-type music while rubbing chest and stomach and crotch. He teasingly lifted his shirt upon his chest while flexing his pecs and then he pulled it over his head and threw it to the floor. His skin was shining with sweat, in the bright lights. He began to tease the audience even more as he turned his back and lowered his shorts over his ass. When he faced the expectant audience again, I could see that he was hung like a little donkey.

Within a few minutes everyone in the first two or three rows was masturbating with eyes focused on the glistening, gyrating dancer. He strode up and down the stage, stopping to pose or stretch for dramatic effect. Standing to one side his profile revealed a lean, taut body and a jutting hard-on. He slowly stroked his cock to work the audience into a frenzy. At the climax of the show, three men in the first row came while the others cheered. After a few minutes the lights went down, several men filed out, and the same tired film played again.

I returned to the hallway behind the screen and went to find out what was going on in the dark space at the end. Upon entering, half a dozen hands approached me from several directions. Unable to see where they were coming from, but sure where they were headed, I backed out of the room. A large naked man fairly covered with lubricant got me in his grasp. I slipped through his greasy fingers and hurried to wash up in the restroom, the only clean place in the theater besides the lobby.

Determined to know what happened in the dark room, I walked back and entered aggressively and defiantly. I kept the hands at bay long enough to realize that there was a lot of sucking and jacking off going on. A passageway connected one dark space with another. Each led to non-discriminating hands and mouths. My pants had been unbuttoned and pulled to the floor within 30 seconds, despite resistance on my part. I escaped un-compromised, but flustered.

One man followed me out, pressed his card into my hand, and told me he'd love to be my boyfriend. I graciously accepted his phone number and said perhaps I'd meet him again at the theater. I moved out to the area in front of the screen and pulled my pants and my thoughts together.

BUSINESS AND RESPONSIBILITY

The city's gay and bisexual men continue to support businesses that pay little attention to the role they might play in encouraging safe sexual behavior. And the city licenses these businesses without stipulations for posting even the most basic risk reduction guidelines.

FIGURE 2. Matrix of Prevention Education by Four Sex Theaters

	CENTURY THEATRE	TEA ROOM THEATER	NOB HILL THEATER	SAVAGES
CONDOMS AND LUBRICANTS	None available.	Condoms available free upon request; lubricants for sale.	Neither available.	Free condoms upon request. Lubricants for sale.
SAFESEX CARDS	None available.	None available.	None available.	None available.
SAFESEX SIGNS AND BROCHURES	"Can We Talk?", and BAPHR's "Note to a Hunk" available in upstairs lounge area. Large wall size bulletin board downstairs with only one small notice on it--about Kevin Collins, the young San Francisco boy missing since February.	Safe sex signs posted. No hygiene-related signs. Warning at entrance that anyone squeamish about gay sexuality the Tea Room is not a good place to visit. No brochures.	No signs posted; no brochures available.	Safe sex signs posted; risk reduction brochures available.
ORGY ROOMS	Former orgy room completely closed off.	Two large orgy rooms, both very dark and very busy in the evening. Primary activities appeared to be jack-off and sucking. Too dark to see very well. Then management shows a video warning against pickpockets but nothing about safe sex.	Orgy rooms with linking passageway. Very darkly lit and fairly busy in the evening. Primary activities appeared to be sucking and jack-off.	(See Glory Holes)
GLORY HOLES	Dimly-lit glory hole area downstairs with ten or so cubicles.	Provided in the orgy room, boarded up in the restrooms.	Booths and stalls with glory holes. Fairly active. Empty liquor bottle found in one booth.	Placed in a complicated maze of doors, passages and booths. Reminds one of an Alfred Hitchcock film. Maze is poorly lit, patrons are unable to give their partners an adequate once over.
AMENITIES	Full-sized theater with large screen, good quality film and video prints. Lounge area upstairs with couch, chair, and coffee table. Snack bar available; staff courteous entryway, pleasant surroundings.	Sex toys and poppers for sale. Poems and prose about sensuality, sexuality and freedom in beautiful calligraphy posted in area behind the screen, quotes from Kierkegaard, Whitman, D.H. Lawrence and others.	Magazines and videos for sale. Erotic male dancers perform at scheduled times. Generally good quality film and video prints. Staff indifferent.	Erotic dancers scheduled twice a day, theater, social area in basement. A few private rooms, lockers, vending machines; a desk furnished with paper in a drawer--perhaps in case you get bored and want to write home.
GENERAL HYGIENE	Theater very clean throughout. Very clean bathroom upstairs and downstairs with sinks, toilets, and urinals. Carpeting and walls clean.	Two sinks and two toilets, one of which was filled up with paper towels. Both areas as clean as your worst experience in a gas station lavatory.	Bathroom facility some distance from orgy room. No papers towels provided, but there is an air dryer--not designed for adequate clean up. Bathrooms clean, orgy rooms not so clean.	The entire facility seemed clean throughout. Toilets and sinks available, but no shower.

The six measures used to compare each facility are the following:
1) CONDOMS AND LUBRICANTS: distribution and availability of condoms and lubricants. 2) SAFE SEX CARDS: availability and distribution of wallet-size cards with risk reduction guidelines. 3) SAFE SEX SIGNS AND BROCHURES: whether signs and brochures are available, where the signs are posted. 4) ORGY ROOMS: whether a facility provides an orgy room, generally an open, dimly-lit area with or without beds where multiple contact, anonymous sex of varying degrees of risk might occur. 5) GLORY HOLES: whether glory hole cubicles for generally anonymous cocksucking are available. 6) AMENITIES: description of what other features or services--sexual and non-sexual--that a facility offers its patrons. 7) GENERAL HYGIENE: the appearance and apparent cleanliness of the facility.

Businesses, their owners and managers, have sole discretion over whether or not to post AIDS awareness and risk reduction guidelines, whether to provide hygiene facilities, or whether to clean the premises. Some are clearly more enlightened than others. One sex club advertises to gay men that it is a club intended solely for jack-off sessions. Another club has signs posted throughout the premises offering free condoms. And yet another posts "Shower After Sex" and "Use Condoms When You Play" signs near sexplay rooms.

There are also bookstores that offer glory holes between video arcade booths, and yet there are no signs that relate to AIDS. Frequently, warnings about pickpockets are the only risk reductions suggested. One major theater that prides itself on its high quality prints and clean premises, had but a few "Can We Talk?" brochures on an upstairs coffee table, unnoticed by the majority of customers. This same business provides a clean bathroom, a dozen dimly-lit glory hole booths, and a very large bulletin board downstairs below the main theater floor. The only thing on the bulletin board was an 8½ × 14 flyer offering a reward for information about Kevin Collins, the San Francisco boy missing since February. To their credit, the management had blocked off a former orgy room.

Bookstore owners might counter that their businesses offer sex toys, magazines, and video booths for individual viewing with possible solo masturbation. One visit to the arcade would expose this pretension. The dozen or so men in any video arcade are not lined up waiting to watch a particularly popular video clip. The majority of the booths are empty at any one time. Most men are there for sex; they wait outside the booths for likely sex partners.

Based on our visits it would be inaccurate to say that *nothing* is being done to discourage high-risk activities. Changes have been made without government intervention, although the *threat* of action may have been a factor. Several business operators have closed orgy rooms, hosted risk reduction forums, increased lighting, promoted safe sex in their advertising, provided free condoms, distributed brochures, and posted safe sex signs. (See Figure 3.)

The variety of these responses parallels the different degrees of change gay customers have made in their sexual behavior.

The attendant checked my card number against those of the members who had already signed in. He handed me a condom, winked, and buzzed me inside. I gave my coat and beer to the hunky man smiling on the other side of the bar. A number of men sat on the barstools or stood chatting quietly by a counter against the back walls. It seemed to be a very friendly place. I noticed that one-time-use lubricants and poppers were available for purchase. There were several signs and posters encouraging safe sex practices.

Rumor had it that the bathtubs had been removed and that there was no longer any watersports action. What was I going to do with my rubber ducky? I first walked to the area where the tubs had once been. The room was pitch black and I could not tell if anyone else was even in there with me. I felt around, blindly and discovered that the tubs were indeed gone. On several later visits to this room I found only a couple of men there. It seemed to be one of the only areas on the premises where one could enjoy privacy with a partner. Men didn't stand around watching in these rooms, because they couldn't see anything.

One room in the back had been blocked off, I stepped gingerly up the back stairs. A bench at the top was a great place to watch the flow of traffic, but I'm always too impatient to see what's happening to wait around just watching others walk by. I walked slowly through the halls and rooms. Three of the rooms were unfurnished and were dimly lit. Each had a dark closet. Another had bunk beds without mattresses and one more was very dark with a couple of stalls that functioned more as partitions.

On my journeys I passed a tall, intriguing man several times. We exchanged glances and sexual energy in the bright hallway. I don't know who followed whom into a side room, but we retired to a small closet to avoid the eyes of others.

We hugged, rubbed, squeezed, twisted and groped. The heat in his hands grew more intense as he felt my cock harden. I pulled his dick out of his pants. We pulled and jerked, all the while feeling the warmth and intimacy of each other's touch. Then a certain shyness came over me, and I began to wonder what he wanted. I moved to leave, but the big man would have none of that. He wanted to play with me and he wanted to play safe. His actions made that very clear.

His arms became a comfortable, secure refuge. I leaned against his broad torso while his anxious hands brought me to a spirited orgasm. He held me tightly for several minutes longer as I relaxed and recovered from my dreamlike state. We parted with a generous hug.

I walked into the bathroom and up to the toilet and pissed. A man who had been sitting there all evening knelt before me and tried to intercept my stream of urine. I stopped and left for the bathroom downstairs.

The above scenario illustrates the dynamic of a business that actually encourages risk reduction in some ways (free condoms, numerous signs and brochures), but not in others (very dark orgy rooms), and customers who insist on safe sex and those who continue with very high-risk behavior.

FIGURE 3. Matrix of Prevention Education by Six Clubs

	THE ACADEMY	THE BOOT CAMP CLUB	1808 CLUB	CIRCLE J	JAGUAR BOOKSTORE	THE SLOT
CONDOMS AND LUBRICANT	Condoms sometimes given upon entry, available upon request. Lubricants available for purchase.	Condoms distributed free upon entry. Available for the asking afterwards. Lubricant for sale.	Available free upon request. Free lubricant available in open containers shared by others.	Available for sale at registration window.	Several brands for sale only.	Not distributed upon registration, but available upon request.
SAFE SEX CARDS	Available on counter before entry.	None available.	No Cards available.	None	Available on counter.	Not distributed and not available.
SAFE SEX SIGNS AND BROCHURES	Numerous posters and signs—both those distributed by SF AIDS Foundation and the club's own which prohibit drug use, sleeping, and watersports. Also posted are several "Free condom" signs. Perhaps the most numerous were the "watch your wallets" signs. Risk reduction brochures available.	Safe sex signs posted in several areas. "Can We Talk?" brochures accessible and prominently displayed.	Signs not noticed, but facility advertises itself as a jack-off club.	"Play Safe" poster as well as one about Hepatitis B posted in main entryway.	"Can We Talk?" and other risk reduction brochures available on counters. "You Can Have Fun" poster on stairwell leading to upstairs rooms. Several signs posted upstairs advising "Use Condoms" and "Shower After Sex"	Poster displayed at top of stairs and on main floor, brochures available, metal signs "Use Condoms," "Shower After Sex" posted.
ORGY ROOMS	Moderately, but not adequately lit. Also several private room areas in basement.	Several moderately to very dark rooms for sex. Very little fucking going on but a lot of cocksucking. Discretion nearly impossible in such dimly lit areas. Many men spend some time in better lit area observing others before following someone into the darker space. No place to lie down comfortably.	The entire facility is a fairly well-lit area for socializing and primarily for jack-off. Advertises itself as a jack-off club. Some sucking observed, but less than 20% of the activity. Fucking observed but only between a pair of lovers who did not include others.	No specific area provided.	Several public rooms available: one with mirrors, one lit only by a bare red light bulb; two others upstairs, one very dark with bunk beds. Maze-like area very dark downstairs. No longer a sling in one of the rooms upstairs.	Two rooms at end of hallways on upper floors, each more darkly lit than hallways, each with beds and mattresses. Patrons visited rooms frequently with some sexual activity ensuing.

	THE ACADEMY	THE BOOT CAMP CLUB	1808 CLUB	CIRCLE J	JAGUAR BOOKSTORE	THE SLOT
GLORY HOLES	About ten glory hole cubicles, generally a busy area. Designed for sucking and for watching through the large holes. Not adequately lit to see partners well.	Only a few glory holes which were not being used during our visits. Upstairs toilets controlled by a very few water sports aficionados. Bathtubs removed.	None.	None.	A few cubicles in maze area are equipped with glory holes.	No area provided. Note: The Slot serves those men who are especially interested in listing and bondage.
AMENITIES	Video room with carpeted, terraced viewing area. Pool table. Friendly, social area with seating; also a bar that served bring-your-own-beer and coffee. Friendly staff. Jacket, clothes check. Poppers for sale. Gay newspapers available. Community bulletin board.	Large areas to sit and socialize. Friendly crowd in bar area. Free coat and clothes check. Bring your own beer. Soft drinks and coffee available. Community newspapers, bulletin boards. Helpful, accommodating staff, even when very busy. Video films at bar.	Free clothes check. Friendly social area with seating available, also a bar. Friendly staff. Adequate and pleasant lighting. Friendly staff. A clear message from the management that encourages safe sex activities.	Friendly attendant during evening. Copies of local gay papers available. Three small video screens, two playing in the same room. Paperback books for sale. Coffee available. Businessman's matinee special at reduced rates during weekdays, noon to 3pm.	Bookstore area out front offers a large selection of magazines and paperback books. Also a large selection of sex toys, dildos, tit clamps, condoms, lubricants, and video cassettes for sale. Gay newspapers available, sometimes community notices are posted. Video viewing room carpeted and tiered for seating. Snacks/beverages, sundries for sale at upstairs juice bar.	Reading/social area, porno video room, rooftop area (undeveloped) but with good view of city, vending machines, rooms and lockers, sign-up blackboard for patrons to list their specialties and room numbers, e.g., tit play--room 231. "Vanilla sex--blank") Generally friendly staff.
GENERAL HYGIENE	Facility very clean throughout. Sinks, toilets and shower available upstairs and downstairs; both clean.	Two clean restrooms without privacy. No showers. Sinks could have been more accessible for cleaning up. Other areas relatively clean.	Restrooms are clean but could be better equipped for cleaning up. Facility generally very clean.	The bathroom floor, sink and toilets were not clean. The carpeting is worn and dirty. The cushions used for seats in the video room had little appearance of being clean.	Bookstore area very clean. Downstairs area of open rooms and maze had an unpleasant odor. Upstairs video room and orgy rooms clean. Upstairs shower, hallway sink, and toilets very clean. Cleaning facilities also available downstairs.	Floors, walls, door handles need to be cleaned (sometimes cruising resembled sliding). A few patrons mentioned that they wished the facility were cleaner.

The six measures used to compare each facility are the following:
1) CONDOMS AND LUBRICANTS: distribution and availability of condoms and lubricants. 2) SAFE SEX CARDS: availability and distribution of wallet-size cards with risk reduction guidelines. 3) SAFE SEX SIGNS AND BROCHURES: whether signs and brochures are available, where the signs are posted. 4) ORGY ROOMS: whether a facility provides an orgy room, generally an open, dimly-lit area with or without beds where multiple contact, anonymous sex of varying degrees of risk might occur. 5) GLORY HOLES: whether glory hole cubicles for generally anonymous cocksucking are available. 6) AMENITIES: description of what other features or services--sexual and non-sexual--that a facility offers its patrons. 7) GENERAL HYGIENE: the appearance and apparent cleanliness of the facility.

Mervyn Silverman of the Department of Public Health has suggested a perspective for analysis of the varying responses to the threat of AIDS. Silverman has frequently lauded the gay community for their major changes in sexual behavior. To city supervisors on August 9th, Silverman said, "It is clear that most members of the gay community have been going to safe sex procedures. The community has responded incredibly." At the same time, Silverman has faced what any proponent of behavior change must acknowledge: for whatever reason some people do not adopt the changes. In a published interview with Stephen Morin, a San Francisco psychologist, the DPH director observed, " . . . no matter what you do or tell them, no matter what, they will not change what they're doing and will continue to maintain a lifestyle at risk . . . It's like with chronic smokers. They know all the problems, and they keep smoking."

NOT SO SERIOUS

It's happening all across the country, and San Francisco has its own versions. The subject is jack-off clubs, and the largest such group is San Francisco JACKS. The club's recent monthly newsletter describes its purpose succinctly:

> The SF JACKS is a meeting of men who wish their primary sexual outlet to be masturbation in the company of other like-minded men. One of the hottest aspects of our club is the mutuality of interest that prevails. Proud as we may be of our club, it is incumbent on us all to discourage visitors whose interest arises merely out of curiosity. If a member or a guest cannot be fully satisfied by j/o alone, then the SF JACKS is not the club for him. Checking of all clothes except shoes is mandatory. The use of poppers is strongly discouraged, but creativity, whim, and non-rule breaking kink during sex play are to be applauded.

There's a quantum leap in ambience, spirit and enthusiasm from the averted glances and nonverbal sex of the bookstores/arcades/glory holes to a roomful of naked men talking and joking with each other, mixing their sex play with their visits.

The SF JACKS and the 5H CLUB, the other major group, are social organizations rather than facilities. Some members would claim that these clubs are really a state of mind. (See Figure 4.)

FIGURE 4. Matrix of Prevention Education by Two Safe Sex Social Clubs

	5H Club (meets weekly at The Academy)	San Francisco Jacks (meets weekly at different clubs and other locations)
CONDOMS AND LUBRICANT	None provided upon entry but available upon request. Stipulation for 5H membership is agreement to engage in jack-off only.	None provided, but stipulation for JACKS membership is agreement to engage in jack-off only.
SAFE SEX CARDS	Provided on counter at door.	None provided but see above.
SAFE SEX SIGNS AND BROCHURES	See section for the Academy.	Depends on where club meets.
ORGY ROOMS	Large, well-lit public room used for individual and group jack-off, rubbing and frottage.	None applicable.
GLORY HOLES	Not applicable; area closed off during club meetings.	None applicable.
AMENITIES	Friendly spirit of camaraderie, welcoming to newcomers, but with some suggestion that applicants be suitable for the city's "premier j/o club." Provides wine, soft drinks, and coffee, plus lubricants and clean-up towels as part of admission price. Free clothes check. Members can stay late for time when regular Academy hours begin. Very sex-positive attitude among club members.	Friendly spirit of camaraderie welcoming to newcomers. Provides beer and soft drinks plus lubricants and clean-up towels as part of admission price. Free clothes check. Sends out weekly newsletter. Very sex-positive attitude among club members.
GENERAL HYGIENE	Lubricants provided in large open containers but used only for jack-off. Members required to wear shoes. Toilet and sink available but no shower. For more information, see section on The Academy.	Depends upon where club meets. But locations are generally clean. Lubricants provided in large, open containers for all to share but used only for jack-off. Members are required to wear shoes.

The six measures used to compare each facility are the following:
1) CONDOMS AND LUBRICANTS: distribution and availability of condoms and lubricants. 2) SAFE SEX CARDS: availability and distribution of wallet-size cards with risk reduction guidelines. 3) SAFE SEX SIGNS AND BROCHURES: whether signs and brochures are available, where the signs are posted. 4) ORGY ROOMS: whether a facility provides an orgy room, generally an open, dimly-lit area with or without beds where multiple contact, anonymous sex of varying degrees of risk might occur. 5) GLORY HOLES: whether glory hole cubicles for generally anonymous cocksucking are available. 6) AMENITIES: description of what other features or services--sexual and non-sexual--that a facility offers its patrons. 7) GENERAL HYGIENE: the appearance and apparent cleanliness of the facility.

A phrase that appears to have settled on the early 80's is "sex-positive." In our opinion the activities that occur in the jack-off parties provide a good example.

The weekly meeting was already underway by the time I entered the rustic barroom. I paid my $5 at the front window and was buzzed through the door. Before me were about 80 men, nearly all naked, except for socks and shoes, Adidas and Nikes. "This could be a gay nudist colony," I thought. Men were standing at the bar, drinking beer or Calistoga, talking freely. Others were walking about visiting, as well as checking each other out.

I walked to the back of the bar, was given a paper sack and a number on a piece of paper. This was the basic clothes check--all clothes went into the sack which was also numbered. I returned to the front room, went to the bar, and asked for a bottle of beer--complimentary with the price of admission. I was a little nervous; I didn't see anyone I knew, and momentarily thought I might be more nervous if I did see a familiar face–or body.

The easy friendliness of the group had a relaxing effect. The mood was positive and upbeat. I felt a consensus asserting pleasure to be gay men enjoying each other's social and sexual company.

Men of all sizes and shapes were there; ages probably ranged from early 20's to late 50's. There were a good number of very handsome men with well-defined muscles and features. But not everyone had just come from the gym.

I couldn't distinguish any one particular type, and that made the atmosphere even more comfortable.

I had been told that tonight was going to be a "theme night." With East Indian instrumental music playing and with several men partly dressed with Native American headdresses, loincloths, cloth bands, and feathers, I was somewhat uncertain of the geographical or cultural focus of the theme. But when I saw one very attractive man walking about with antlers on his head, I sensed that this was a "Primal" night with faerie/earthspirit/Druid influence. The whole evening I never quite managed to "get the spirit" but others enjoyed the possibilities of mixing fantasy with their sex play. The room, in fact, was bristling with high and hot sexual energy. It didn't take long for things to get down to business.

When Dr. Mervyn Silverman, director of the Department of Public Health, held his news conference in April and issued his proposed ban on "sex between individuals," some of the nongay media people snickered at the tortured phrase. One TV reporter commented, "So what's he want, 'sex between groups'?" The sex play that occurs at jack-off clubs sometimes meets Silverman's restrictions, but most often not. Usually the action is among individuals; and frequently it just might appear as sex between groups.

The nature of the action in jack-off clubs is one of "hot spots," spontaneous combustions that ignite between two men who are joined by others who, in turn, attract several more, all drawn together by the desire to be in the midst of hot sexual action. Such a hot spot was about to form when I entered one of the club's side rooms.

Two men had gone into the empty room together. Both naked, they sat close together on a bench, looking at each other's erect cock. Both cocks were jutting out several inches beyond average, one already had a little fluid gleaming at the tip. One man was blond, the other dark;

both very attractive. The blond reached over and started pumping his companion's cock. He followed this by leaning over and flicking his tongue against the man's extended right tit. Both actions elicited groans as the dark man leaned his head back against the wall. Two men joined the scene, just watching at first, pumping on their own cocks. One tentatively reached to touch the blonde's unattended cock. After a moment of silent permission, he began to pay more active attention to it. The other newcomer stepped over and gently slapped his own hard cock against the cheek of the dark man. The scene was getting very hot. Within minutes there were eight men in the room, and then there were a dozen all standing close together facing the two on the bench. Quickly the variations of body contact became too numerous to think of the group as anything less than an erotic energy force of male sexuality. The peak moment came when both the blond and his darker friend climaxed together, spurting cum on each other's thighs.

What is the risk involved among participants of these jack-off events? One gay doctor has suggested that mutual jack-off is not absolutely safe because a man may have a hangnail on his toe and some cum might splatter on it, constituting an "exchange of bodily fluids." With an illness as serious as AIDS, extensive precautions are clearly in order. However, some commentators have placed such a narrow perspective on AIDS risk reduction, that they have begun to advise that "if only one life is saved, then any action is worthwhile." This reasoning has most recently been applied to bathhouse closure. It will be a very long time before the incidence of AIDS fatalities nears the terrible toll taken on the nation's freeways, and yet no one would suggest that the highways be closed. Without anxiously gazing at toenails, the intent of the doctor's advice appears to be an awareness of any open cuts on the body's surface.

We consistently found that gay and bisexual men in the city continue to grapple with behavior changes required by the AIDS epidemic.

The young man in the white T-shirt put an aggressive grip on my cock as I took hold of his. For a few minutes we played, squeezing and stroking the slick, hard dicks. He was uncut and had a natural sheath for rubbing up and down. He jerked me with great relish and skill. We were right on the verge of popping when instinctively our hands dropped, not a moment too soon. Neither of us had been there more than ten minutes, and we had the whole evening ahead of us.

We separated, but a few minutes later I saw him sitting alone on a couch in the lounge area. I moseyed over rather nonchalantly and plopped myself down.

"Come here often?" I asked.

"I beg your pardon," he re replied in a funny accent. He cocked his head forward and screwed up his face.

"I just wanted to know if this is a place you frequent." Then I told him my name, and we shook hands.

"Well, mine's Richard. I came here last night, but I've only been in San Francisco two days. I'm visiting from England."

He had been to half a dozen major American cities, and this was his last stop before returning to Liverpool. He was having a terrible time, he said; he thought he would go home a week early.

Richard had ruffled the feathers of my civic pride. How could anyone want to leave this city? Much less to return to Liverpool?

"What don't you like about San Francisco?"

The sole concern of Richard's visit was men. He didn't care to see museums, parks, theaters, or anything except bars, baths, and clubs. He went to South of Market during British pub hours, 7 to 9 pm. Richard wanted to know if it was always so quiet. I explained that Folsom doesn't get busy until after 10 pm and usually later. His ignorance of proper timing made San Francisco seem like a ghost town. I gave him some suggestions about when to go to different places and advised that the sex scene had calmed down considerably over the last couple of years.

Richard looked around rather nervously. "My friends think I'm crazy to come to America. The pubs in England have these 'safe sex' posters too. They say, 'Don't sleep with an American or anyone who's been to America in the last two years.'"

"That seems a little harsh."

"It's true. If I go home with somebody here and he doesn't ask me to use a rubber, I just leave. I know the guy would use one if I asked, but I want to find out what his habits are. They're not safe as far as I'm concerned if he doesn't suggest it himself."

"So you won't fuck here without a condom. What about in Liverpool?"

"I think things could change in England too. But I know men will be afraid to sleep with me when they find out where I've been."

"What do you think of the club?"

"I'm feeling very comfortable here. All these naked men running around, beating off together. It's hot and I feel safe here. You'd never see anything like this in England. Everyone there expects you to fuck.

There aren't many AIDS cases. No one uses rubbers and they'd get really insulted if you wanted to use one. The men there would have a really hard time changing."

Richard and I talked for awhile longer about things to see and do in the city and about having good, safe sex. We connected again later in the evening while standing in an excited group clustered to one side of the main room. Richard gasped as he pumped his cock, screamed in ecstasy, and collapsed into my arms. Happy to be together again, we sat down and just held on for a few minutes. Later, I drove Richard back to his hotel.

The men at the jack-off clubs say they have found a means of healthy sexual expression to help them live through these difficult times. One man, a recent arrival from the East Coast, explained that he used the club meetings as an opportunity to meet new friends as well as to enjoy safe sex.

"T.S.," an enthusiastic member of SF JACKS submitted the following letter to the club's March newsletter: "The JACKS have literally saved my sex life . . . I have been enriched by attending JACKS. I have learned much about the giving and cooperative nature of gay men, about freedom; I have experienced complete letting go, blending hot sex and happiness."

FUTURE DIRECTIONS

Most of the sex action observed in the clubs, theaters, and bookstores involved enthusiastic variations of mutual masturbation and cocksucking. While there were a few incidents of fisting and fucking and some preparations for bondage and watersports, gay men who frequent these businesses appear to have narrowed their sex play to jacking off and sucking cock. While the former is thought to bring very minimal risk, the latter, cocksucking, still poses a challenge to men trying to change their behavior and to educators trying to encourage that change.

The darkened orgy rooms and glory holes offer a sense of mystery, intrigue, and a flush of excitement. Some men seek sex in these environments for the thrill of it; others welcome the anonymity and privacy that darkness provides. Our observations indicate that activities in these places have changed dramatically already. Not only does the current turnabout in sex behavior pose fewer risks, it potentially prompts a greater acceptance of shared sexuality with other men.

As 2 am drew near, more and more men filed into the club. Many of them had just left the closing bars. Most checked their jackets, sometimes their shirts, but otherwise remained clothed. I walked to the upstairs and looked into the video room. It was a small, cozy room resembling a little den. Ten men sat on the carpeted, tiered platforms. Lighting the room was a small inset TV showing sex videos. On the screen were two very muscular men grappling as if in a wrestling match, only to reach a point where one began sucking the other's cock.

A slender, dark-haired, and very attractive man wearing Levi's and a white tank top sat at the center of the upper tier. The other men had their cocks out and were slowly jacking them while watching the video. There was no talking in the room. The attractive man began to rub his crotch; he had become the center of attention. He appeared to be one of those seemingly "untouchable pretty boys" but he had a different air about him. His attitude seemed more inclusive *than* exclusive. *He maintained eye contact with the other men, seductively pulling them into his sexual aura. He basked in the attention but also shared it, sending it back as well. His steady gaze brought one man from across the room to squeeze in beside him. Next he pulled out his cock; it was hard and erect, not huge but average. He reached over to both men on either side of him. They already had their cocks out. Both were very large, probably 9 or 10 inches, and stood erect. Neither of them were exceptionally attractive, but they received full attention from the man between them.*

He pushed up his tank top, running his left hand over his hairy chest, stopping to squeeze his tits. He reached to his left and felt the stomach, chest, and hard cock of his one partner. When he lifted his ass to shove his pants down to his ankles, the other two men followed suit. All the men in the room focused on the action of the three. No one watched the video. The center of attention kept drawing the others into his scene, making everyone very excited.

An older man, perhaps in his 50's, knelt in front of the younger, feeling his calves and thighs, squeezing his balls. At one point the older one tried to go down on the other's cock, but was prevented from this attempt to change the nature of this group jack-off. It wasn't a rebuke from a younger man to an older man; just a commitment to the sexual scene he had established.

The center continued to gaze around the room. The tension rose; one man sitting on a lower tier came with a cry and a moan. The three men who sat together began to vigorously jerk on each other's cocks, knowing the time was near. The center man shifted to his right and squeezed the tits of the man on that side. The extra sensations carried him over the brink and he also shot his cum. The center man continued to rub the throbbing cock. Then the man on the left began to breathe heavily, gasping and his cum shot straight up in spurts.

Having waited for the others, the center man took his turn. He looked around the room, pulling the energy in. He let others squeeze his balls and play with his tits, and then he came, spilling his cum on his hairy chest and stomach.

The tension broke; the focus relaxed. The cute man grinned at the two on either side. Seeming a little shy for the first time, he pulled his shirt down and his Levi's up, stood up and left the room.

Not too long ago jack-off was generally dismissed among gay men as the "Sex of last choice." Now, in the midst of so many health advisories, jack-off has merited another look. The renewed interest has resulted in sex play patterns that suggest there's more than one way to jack-off. Men who are into bondage and restraint and those who prefer S&M may conclude a two-hour sexually charged session with solo or mutual jack-off. The psychological and physical foreplay for these men frequently equals or surpasses the excitement of final orgasm. Our report does not include examples of such activities only because we did not observe them during any of our visits at the sex clubs, theaters, and bookstores.

For some men jack-off has been their preference all along; they find their choice now to be all the rage. For most others, the adoption of jacking off as a low-risk activity with others is an adaptation to the times, easier for some than others. It has also become symbolic of gay men's refusal to deny their enjoyment of sex and an affirmation of bonds of camaraderie.

PERSONAL CONCLUSIONS AND RECOMMENDATIONS

1. Owners of sex businesses that cater to gay and bisexual men have a long way to go before they can accurately claim that all efforts are being taken to encourage low risk activities. Needed actions include increased lighting, free condoms, and safe sex signs and brochures.

    Whereas the San Francisco AIDS Foundation once took a more aggressive advocacy role to encourage changes by bathhouse owners, that organization appears to have retreated from this position. To our knowledge no other representative from the Mayor's office or the Public Health Department has filled this void. A commitment to preventive education and risk reduction must include, in our opinion, an ongoing dialogue with the owners and the managers of the sex businesses. Only with some rapport established will the business owners be likely to implement stepped-up prevention and education efforts in their facilities. At the same time there is nothing stopping these businesses from taking the initiative to contact the health department or the AIDS Foundation to determine what more can be done.

2. However government officials choose to continue their public debate about sex businesses, substantial efforts to encourage risk reduction remain. Actions need not interfere with an individual's right to privacy and free choice. For example, Dr. Silverman could shift some of his attention to requiring sex businesses to post risk reduction guidelines and health advisories and to enforcing basic standards of hygiene.

3. Use of condoms should be encouraged at all facilities. Condoms should be given to customers directly along with the new safe sex cards upon registration or entry.

4. Businesses that do not provide toilets and sinks for cleaning up should provide these minimal amenities to their customers. Those that already do should keep them clean.

5. City government should be encouraged and challenged to bring Sexually Transmitted Disease testing and treatment on a regular basis to the city's bathhouses and clubs. Very little has been heard from the public health department about the serious incidence of Hepatitis B and parasites in the gay community. Several hundred thousand dollars had been budgeted for public service announcements about AIDS on TV and radio. There is no reason not to commit similar funds for the medical screening and treatment that would bring an end to the parasite epidemic in the city.

6. Researchers and physicians now suggest that if ever there was a disease affected by contributing factors, it's AIDS. They say it appears likely that a great number of gay men have been exposed to the AIDS agent, and yet a small percentage have developed "full blown" AIDS. An already compromised immune system–weakened by other illness, frequent STDs, substance abuse–may be a more determining factor for contracting AIDS symptoms than exposure to the probable virus itself.

The problem of substance abuse among lesbians and gay men is very extensive and serious. Ignored for too long by the community and recently overshadowed by the dramatic presence of AIDS, substance abuse may ironically receive needed attention because of its possible contribution to AIDS symptoms.

Whatever its relationship to AIDS, substance abuse is a serious problem demanding preventive measures, extensive education efforts, and community support for those personally affected. Local business groups–Golden Gate Business Association, the Tavern Guild, Bay Area Career Women, Eureka Valley Merchants Association–could take the lead to increase awareness and support of substance abuse programs.

7. During the last several months of debate regarding the baths and other sex businesses, very little attention has been paid to the sexual needs of those men who frequent these places without any genuine expectations of having a sexual exchange of any sort with another man. The lack of concern or attention granted to these men borders on callous disregard.

8. The development of safe sex videos remains problematic at this point. Producers are evidently uncertain of their marketability; the health department and its contract agencies are skittish about such a use of public funds. At this point, safe sex messages–in print or photographs–could be made and distributed to the city's video arcades and sex theaters.

9. The San Francisco AIDS Foundation not only receives considerable funding from the city for its formidable tasks; it also continues to receive donations from gay and lesbian businesses and individuals. The organization should continue to develop its bonds of trust and accountability with the lesbian/gay community by regular reports of expenditures and income as well as detailed plans for community education and prevention programs. The Foundation last published such a public accounting of its financial standing and its proposed programs in December of 1983.

Designing an HIV Counseling and Testing Program for Bathhouses: The Seattle Experience with Strategies to Improve Acceptability

Freya Spielberg, MD, MPH

University of Washington

Bernard M. Branson, MD

Division of HIV/AIDS Prevention, National Center for HIV,
STD and TB Prevention Centers for Disease Control and Prevention

Gary M. Goldbaum, MD

University of Washington and Department of Public Health–Seattle and King County

Ann Kurth, CNM, PhD

University of Washington

Robert W. Wood, MD

University of Washington and Department of Public Health–Seattle and King County

Correspondence may be addressed to Dr. Freya Spielberg, Center for AIDS and STD, Box 359931, 325 9th Avenue, 3EC44 Seattle, WA 98104-2499 (E-mail: freya@u.washington.edu).

[Haworth co-indexing entry note]: "Designing an HIV Counseling and Testing Program for Bathhouses: The Seattle Experience with Strategies to Improve Acceptability." Spielberg, Freya et al. Co-published simultaneously in *Journal of Homosexuality* (Harrington Park Press, an imprint of The Haworth Press, Inc.) Vol. 44, No. 3/4, 2003, pp. 203-220; and: *Gay Bathhouses and Public Health Policy* (ed: William J. Woods, and Diane Binson) Harrington Park Press, an imprint of The Haworth Press, Inc., 2003, pp. 203-220. Single or multiple copies of this article are available for a fee from The Haworth Document Delivery Service [1-800-HAWORTH, 9:00 a.m. - 5:00 p.m. (EST). E-mail address: docdelivery@haworthpress.com].

SUMMARY. Bathhouses are important venues for providing HIV counseling and testing to high-risk men who have sex with men (MSM), yet relatively few bathhouses routinely provide this service, and few data are available to guide program design. We examine numerous logistic considerations that had been identified in the HIV Alternative Testing Strategies study and that influenced the initiation, effectiveness, and maintenance of HIV testing programs in bathhouses for MSM. Key programmatic considerations in the design of a bathhouse HIV counseling and testing program included building alliances with community agencies, hiring and training staff, developing techniques for offering testing, and providing options for counseling, testing, and disclosure of results. The design included ways to provide client support and follow-up for partner notification and treatment counseling and to maintain relationships with bathhouse management for support of prevention activities. Early detection of HIV infection and HIV prevention can be achieved for some high-risk MSM through an accessible and acceptable HIV counseling and testing program in bathhouses. Keys to success include establishing community prevention collaborations between bathhouse personnel and testing agencies, ensuring that testing staff are supported in their work, and offering anonymous rapid HIV testing. Use of FDA approved, new rapid tests that do not require venipuncture, centrifugation, or laboratory oversight will further decrease barriers to testing and facilitate implementation of bathhouse testing programs in other communities. *[Article copies available for a fee from The Haworth Document Delivery Service: 1-800-HAWORTH. E-mail address: <docdelivery@haworthpress.com> Website: <http://www.HaworthPress.com>* © 2003 by The Haworth Press, Inc. All rights reserved.]

KEYWORDS. HIV, bathhouse, HIV counseling and testing, HIV prevention

Human immunodeficiency virus (HIV) counseling and testing can be a powerful motivator for behavior change among men who have sex with men (MSM), especially those who learn they are HIV-positive (Kelly, 2000; Valdiserri, 1997). Testing early in the course of HIV disease is increasingly important because it allows access to life-prolonging treatments (Carpenter et al., 1997). Yet many persons at high risk do not seek testing in clinics (Anderson, Carey, & Taveras, 2000), and as many as one-third of the 800,000 to 900,000 people estimated to be infected with HIV in the United States are unaware of their HIV status

(Centers for Disease Control and Prevention [CDC], 1999, 2001b). Although most MSM have been tested for HIV, many are not tested regularly, despite ongoing risks (MacKellar et al., 2002). Given that large numbers of MSM are still becoming infected with HIV (CDC, 2001a; Valleroy et al., 2000), the CDC now recommends annual HIV testing for all sexually active MSM (CDC, 2002). New approaches may be required to bring acceptable HIV counseling and testing to this population (Spielberg, Kurth, Gorbach, & Goldbaum, 2001).

Bathhouses have long been recognized as venues where prevention interventions could reach MSM at high risk for sexually transmitted diseases (STDs) (Judson, Miller, & Schaffnit, 1977; Merino, Judson, Bennett, & Schaffnit, 1979; Merino & Richards, 1977; Ritchy & Leff, 1975; Turner, Miller, & Moses, 1989). However, current prevention interventions in bathhouses typically involve only the display of posters and occasional opportunities to talk with outreach workers and obtain condoms and lubricants. According to a national survey, HIV counseling and testing were offered in only 40% of bathhouses (Woods, Binson, Mayne, Gore, & Rebchook, 2000; Woods et al., 2000; Woods, Binson, Mayne, Gore, & Rebchook, 2001) and, in some of these, no more than once a month. Barriers to, and facilitators of, the implementation of HIV counseling and testing in bathhouses have not been well described, and many questions remain about how best to design such a program to appeal to clients.

In the HIV Alternative Testing Strategies (HATS) study (Spielberg et al., 2001; Spielberg, Branson, Goldbaum, Lockhart, Kurth, Celum et al., 2002; Spielberg, Branson, Goldbaum, Lockhart, Kurth, Rossini et al., 2002; Spielberg, Jackson et al., 2002), we studied barriers to HIV counseling and testing and preferences for alternative HIV counseling and testing strategies among MSM in a bathhouse and a sex club (referred to here as bathhouses) and at two other venues for clients at high risk (a needle exchange program and an STD clinic). The results of interviews and focus groups with 100 participants and survey responses from 460 participants suggested several possibilities for improving the acceptability of HIV counseling and testing among people at these venues (Spielberg et al., 2001; Spielberg, Branson, Goldbaum, Lockhart, Kurth, Celum et al., 2002). Some of the 160 MSM who participated in the survey described barriers that could be influenced by the design of the counseling and testing program. A significant proportion of the bathhouse patrons said they had delayed HIV testing because they did not like the anxiety associated with the 1-week wait for test results, were concerned about having their names reported if the results were positive, or were unable to find convenient testing sites. Some delayed testing because they did not want to have blood drawn or did not want to speak with an HIV counselor. Many of the MSM surveyed at the bathhouses expressed preferences for rapid testing, oral fluid tests, or urine tests instead of standard blood testing for HIV and for receiving test results by telephone instead of coming in for a second visit.

Using the survey responses, we designed a program located in bathhouses. We offered the option of anonymous testing for those worried about confidentiality and the option of receiving test results by telephone. In the randomized trial (Spielberg, Branson, Goldbaum, Lockhart, Kurth, Rossini et al., 2002), we compared several HIV counseling and testing strategies (rapid testing, oral fluid testing, and counseling options) on the acceptability of testing and on the number of clients receiving results. The HATS study found that alternative counseling and testing strategies were more acceptable, more effective, and less costly than standard counseling and testing. In this paper, we describe the process through which HIV testing was initiated at bathhouses in Seattle, what we learned, and make recommendations for the optimal design of an HIV counseling and testing program in a bathhouse.

SETTING THE STAGE FOR HIV COUNSELING AND TESTING IN BATHHOUSES

Our experience in Seattle demonstrated that first-hand knowledge of successful testing collaborations and strong relationships between bathhouse owners and testing providers were necessary before bathhouse testing could be widely implemented. Community organizations, the public health department, and bathhouse owners in Seattle have been engaged in a partnership for HIV prevention for some time. In the late 1980s, the North West AIDS Foundation (NWAF, now Lifelong AIDS Alliance) developed a prevention outreach program in the three bathhouses in Seattle. At that time, outreach workers mainly provided information on HIV/AIDS and distributed condoms and lubricant. Discussions between the organizations focused on the mutual benefits of providing HIV prevention in bathhouse venues. The Department of Public Health Seattle & King County first offered HIV testing at the bathhouses in 1992 as part of an NWAF prevention event featuring a local porn star who did safer-sex demonstrations that attracted a large number of patrons. After this success, testing was conducted intermittently at similar events. However, routine HIV testing was not implemented until 1996, when the health department, noting declining rates of testing in county clinics, undertook an outreach effort to reach populations that may not have sought testing in clinics. Because of its established relationships with bathhouse owners, NWAF was able to initiate discussions about coordinating a collaboration for HIV testing with the bathhouses and the health department.

Implementation of such testing took place slowly. Initially, the management of only one bathhouse was willing to allow routine HIV counseling and testing, provided that most of the patrons valued the service. The second bathhouse was unwilling because of concerns about the potential negative effect on the social climate at the bathhouse, and the third did not have suitable space for testing. For 2 years, a single bathhouse offered HIV testing 1 night a week. In 1998, the health department and NWAF set up a meeting at which that bathhouse owner shared positive experiences with the other bathhouse owners, and the second bathhouse owner decided to allow weekly testing. A year later, the third bathhouse relocated to a new space and began to offer HIV testing in a room that had been set aside for HIV prevention efforts. Thus, by 1999, all three bathhouses offered HIV counseling and testing 1 or 2 nights per week. During that time, the NWAF initiated a prevention group at which community prevention workers, researchers, and bathhouse owners met periodically to discuss experiences and plan prevention efforts. That group and its leader continue to be instrumental in maintaining good relationships, communication, and coordination among HIV prevention community groups, clinical trial networks, researchers, and bathhouse owners and staff.

The implementation of rapid testing in bathhouses required additional collaboration with the public health department laboratory. The rapid HIV test that we used (Single Use Diagnostic System for HIV-1 [SUDS], Abbott-Murex, Abbott Park, IL) is categorized under the Clinical Laboratory Improvement Amendments (CLIA) as a moderately complex test. In Seattle, staff with at least a high school education performed the test at bathhouses. However, to comply with CLIA, the testing must be done under the oversight of a CLIA-certified laboratory. In Seattle, the public health laboratory agreed to provide this oversight.

In November 2002, a new rapid finger-stick was approved by the FDA (OraQuick Rapid HIV-1 Antibody test, OraSure Technologies Inc., Bethlehem, PA). In January 2003 this test received a CLIA waiver that allows use without the supervision of a CLIA certified laboratory. With this waiver HIV prevention organizations that have traditionally been limited to outreach will now be able to provide testing, so that access to testing in outreach venues where people at high risk congregate could be greatly expanded.

STAFFING

It is difficult to maintain HIV counseling and testing staff in bath-house settings because of the special demands of the job. To reach the greatest number of clients, testing is usually provided at peak atten-dance hours (typically Friday to Sunday, evenings to early mornings). Bathhouses are typically smoky, and the space for testing is usually cramped and poorly lit. Although optimal staffing demands that several persons working part-time provide these services, the pool of candi-dates is limited (many bathhouses do not permit women to work on the premises). Furthermore, having staff work in a sexually charged envi-ronment with clients who are scantily clad raises issues about the need for supervision.

Training for bathhouse staff included the CDC-recommended train-ing in HIV client-centered counseling and testing. In addition, staff needed to learn how to recruit clients in challenging environments, how to interact with clients who have been drinking or using recreational drugs, and how to fend off sexual advances. When giving positive test results in the bathhouses, staff must also learn how to deal with dis-traught clients and, if desired, escort them off site to a mutually agree-able space for additional counseling. After experiencing the challenges of outreach testing, the staff of the health department developed training in these areas. It was also useful to have at least two staff members at the bathhouses when testing was offered so that one staff member could continue to recruit for testing and manage client flow while the other conducted the counseling and testing session. More recently, the health department has been partnering with community groups to provide out-reach and recruitment so that disease intervention specialists can focus their efforts on providing HIV/STD counseling and testing while part-ner groups interact with clients and encourage testing. Ongoing staff meetings have been helpful in allowing staff to discuss the challenges of, and successful strategies for, working in bathhouses, for assessing the quality of recruitment logs and counseling notes, and developing plans to meet additional training needs.

TECHNIQUES FOR OFFERING TESTING

Before the HATS study, the testing staff of the health department an-nounced the testing services at the bathhouses through loudspeaker an-nouncements and then waited for clients to come for testing. During the study, we enlisted a recruiter to approach each man who entered the bathhouse. The recruiter asked patrons when they had most recently been tested for HIV and then offered free HIV testing. Although there was initial concern from testing staff and bathhouse management that patrons would find this approach off-putting, we found that rates of nonresponse to testing staff dropped significantly as patrons (and staff) became comfortable with this recruitment technique. Recruiters also noted that many patrons would refuse testing on several occasions before they accepted. In addition, staff became adept at avoiding the handful of patrons who were hostile and found that even those patrons would, at times, approach staff to find out why they had not been offered HIV testing and would finally accept. Compared with loudspeaker announcements, approaching individual patrons promoted more personal HIV testing discussions, did not result in patron complaints to management, and increased acceptance of testing.

To evaluate the testing process and the effect of changes in the design of the counseling and testing program, staff used recruitment logs to record the age, race/ethnicity, date of most recent HIV test, and testing decisions of each patron approached. To determine staffing needs, information on the number of persons who visited the venue during testing hours was also obtained from bathhouse management. More recently, community-based outreach counseling and testing programs have also started collecting information on the recruitment log on the timing and the nature of the most recent HIV risk and whether HIV was discussed with their most recent partner–information intended to facilitate discussions about HIV and to allow recommendations for counseling and testing services. In addition, this information allows the design of acceptable testing services and better targeting of counseling and testing efforts to people at high risk, as well as the monitoring of community risk behaviors and testing needs. We suggest that other testing programs adopt such recruitment logs so that the success of program innovations can be evaluated with data that are routinely collected.

BATHHOUSE CLIENTS REACHED THROUGH ON-SITE HIV TESTING PROGRAM

Most of the clients who accepted HIV testing and responded to staff interviews in the HATS study were more than 24 years old, white, educated, and had incomes above the poverty level, homes, and health insurance (Table 1). Although 92% had been tested for HIV, nearly a third

TABLE 1. Characteristics of MSM Tested at Bathhouses, HATS Study

	n = 437 (%)
Demographics	
Gender	
Male	437 (100)
Age	
< 20	2 (0.5)
20-29	115 (26)
30-39	123 (28)
≥ 40	194 (44)
Race/Ethnicity	
White	359 (82)
Black	15 (3)
Hispanic	27 (6)
Other	32 (7)
Education	
High school diploma or below	47 (11)
Some college	124 (28)
College degree or above	248 (57)
Has health insurance	360 (82)
Substance Use	
Recreational drug use past year	159 (36)
≥ 5 drinks per night past month	118 (27)
Last HIV Test	
< 6 months	91 (21)
6-12 months	211 (48)
> 12 months	101 (23)
Never tested	34 (8)
HIV risks	
≥ 4 sex partners, past year	322 (74)
Unprotected anal sex, past 2 months	110 (25)
Sex with known HIV-positive person, ever	111 (25)
Engaged in unsafe sexual behavior while on drugs or alcohol, past 2 months	159 (36)
Traded sex for money or drugs, ever	17 (4)
Injected drugs, ever	20 (5)
HIV risks since last test	
Unprotected anal sex	158 (36)
Unprotected anal or oral sex	353 (81)

had not been tested during the past year. Most reported having engaged in risks for HIV since their most recent test: 77% had had more than four sex partners in the past year, and 25% reported that they had had unprotected anal intercourse during the past 2 months. Substance use was common. Among bathhouse clients, 27% reported binge drinking (5 drinks or more in a day) during the past month, 36% reported recreational drug use during the past year, 5% reported having injected drugs in their lifetime, and 36% reported having taken more sexual risks while drinking alcohol or taking drugs during the past 2 months. These data confirm that bathhouse testing programs can reach clients who are likely to benefit from HIV counseling and testing.

COUNSELING AND TESTING LOGISTICS

One of the biggest challenges for a bathhouse testing program is to ensure that clients receive their test results. Among the bathhouse clients in the HATS study who accepted HIV testing, 97% chose to be tested anonymously. Thus, it would not be possible to notify HIV-positive clients who did not return for their test results. In general, testing in bathhouses, like other HIV testing, has been done with the standard blood enzyme immunoassay and Western blot. These tests require a blood sample, which is sent to a laboratory. Typically, a week or more elapses before test results are available. Standard tests can also be done on oral fluids (Table 2), collected with the OraSure collection device (OraSure Technologies, Bethlehem, PA), which allows easier specimen collection and increases acceptability among clients who prefer not to have their blood drawn. However, oral fluid test results are not available for a week or more. Because of the time lag between testing and results, 25% to 33% of persons who receive standard testing with either blood or oral fluids in public testing venues do not return for their test results (Anderson et al., 2000).

In the HATS study, we provided clients with CDC-recommended client-centered pretest risk-reduction counseling (CDC, 2001b; Kamb et al., 1998) with standard, oral fluid, and rapid testing and evaluated the acceptability of providing the option of written materials instead of counseling. In this setting, offering the option of written materials resulted in 80% fewer clients receiving counseling, but did not improve testing acceptance or increase the number of clients who received test results. Thus, we do not recommend providing the option of written materials with HIV testing when face-to-face counseling is feasible. However,

TABLE 2. Logistical Requirements for HIV Counseling and Testing in Bathhouses

	Standard Blood Testing	Oral Fluid Testing (OraSure)	Rapid Blood Testing (SUDS)
Staff training			
Anonymous testing	Yes	Yes	Yes
Recruiting for testing	Yes	Yes	Yes
Venipuncture	Yes	**No**	Yes
HIV counseling	Yes	Yes	Yes
Telephone results disclosure	Yes	Yes	**No**
Performing rapid test	**No**	**No**	Yes
Positive results disclosure	Yes	Yes	Yes
Partner notification protocol	Yes	Yes	Yes
STD education and referrals	Yes.	Yes	Yes
Manpower			
Recommended	2	2	2
Feasible	1	1	1
Facility requirements			
HIV counseling 1st visit	Private space	Private space	Private space, outlet for small centrifuge
HIV counseling only with results	Clipboard, chair	Clipboard	Private space, outlet for small centrifuge
Specimen/kit storage	Room temp. while testing, Refrigerate overnight	Room temp.	Room temp. while testing, Refrigerate controls overnight
Laboratory			
Screening test	Public health	Commercial	On-site testing
Confirmation	Public health	Commercial	Public health
Wait for test results	1 week	1 week	20 minutes
Cost of purchasing test	$8	$24	$18*
Total cost of providing test results to one person	$118	$111	$74

*Includes cost of controls required with each test.

providing client-centered counseling requires a private room, which is not feasible in all bathhouses. When a private room is not available, it would be possible to offer oral fluid testing with written materials and a second appointment for counseling and the disclosure of results.

With standard blood and oral fluid testing, we also routinely offered clients the option of receiving their test results by telephone. This option has been standard practice in anonymous testing at the health department clinic since 1999, and data confirm that a greater proportion of clients receive their test results when offered the option of telephone counseling (Tsu, Burm, Gilhooly, & Sells, 2002; Schluter et al., 1966). In the HATS study, 93% of the bathhouse clients receiving standard testing chose to receive their results by telephone, and 246 of 334 (74%) received their test results. Those who preferred receiving their test results face-to-face were given the option of returning to the bathhouse 1 week later or scheduling a follow-up appointment at the health department clinic (which most chose). Thus, if bathhouse testing programs offer standard blood or oral fluid HIV tests, we recommend routinely offering the option of receiving test results by telephone.

After rapid HIV testing, clients can learn their test results within 30 minutes. The HATS study was the first program to attempt rapid blood testing in bathhouses (Single Use Diagnostic System for HIV-1 [SUDS], Abbott-Murex, Abbott Park, IL). To perform the rapid test, staff carried a small centrifuge to a room set aside in the bathhouse for counseling and testing. In this setting, sometimes with dim lighting and little space, the staff member drew the blood (into a tube with a serum separator to avoid the need for clotting time) at the beginning of the visit and let it centrifuge (on the floor) while conducting the HIV counseling. At the end of the 20-minute counseling session, the counselor would ask the client to step out of the room for 10 minutes while the test was performed. The client would then return to the room for posttest counseling and test results. With rapid testing, 102 of 103 (99%) of clients received their test results. Because of the much higher number of clients who receive test results with rapid testing as compared to standard blood and oral fluid testing, in bathhouses this strategy was the most effective, as well as the most cost-effective (Spielberg, Jackson et al., 2002).

The new OraQuick rapid finger-stick test offers additional advantages to the SUDS test in that it does not require venipuncture training, a centrifuge, or an electrical outlet to perform. The lateral flow design also simplifies the test procedure in that once the finger-stick specimen is collected with a plastic loop and mixed into the test buffer, one simply needs to place the device in the buffer and incubate for 20 minutes, during which time counseling can be conveniently provided. In places where lighting is poor we recommend having a flashlight on hand to read the test results. As with the SUDS, all reactive rapid tests must be confirmed with Western blot or Immuno Flourescence Assay, which optimally should be done on venipuncture specimens. However, if venipuncture is not possible, it would be acceptable to collect a second finger-stick specimen on filter paper or oral fluid for western blot. The OraQuick test will also likely be more cost-effective than the SUDS test. Although the price of one OraQuick test ($9.10) is more than the SUDS test ($6), when the cost of controls is included the cost of the OraQuick test is less ($11.20 vs. $18), because the internal negative control allows external controls to be run as infrequently as once with each new 25 test kit, whereas with SUDS it is necessary to run controls each time.

At the time that the study implemented rapid testing for HIV in the bathhouses, the owner of one of Seattle's three bathhouses was not comfortable with revealing positive results at the bathhouses, fearing that the emotional response might be disruptive. Thus, only two bathhouses participated in the randomized trial. Before implementing rapid testing, we found that staff were uncomfortable with the idea of giving rapid test results. However, after training and experience, the comfort level of staff with rapid testing increased dramatically. Several measures helped to reassure staff and clients. When testing was offered, we routinely advised clients that if the HIV test results were positive, we would escort them to a comfortable private setting of their choice (the clinic, their home, the home of a friend or family member) for additional counseling. Results to confirm positive rapid test results were available within 3 days. To further minimize the possibility of adverse outcomes of testing, clients who acknowledged a risk for suicide or violence to others would be referred for additional mental health services and advised to wait for testing. As mentioned, a second staff member was also present for logistical and emotional support. If it is not possible to have a second staff present, we recommend establishing on-call support and linkages with mental health professionals in nearby emergency rooms. Given these precautions, our experience with rapid testing for HIV in the bathhouses was very good. Staff quickly became comfortable performing the test and providing test results in the bathhouses, and the accuracy of the test was equivalent to that claimed in the product insert (sensitivity 100%; specificity 99.6%).

An unexpected benefit of rapid testing was an increase in the proportion of clients who returned for partner notification and early treatment counseling (compared with clients who received their confirmed test results after standard oral fluid or serum testing). Overall, 22 persons tested HIV-positive during the study. The 5 who received positive rapid-test results returned for a second face-to-face counseling visit for their confirmed test results. Because they had time to consider the possibility that the positive test result would be confirmed, they seemed emotionally prepared at the second visit to discuss partner notification and to receive early treatment counseling. In contrast, only 9 of 17 persons who had a standard HIV test and who tested positive received their test results. Those who did receive their confirmed positive test results were too upset to accept substantive additional counseling for early treatment or for partner notification at that visit and were less likely to return for a second face-to-face counseling visit: only 4 received counseling for early treatment and partner notification at the health department.

Rapid HIV tests offer many advantages for bathhouse testing programs. Now that the FDA has approved the new OraQuick rapid HIV-1 finger stick test for the point of care testing, it should be feasible for many more bathhouse testing programs to implement rapid testing and reach populations of high-risk MSM who may not access testing elsewhere. In the future it is anticipated that the Federal Drug Administration will approve an oral fluid rapid test that will likely receive even greater acceptance. Until that time, the OraQuick finger-stick test, if implemented, will likely result in significant increases in testing acceptance and receipt of test result among bathhouse populations.

DEVELOPING PREVENTION PARTNERSHIPS AND BRINGING RAPID TESTING TO BATHHOUSES

At the end of the randomized trial, the results of the HATS study demonstrating the acceptability and feasibility of rapid testing in bathhouses were given to the bathhouse prevention group and shared with community HIV counseling and testing providers, bathhouse owners, and staff. Owners who became familiar with rapid testing during the HATS study were able to share their positive experiences with other staff and the bathhouse owner who had been hesitant to allow rapid testing in the bathhouse. Involved bathhouse managers and owners reported that clients viewed the presence of testing in the clubs as a valuable service. One bathhouse manager said, "Testing isn't intrusive in clubs; people call up in advance to see if the testers will be there. People like the convenience." The owner of another bathhouse said, "Very few people were upset at the testing presence; more people applauded our participation. It's valuable and important that the testing groups come regularly and consistently." By the end of the discussion, there was overall agreement that rapid testing was the best testing choice for bathhouses, and the owner who had been hesitant expressed interest in implementing rapid testing. After a similar forum for bathhouse owners and HIV testing providers in the San Francisco area, participants expressed support for instituting rapid HIV testing in bathhouses.

However, barriers to implementation of rapid testing exist. For example, in some cities, it may be difficult to find a CLIA-certified laboratory to supervise rapid testing for bathhouse testing programs. In Seattle, the health department lab accepted responsibility for CLIA compliance with quality assurance standards and notified our testing team when the required proficiency panels arrived. Masked panels of sera had to be ordered three times a year (Wisconsin State Laboratory of Hygiene, Madison, WI, $302/year) and tested by one of the study staff. Because the proficiency panels were frozen and required pretest centrifugation with a high-speed centrifuge, it was necessary to test the specimens at the health department lab. Results were then returned to the company; if they were accurate, we were given approval to continue using SUDS for another 4 months. If the results of the proficiency panel were inaccurate (which never happened), we would have had to stop using the SUDS until the problems could be resolved and the proficiency panel was performed accurately. Given that the only requirements were to review Quality Assurance protocols and make space available three times a year for one of our staff to perform the proficiency panel, the health department laboratory director did not find oversight to be a burden. In other cities, it may be more difficult to find a laboratory to accept responsibility for oversight, which is why the recent CLIA waiver of the OraQuick test is so important. With this new CLIA waived rapid test States are now developing plans for training and quality assurance. Ideally, laboratory oversight will not be a requirement, as that would impose a significant barrier to implementation of rapid testing in outreach venues. For rapid tests that are assigned the CLIA designation of "Moderately Complex," like the SUDS test, the first step in implementation is for persons involved in the design of the testing program to meet with local laboratory directors to discuss the benefits of rapid testing and to develop a specific plan for laboratory supervision. Companies that develop future rapid HIV tests should seek, and be granted, CLIA waivers to eliminate this barrier to implementation of rapid testing in outreach venues.

CONCLUSION

Bathhouses provide an opportunity for HIV prevention interventions that can reach MSM at highest risk (Binson et al., 2001). Although our experience may not be applicable to all communities, the increased acceptability and effectiveness of anonymous rapid testing was demonstrated in two bathhouses. An important first step in the design of a rapid HIV testing program in bathhouses is to convene meetings that include all key stakeholders (Table 3)–HIV counseling and testing providers; bathhouse owners, managers and staff; prevention outreach workers; and laboratory directors–to discuss the potential benefits of such a program and to identify barriers and consider how to overcome them.

TABLE 3. Implementing HIV Counseling and Testing in Bathhouses: Keys to Success

Topic	Recommendation
Developing partnerships between: HIV testing providers Bathhouse owners and staff Community prevention staff Laboratory directors	Hold planning meetings with key stake holders to discuss benefits, and how to overcome barriers, to providing testing in bathhouses
Staffing	Hire multiple part-time staff Work in pairs Hold weekly meetings for clinical support, quality assurance and on-going training
Recruitment	Engage in active recruitment rather than self-referral with loud speaker announcements
Counseling	Provide CDC-recommended client-centered risk reduction counseling
Testing	Provide anonymous and confidential testing Provide rapid testing When FDA approved, use new rapid tests that do not require venipuncture, centrifugation or laboratory supervision
Results disclosure	Offer telephone results when rapid testing is not available
Partner Notification and Referral	Coordinate services with visit for confirmatory results
Evaluation	Use: Recruitment logs HIV counseling and testing risk assessment and clinical note Testing logs Positive referral logs Partner notification forms
Sustaining and expanding bathhouse testing programs	Hold on-going meetings between testing providers, bathhouse management and staff, community prevention workers, and laboratory directors to discuss benefits and concerns of bathhouse testing programs, and to plan and coordinate future prevention activities

In the implementation of anonymous rapid testing in bathhouses, key programmatic considerations include building alliances with community agencies; hiring and training multiple part-time staff who work in pairs; holding weekly meetings to discuss difficult clinical situations, review charts for quality control, and identify training needs; using active recruitment strategies with one-on-one outreach rather than loudspeaker announcements; and providing the option of receiving results by telephone for those who do not choose rapid testing. For clients who have positive rapid-test results, coordinating partner notification and treatment counseling to coincide with the follow-up visit for confirmed test results will increase the number of clients who receive these services. Sharing feedback and experiences is essential to sustaining the program and to recruiting other bathhouses. Use of FDA approved, new simple rapid tests that do not require venipuncture, centrifugation or laboratory oversight will improve the acceptability and feasibility of bathhouse HIV counseling and testing programs. The wider implementation of acceptable and effective HIV counseling and testing programs in bathhouses could lead to substantial advances in HIV prevention and to the early diagnosis and treatment of HIV infection among MSM.

ACKNOWLEDGMENTS

The authors thank Kevin Henderson, the HIV Alternative Testing Strategies study staff, and staff from the bathhouses for their hard work and support.

The HIV Alternative Testing Strategies (HATS) study was supported by a grant from the University of Washington Center For AIDS Research New Investigator Award AI27757 and from cooperative agreement R18/CCR015258-01 with the Centers for Disease Control and Prevention (CDC). Time to prepare this manuscript was supported by a grant from the National Institute for Drug Abuse (K08 DA00472-01). This work was approved by the University of Washington Human Subjects Committee (27-0287-C/B) and by the CDC Institutional Review Board (2209).

REFERENCES

Anderson, J. E., Carey, J. W., & Taveras, S. (2000). HIV testing among the general US population and persons at increased risk: Information from national surveys, 1987-1996. *American Journal of Public Health, 90*, 1089-1095.

Binson, D., Woods, W. J., Pollack, L., Paul, J., Stall, R., & Catania, J. A. (2001). Differential HIV risk in bathhouses and public cruising areas. *American Journal of Public Health, 91*, 1482-1486.

Carpenter, C. C., Fischl, M. A., Hammer, S. M., Hirsch, M. S., Jacobsen, D. M., Katzenstein, D. A., Montaner, J. S., Richman, D. D., Saag, M. S., Schooley, R. T.,

Thompson, M. A., Vella, S., Yeni, P. G., & Volberding, P. A. (1997). Antiretroviral therapy for HIV infection in 1997: Updated recommendations of the International AIDS Society-USA panel. *Journal of the American Medical Association, 277,* 1962-1969.

Centers for Disease Control and Prevention (1999). Guidelines for national human immunodeficiency virus case surveillance, including monitoring for human immunodeficiency virus infection and acquired immunodeficiency syndrome. *MMWR Recommendations and Reports, 48*(RR-13), 1-27, 29-31.

Centers for Disease Control and Prevention (2001a). HIV incidence among young men who have sex with men–seven U.S. cities, 1994-2000. *MMWR Morbidity and Mortality Weekly Report, 50*(21), 440-444.

Centers for Disease Control and Prevention (2001b). Revised guidelines for HIV counseling, testing, and referral. *MMWR Recommendations and Reports, 50*(RR-19), 1-57.

Centers for Disease Control and Prevention (2002). Sexually transmitted disease treatment guidelines. *MMWR Recommendations and Reports, 51*(RR-6), 1-84.

Judson, F. N., Miller, K. G., & Schaffnit, T. R. (1977). Screening for gonorrhea and syphilis in the gay baths–Denver, Colorado. *American Journal of Public Health, 67,* 740-742.

Kamb, M., Fishbein, M., Douglas, J. M., Jr., Rhodes, F., Bolan, G., Zenilman, J., Hoxworth, T., Malotte, C. K., Iatesta, M., Kent, C., Lentz, A., Graziano, S., Byers, R. H., & Peterman, T. A., for the Project Respect Study Group (1998). Efficacy of risk-reduction counseling to prevent human immunodeficiency virus and sexually transmitted diseases. *Journal of the American Medical Association, 280,* 1161-1167.

Kelly, J. A. (2000). HIV prevention interventions with gay or bisexual men and youth. *AIDS, 14*(Suppl. 2), S34-39.

MacKellar, D. A., Valleroy, L. A., Secura, G. M., Bartholow, B. N., McFarland, W., Shehan, D., Ford, W., LaLota, M., Celentano, D. D., Koblin, B. A., Torian, L. V., Perdue, T. E., & Janssen, R. S., for the Young Men's Survey Study Group (2002). Repeat HIV testing, risk behaviors, and HIV seroconversion among young men who have sex with men: A call to monitor and improve the practice of prevention. *Journal of Acquired Immune Deficiency Syndromes, 29,* 76-85.

Merino, H. I., Judson, F. N., Bennett, D., & Schaffnit, T. R. (1979). Screening for gonorrhea and syphilis in gay bathhouses in Denver and Los Angeles. *Public Health Reports, 94,* 376-379.

Merino, H. I., & Richards, J. B. (1977). An innovative program of venereal disease casefinding, treatment and education for a population of gay men. *Sexually Transmitted Diseases, 4*(2), 50-52.

Ritchey, M. G., & Leff, A. M. (1975). Venereal disease control among homosexuals: An outreach program. *Journal of the American Medical Association, 232,* 509-510.

Schluter, W. W., Judson, F. N., Baron, A. E., McGill, W. L., Marine, W. M., & Douglas, J. M., Jr. (1996). Usefulness of human immunodeficiency virus post-test counseling by telephone for low-risk clients of an urban sexually transmitted diseases clinic. *Sexually Transmitted Diseases, 23*(3), 190-197.

Spielberg, F., Branson, B., Goldbaum, G., Lockhart, D., Kurth, A., Celum, C., Rossini, A., Critchlow, C., & Wood, R. (2002). Overcoming barriers to HIV testing: Preferences for new strategies among clients of a needle exchange, an STD clinic and sex venues for MSM. *JAIDS* 2003; 32(3): 318-327.

Spielberg, F., Branson, B., Goldbaum, G., Lockhart, D., Kurth, A., Rossini, A., & Wood, R. (2002, March). *Acceptance of alternative HIV counseling and testing strategies (rapid, oral fluid, and optional pre-test counseling)* [abstract P64]. 2002 National STD Prevention Conference, San Diego, CA.

Spielberg, F., Jackson, S., Varghese, B., Branson, B., Reed, S., Goldbaum, G., & Sullivan, S. (2002, March). *HIV testing with oral fluids and rapid tests is more effective and less costly* [abstract P63]. 2002 National STD Prevention Conference, San Diego, CA.

Spielberg, F., Kurth, A., Gorbach, P. M., & Goldbaum, G. (2001). Moving from apprehension to action: HIV counseling and testing preferences in three at-risk populations. *AIDS Education and Prevention, 13*, 524-540.

Tsu, R. C., Burm, M. L., Gilhooly, J. A., & Sells, C. W. (2002). Telephone vs. face-to-face notification of HIV results in high-risk youth. *Journal of Adolescent Health, 30*(3), 154-160.

Turner, C. F., Miller, H. G., & Moses, L. E. (1989). *AIDS: Sexual behavior and intravenous drug use.* Washington, DC: National Academy Press.

Valdiserri, R. O. (1997). HIV counseling and testing: Its evolving role in HIV prevention. *AIDS Education and Prevention, 9*(Suppl. 3), 2-13.

Valleroy, L. A., MacKellar, D. A., Karon, J. M., Rosen, D. H., McFarland, W., Shehan, D. A., Stoyanoff, S. R., LaLota, M., Celentano, D. D., Koblin, B. A., Thiede, H., Katz, M. H., Torian, L. V., & Janssen, R. S., for the Young Men's Survey Study Group (2000). HIV prevalence and associated risks in young men who have sex with men. *Journal of the American Medical Association, 284*, 198-204.

Woods, W. J., Binson, D. K., Mayne, T. J., Gore, L. R., & Rebchook, G. M. (2000). HIV/sexually transmitted disease education and prevention in US bathhouse and sex club environments. *AIDS, 14*, 625-626.

Woods, W. J., Sabatino, J., Bauer, P. L., Adler, B., Dilley, J. W., & Binson, D. (2000). HIV testing in gay sex clubs. *International Journal of STD & AIDS, 11*(3), 173-175.

Woods, W. J., Binson, D., Mayne, T. J., Gore, L. R., & Rebchook, G. M. (2001). Facilities and HIV prevention in bathhouse and sex club environments. *Journal of Sex Research, 38*(1), 68-74.

Comparing Sexual Behavioral Patterns Between Two Bathhouses: Implications for HIV Prevention Intervention Policy

Matt G. Mutchler, PhD

AIDS Project Los Angeles

Trista Bingham, MPH, MS

Los Angeles County HIV Epidemiology Program

Miguel Chion, MD, MPH

AIDS Project Los Angeles

Richard A. Jenkins, PhD

Centers for Disease Control and Prevention

Lee E. Klosinski, PhD

AIDS Project Los Angeles

Gina Secura, MPH

Centers for Disease Control and Prevention

Correspondence may be addressed to Matt G. Mutchler, AIDS Project Los Angeles, 3550 Wilshire Boulevard, Suite #300, Los Angeles, CA 90010.

[Haworth co-indexing entry note]: "Comparing Sexual Behavioral Patterns Between Two Bathhouses: Implications for HIV Prevention Intervention Policy." Mutchler, Matt G. et al. Co-published simultaneously in *Journal of Homosexuality* (Harrington Park Press, an imprint of The Haworth Press, Inc.) Vol. 44, No. 3/4, 2003, pp. 221-242; and: *Gay Bathhouses and Public Health Policy* (ed: William J. Woods, and Diane Binson) Harrington Park Press, an imprint of The Haworth Press, Inc., 2003, pp. 221-242. Single or multiple copies of this article are available for a fee from The Haworth Document Delivery Service [1-800-HAWORTH, 9:00 a.m. - 5:00 p.m. (EST). E-mail address: docdelivery@haworthpress.com].

SUMMARY. There is a glaring lack of data to inform culturally appropriate HIV prevention interventions targeting environments such as bathhouses where men who have sex with men (MSM) practice sexual risk behaviors. This study compares sexual behavioral patterns across two bathhouse sites in order to identify important themes to address when tailoring HIV prevention interventions to bathhouse environments. We analyzed semi-structured interviews with workers and patrons at two bathhouses to explore similarities and differences. A coding scheme was established and data were organized according to conceptual themes. We found that differences between the two sites emerged in six key areas: bathhouse clientele, attraction to particular sites, sexual practices and condom use, communication about sex and HIV status, bathhouse rules, and substance use. Implications for HIV prevention intervention policy are discussed. *[Article copies available for a fee from The Haworth Document Delivery Service: 1-800-HAWORTH. E-mail address: <docdelivery@haworthpress. com> Website: <http://www.HaworthPress.com> © 2003 by The Haworth Press, Inc. All rights reserved.]*

KEYWORDS. Gay men, MSM, HIV/AIDS, sexual risk behaviors, HIV prevention intervention policy, bathhouse, public sex venues

INTRODUCTION

Over twenty years have passed since the first HIV/AIDS cases were diagnosed in Los Angeles. In the mid-1990s, new treatments known as highly active antiretroviral therapy (HAART) brought some hope for people living with HIV and led to dramatic declines in AIDS incidence rates and HIV-related mortality (*HIV/AIDS Surveillance Report*, 1999). Recent research suggests that HIV incidence rates once stable among men who have sex with men (MSM) may be increasing for particular populations such as African American and Latino MSM (*HIV/AIDS Surveillance Report*, 2000). Continued HIV transmission combined with decreased mortality for those on improved treatment regimens translates into more people living with HIV and AIDS.

Recent investigations have suggested that HIV risk behavior and transmission have been increasing among MSM populations nationally (Stall et al., 2000; Wolitski et al., 2001). As the epidemic enters its third decade, there are over 16,000 people living with AIDS in Los Angeles County. The most common mode of transmission in Los Angeles

County continues to be male-to-male sexual contact, representing 71% of the cumulative AIDS cases. In Los Angeles, outbreaks of syphilis among MSM have recently been reported (CDC, 2001). In response to the evidence of increasing HIV risk among MSM, there are efforts to take research and prevention activities closer to the social environments where MSM congregate and to better understand these environments. Bathhouses provide a potentially important setting for this kind of research and intervention for reasons discussed below.

For more than one hundred years, bathhouses have been an important part of gay sexual cultures in the United States; from bathhouses where men occasionally had sex in the late 1890s to the modern bathhouses that exclusively cater to social and sexual needs of gay men (Bérubé, 1996). There have been recurring public health debates over the role of bathhouses in the proliferation of STDs such as HIV (Alexander, 1996; Bérubé, 1996). In the mid-1980s, San Francisco experienced a controversy over closing bathhouses that is not atypical of other debates (see Disman, this volume). During the San Francisco debate, some argued bathhouses should be shut because they encouraged activity that drove the HIV epidemic. Others promoted them as unique venues that facilitated outreach to populations with high-risk behaviors. Still others made bathhouses symbols of gay and civil rights (Shilts, 1987). Given their niche in gay sexual history, surprisingly little research has been conducted with respect to sexual risk behaviors within bathhouses.

Clearly, sexual behaviors that may transmit HIV do occur in bathhouses. For instance, Richwald (1988) interviewed 807 men as they left seven bathhouses in Los Angeles County; 10% reported having had unprotected anal intercourse (UAI) in bathhouses. The men who were having UAI were more likely to report 5 or more male partners in the past month than those who did not have UAI. Elwood et al. (1998) found that while many bathhouse patrons reported knowledge of HIV and safer sex practices and avoided penetrative sex or used condoms, a minority of this sample also reported complete disregard of risks of HIV infection or sexual prevention. Sey and Harawa (2001) found that 63% of HIV seropositive (+) MSM diagnosed with acute/primary or recent HIV infection had sex in public sex environments; at 12-month follow-up, 36% reported sex at bathhouses (personal communication with Harawa, 3/25/02). Binson and colleagues (2001) found that people using bathhouses are more likely to be HIV positive compared to men who cruised for sex only in cruising areas such as parks, tearooms, beaches, or bookstores.

Recent studies have begun to illustrate that differences may exist among bathhouse patrons. For example, Elwood and Williams (1998) found that men who frequent bathhouses were not a homogeneous group; attendees varied in terms of sexual identities and sexual behaviors. Another study found differences in the prevalence of sexually transmitted diseases, drug use, and risky sexual practices among men who frequent gay sex venues by type of venue (e.g., bathhouse, cruising areas, and multiple venues) (Binson et al., 2001). Previous bathhouse studies have not examined differences between patrons and their sexual activities across bathhouse sites (Richwald et al., 1988). Still, policy discussions regarding HIV prevention interventions targeting bathhouse settings continue to presume that one size fits all. If differential risk patterns exist across bathhouse sites, this nonspecific prevention policy model may be flawed and may inhibit efforts to intervene appropriately to reduce bathhouse sexual risk activities. Therefore, exploring whether or not differential behavioral patterns do exist between bathhouses is important for considering how to conceptualize HIV prevention policy and develop HIV interventions in these special settings.

We conducted a qualitative study of bathhouse sexual behavioral patterns and HIV risk behavior in two Los Angeles County bathhouses in order to identify themes that may be relevant for designing HIV prevention interventions targeting bathhouses. We found that differences as well as similarities emerged around the following themes that may be important to consider for assessing such efforts in other venues: perceptions of behavioral patterns and rules governing sexual and HIV risk behaviors such as clientele's attraction to particular bathhouses, condom use and sexual activities, the customary interpersonal processes involved in negotiating sex and condom use (communication about sex and HIV), and substance use. We also were interested in better understanding differences in clientele demographics and the formal and informal processes that were used by management and patrons to regulate sexual behavior and HIV risk.

The study included two bathhouses which, at the outset, were characterized by their management as having very different clientele: Bathhouse A clientele was seen as predominantly Caucasian, relatively young, affluent, and "out" with regard to sexuality. Bathhouse B was characterized as having a clientele that was predominantly ethnic/racial minority, more mixed in age and largely working class in economic background, with a greater proportion of closeted men (men who are not "out" or open about being gay or bisexual) than Bathhouse A. Though the number, location, and behavioral patterns of bathhouses evolve constantly, there were eight bathhouses and two sex clubs operating in Los Angeles County at the time we started collecting these data (1999). The two participating bathhouses were chosen because of their differing clientele demographics and their managers' willingness to commit to this formative research as well as to a subsequent epidemiological study. The differences in location and clientele in these two settings provide a useful example for examining how the specific behavioral pattern that develops in a setting may be related to the patterns of risk behavior there and the considerations needed in developing setting-specific interventions to reduce HIV risk behavior in bathhouses.

METHOD

Study staff conducted face-to-face, qualitative interviews (Goldbaum et al., 1996) with individuals who worked at the two bathhouses and, subsequently, with bathhouse patrons, or "key participants" between November 1999 and April 2000. Respondents were selected using a purposive nonprobability method (Kuzel, 1992; Patton, 1990). For both the bathhouse worker and patron samples, we attempted to obtain a broad cross-section of perspectives, experiences, ages, and racial/ethnic groups. Bathhouse workers were referred to study staff by the bathhouse management. Bathhouse patrons were recruited in a number of ways, including referrals from bathhouse management or outreach workers, promotional activities such as posting of flyers in the bathhouses, and by study staff directly approaching patrons during their visit.

Participants

The participants included 16 bathhouse workers and 24 bathhouse patrons. The 16 bathhouse workers included 2 managers, 8 staff (cashiers, cleaners, etc.), and 6 outreach workers who were employed by local community-based HIV prevention organizations. Seven workers from Bathhouse A were interviewed and 9 workers from Bathhouse B were interviewed. These interviews provided a staff perspective and an overview of bathhouse operations. The patrons included 13 from Bathhouse A, 10 from Bathhouse B, and 1 individual who did not identify with either bathhouse. This "unaffiliated" patron was excluded from further analysis of the data because of our interest in looking at possible differences between the two bathhouses. These interviews provided a first-hand description of the behavioral patterns and functions of the two Los Angeles-area bathhouses.

Characteristics of Participants

Workers. Sixteen bathhouse workers were interviewed. All of the bathhouse workers interviewed were male. Their average age was 34 (range = 21-52, s.d. = 8.2); 31.3% were white, 31.3% were Latino, 25% were African American, and 12.5% were unknown (missing data). The average education level was 12 years (high school equivalent). No data were collected on the sexual orientation of bathhouse worker respondents.

Patrons. Among the 23 bathhouse patrons interviewed, the majority at both bathhouses reported being primarily gay and the average age reported at both sites was in the upper-thirties. Of patron respondents at Bathhouse A, 84.7% were self-identified gay while 15.4% were self-identified as bisexual. The mean age of patron respondents at Bathhouse A was 36 (range = 22-45; s.d. = 8.6). Most of the patrons at Bathhouse A were Caucasian and reported having 4 or more years of college education. The racial/ethnic composition of patrons interviewed at Bathhouse A was 41.7% Caucasian, 33.3% Latino, 16.7% African American, 8.7% unknown, and 0% Asian/Pacific Islander.

Patrons interviewed from Bathhouse B were mostly African American or Latino, and reported having some college education. The racial/ethnic breakdown at Bathhouse B was 44.4% African American, 33.3% Latino, 11.1% Caucasian, and 11.1% Asian/Pacific Islander. At Bathhouse B, 88.9% self-identified as gay, 0% self-identified as bisexual, and 11.1% did not report a sexual identity. The mean age of patron respondents at Bathhouse B was 39 (range = 25-52, s.d. = 8.5).

Procedures

All qualitative research participants were enrolled after giving written, informed consent. The research protocol and consent forms were approved by the Los Angeles County-University of Southern California Institutional Review Board (IRB) and the Centers for Disease Control and Prevention (CDC) IRB. Four interviewers collected the qualitative data after they attended a standardized three-day training workshop and completed a series of practice interviews. The workshop focused on methods for conducting face-to-face, semi-structured interviews. The interviewers were self-identified gay or bisexual men, ages 22 to 38, who had prior work experience in clinical or community outreach settings.

Interviews were conducted at either of the bathhouses or at another mutually agreed-upon place that provided a quiet and private environment (e.g., community-based agencies, homes). The interviews were audio taped and transcribed verbatim into a computer database for analysis of qualitative data (CDC-EZ-Text, version 3.06C; Carey et al., 1998). The study coordinator performed quality assurance checks by comparing the transcribed interview documents with the tapes. The tapes were destroyed after quality assurance was completed. The interviews were confidential and no names or other identifying information were included in the transcripts. Respondents were compensated $35 for travel or other out-of-pocket costs related to participation.

The respondents' beliefs, opinions, and behaviors described in the transcripts were assigned thematic codes by two CDC research staff in Atlanta who had not been involved in the collection of data. They defined codes in a codebook (MacQueen et al., 1998; Miles et al., 1994). Coding of the text passages was done using CDC EZ-Text, version 3.06C (Carey et al., 1998). To ensure consistent, thorough, and replicable coding between the two coders, a series of inter-coder reliability checks were undertaken, which used methods recommended for analysis of semi-structured qualitative data (Carey et al., 1996). Final intercoder reliability was excellent: 338 of the 396 codes (85.4 percent) defined in the final codebook used for the bathhouse patron database had Cohen's *kappas* ≥ 0.90, and 283 of these 338 codes had a *kappa = 1.00* indicating complete agreement between the two coders. Similar high intercoder reliability was attained for the bathhouse workers (83.3% of the codes had a *kappa > 0.90*). After completing this process, remaining coding disagreements were resolved by the two coders discussing their divergences and arriving at a consensus for the final coding of the entire data set.

Coding was iterative and began with a content analysis of the qualitative interview questions and probes, with subsequent adjustments based on codes that emerged from subsequent content analysis of the interviews and reconciliation of these codes between the two raters (MacQueen et al., 1998). Themes were also allowed to emerge from the initial coding of the data (Buroway et al., 1991). Where visual inspection of the data suggested differences between the bathhouses, themes were identified and labeled. Axial coding was used to organize themes into concepts that clustered together around six major categories (Strauss, 1987). Illustrative quotes were obtained for each bathhouse site to demonstrate differences and similarities across sites. No statistical tests for significance were conducted because the "n" for participants (patrons and workers) was very small (23 and 16, respectively). Bathhouses were coded as A and B to protect the confidentiality of these institutions. Interviewees were given pseudonyms to ensure confidentiality and these pseudonyms are used in the reporting of results here.

Measures

The interviews used a semi-structured format, with a standard protocol of open-ended questions and probes. The worker and patron interviews were parallel in content and queried respondents regarding the clientele of the individual bathhouses (e.g., demographics; characteristics of popular patrons; popular times for patronage; the normal routine for bathhouse patrons; reasons for attending bathhouses; common sexual practices; verbal and nonverbal negotiation of sex; drug and alcohol use; condom use; disclosure of HIV status by patrons; and a number of questions regarding HIV counseling and testing). The results of the worker interviews informed development of specific items for the patron interview questionnaire, although topical areas of the two protocols were similar. The interviews were pretested with 4 gay-identified men working on different research projects.

RESULTS

As stated previously, our purpose was to explore differences in the perceived and actual behavioral patterns of patrons at these two bathhouses in order to better understand how HIV prevention interventions may need to be targeted to specific bathhouse sites. We analyzed how the sexual norms, rules, and risk behaviors varied between Bathhouse A and Bathhouse B. In our analysis, we found that the patrons' proximity to fellow patrons and to the activities occurring behind closed doors at each bathhouse allowed for a richer characterization of the bathhouse clientele. For this reason, we have focused our presentation of results on the patron interviews with an occasional reference to the worker data set. Six categorical themes emerged that indicated differences: perceptions of bathhouse clientele, attraction to particular sites, bathhouse sexual practices (perceived and self-reported sexual activities and condom use), communication about sex and HIV status, bathhouse rules, and perceived substance use practices among patrons. First, we will highlight the similarities across each site vis-à-vis these themes. We illustrate differences in how these categorical themes played out in our descriptions of each bathhouse site below in order to provide a sense of behavioral and demographic patterns reported at each bathhouse. A summary of similarities and differences between behavioral and demographic patterns reported at the two sites concludes this results section.

Similarities Between Bathhouse A and Bathhouse B

The typical routines of patrons were consistent across sites. Such routines are characterized by patrons renting lockers or rooms, walking around to look for sex, and engaging in other secondary activities (e.g., socializing, taking showers, and using the spa or steam room). However, all patrons from both bathhouses perceived that they and other patrons were there primarily to have sex. Some patron respondents mentioned other motives such as "blowing off steam," being in a "gay" environment and relaxing with acquaintances. Seeking multiple sexual partners, either successively or simultaneously, was believed to be very common in both bathhouses.

Sexual and condom using behaviors. Most patrons perceived that fellow patrons were less likely to use condoms for oral sex versus anal sex in both bathhouses (indeed, condoms were rarely reported to be used for oral sex). Patron interviewees also self-reported being more likely to use condoms for anal sex than oral sex. When asked how they decide to use condoms, the most common response among all patrons interviewed was that the participant let his partner decide whether or not condoms would be used.

Communication about sex and HIV. Patron respondents at each bathhouse were likely to state that indirect, nonverbal communication about sexual interests was more common than direct communication. Paul, a patron from Bathhouse B, said:

> A lot of times, there is not a lot of verbal communications . . . it is common in my experience that people would try to start doing something . . . they would try to start penetrating you . . . or I will start licking a guy's anus . . . guys know what you are trying to do and if they don't like it they will just gently stop you . . . just put their hand on your head or on your penis or your hand . . . "

Many patrons interviewed shared their observation that men who like to receive anal sex will lie on their stomachs on their beds with the door open and wait for someone they like to enter the room; alternatively, men who prefer to be the insertive partner will lie on their backs and wait for a partner. At the same time, the majority of each group stated that direct verbal communication and eye contact were also common forms of communication. For instance, Phil from Bathhouse A shared how he communicates with potential sexual partners:

> I usually say, um . . . Hi . . . my name is . . . and they will tell me their name and then I can tell if they are still interested . . . then I will . . . give them a compliment and they will usually like look at my body and then . . . do you have a room? . . . and we will go somewhere.

While a few patrons stated that some direct verbal communication about sex happens, their perceptions of how other patrons communicate at both bathhouses emphasized indirect communication.

The majority of patrons interviewed at both bathhouses stated that other patrons also tend to make assumptions about HIV status based on top/bottom roles ("top" refers to being the insertive partner in anal sex and "bottom" refers to being the receptive partner). For instance, George, a patron from Bathhouse A stated:

> I don't think either of them really think about it, but if anyone's going to think about, especially not a top. Because if they're going to be doing the fucking they're going to think, you know, my chances of being infected are, are little. Bottoms, it might cross their mind more.

This "top/bottom" myth that tops are not HIV infected was consistent across sites.

Bathhouse rules. Patrons at each site perceived management's enforcement of bathhouse rules similarly. For instance, both sites were perceived by most patrons to include rules such as "No Public Sex" and "Use Condoms and Lube (encouragement of safer sex)"; these rules were perceived by some at each site to be enforced by signs and by employees who patrolled public areas. At both sites, a smaller proportion of patrons also perceived that there were no rules. Interviews with workers at both bathhouses reveal very similar perceptions of the rules compared with interviews with patrons (no public sex, encouragement of safer sex, and no substance use), with the exception that the majority of workers at both sites also stated that bathhouse management enforced rules by providing information such as posters about safe sex and testing information (whereas only one patron mentioned these posted materials).

Substance use. Patrons at both sites indicated that other patrons use poppers (inhalants such as amyl or butyl nitrate) and many also indicated that substances were used to relax and enjoy sex more. Patron respondents also perceived that fellow bathhouse patrons sometimes came to the bathhouse already intoxicated either from a party or the bars. Almost all patrons at each bathhouse said that substance use contributes to unsafe sexual behaviors.

Bathhouse A

Perceptions of bathhouse clientele demographics. Our descriptions of Bathhouse A and Bathhouse B reveal unique characteristics of each site regarding clientele and behavioral patterns that cluster around the six categorical themes. Workers at Bathhouse A most frequently said that their patrons were openly gay or bisexual. Bathhouse A workers also described their clientele as white or representing a variety of racial/ethnic backgrounds. Patrons at Bathhouse A were also most likely to state that other patrons were from diverse racial/ethnic backgrounds (without one race/ethnicity being predominant). Chris, a patron respondent, described other patrons at Bathhouse A:

> R: Well, like I came here on a Tuesday on a Latin-night and it was mostly Latinos, so it usually fits the bill pretty well. Sometimes there's a mix and sometimes there's more Caucasians than not.
> I: And do you think most of these guys would describe themselves as gay, or either like straight guys, closeted guys?
> R: Mostly gay, I've met a couple of bi ones, I've met like one that just came here before he came home from work to his wife.

This assessment of patrons at Bathhouse A typifies perceptions at this site.

Communication about sex and HIV. As stated above, patrons reported similar patterns of indirect (nonverbal) communication about sex at both sites. HIV status is also never or rarely directly discussed at either site as reported by most patron respondents, but patrons from Bathhouse A and B reported different assumptions about how other patrons perceive the HIV status of sexual partners. Among patrons interviewed from Bathhouse A, the most common perceived assumptions regarding HIV status of sexual partners were: (1) other patrons are all HIV+ and (2) other patrons are HIV-negative. Some Bathhouse A patrons perceived that other patrons either make no assumptions about HIV status or make assumptions about HIV status based on criteria other than reported HIV status.

Patrons' attraction to site. Patrons at Bathhouse A most often mentioned being drawn to that site by good-looking, muscular patrons. For instance, one Bathhouse A patron, David, stated that he liked, "Attractive, butt, no fat people, or my frame, or nice looking (men)." Some of the patrons at Bathhouse A also said that they were in the frame of mind to party (use recreational substances) when they came to the bathhouse.

Sexual and condom using behaviors. Patrons at Bathhouse A perceived that both oral sex and anal sex were very common practices on site. While the practice of using condoms more frequently for anal sex compared to oral sex was consistent across bathhouses, we found that patrons at Bathhouse A were perceived to be very likely to be seeking anal sex at that site. Some of the patrons interviewed there said that they did not like using condoms. For instance, Rick, a patron from Bathhouse A, said that, "Having to fucking deal with them (condoms) right in the middle of a passionate moment, and everything is (discouraging)." Most patron respondents at Bathhouse A also reported that other patrons there use substances in order to lower inhibitions and to enjoy sex.

Substance use. Rafael, a patron interviewed from Bathhouse A, shared his perception of why patrons use substances such as crystal, ecstasy, and poppers in order to be uninhibited and enjoy sex at Bathhouse A:

> I: Approximately what percent of people would you say have sex here at the bathhouse while under the influence of drugs or alcohol?
> R: I'd say eighty-five to ninety.
> I: Okay, why do you think they use that, the drugs or the alcohol? . . .
> R: Uninhibited.
> I: Like less, like they feel more open?
> R: They're just more relaxed and they're not so conscious of, how can I put it, they're not in cue with what's really important, it just comes as a fantasy thing here, and it's just for fun and to let, you know.

Patron respondents reported substance use at both bathhouses; yet the use of ecstasy, cocaine, GHB, and crystal methamphetamine was frequently reported by patron interviewees at Bathhouse A. At the same time, when probed, most patrons interviewed at Bathhouse A cited rules about not using drugs and alcohol; many also stated that patrons at Bathhouse A were kicked out if they did not follow rules. If the perceptions of patron interviewees at Bathhouse A are true, clientele (predominantly from diverse racial/ethnic backgrounds and gay) there may be engaging in high risk anal sex activities under the influence of multiple substances.

Bathhouse B

Bathhouse clientele demographics. When asked to describe their patrons, some workers at Bathhouse B stated that their clientele were alternatively married, straight, gay, bisexual or closeted. Workers at Bathhouse B were most likely to state that black and Latino MSM patronize their establishment. The Bathhouse B patrons' perceptions of the race/ethnicity of other patrons were similar to the workers' perceptions, i.e., they were also most likely to state that patrons there were Latino or black. Many patrons at Bathhouse B also mentioned that some portion of fellow patrons there were married or closeted. For example, consider Mario's response, a patron interviewed at Bathhouse B, when asked about the typical patrons there:

> I: Okay. And race, how would you describe the customer's race here?
> R: I'd say a high percentage of them are Black, next would be probably Latinos, and probably less white people . . .
> I: Okay. How would you describe the customer's degree of outness, you know, in terms of are they gay identified or are they more closeted, or is it a mix?
> R: It's a mix, I would say it's a mix . . . I would say maybe at least seventy percent are totally gay, and probably out and the rest are probably like closeted.

The behavior of the closeted men at Bathhouse B is perceived by a comment by Jose, also a patron at Bathhouse B, "Closet case men, they feel they're at risk if they're going to give their name or their telephone number. They want to forget, they want to remain anonymous."

Communication about sex and HIV. As mentioned above, HIV status is never or rarely discussed at either site as reported by most patrons at Bathhouse A and B. Bathhouse B patrons were most likely to report that their fellow patrons make no assumptions about HIV status or that other patrons are HIV+. Some perceived that patrons make assumptions based on other criteria of potential sexual partners, whereas assuming that other patrons were HIV-negative was not a common theme among patrons interviewed from Bathhouse B.

Patrons' attraction to the bathhouse. Patrons at Bathhouse B mentioned multiple reasons (e.g., convenient location, erotic videos, or other sexual scenes such as exhibitionism) as the primary feature that attracted them to that bathhouse. For instance, Paul shared the following reasons for being attracted to Bathhouse B:

> I: Are there particular scenes or kinds of partners here that make the bathhouse attractive to you?
> R: Yes . . . um going back to how the men are more real . . . they are not the West Hollywood young boys with the perfect bodies . . . but they ah . . . they don't even have to be overweight . . . they just have to have a regular body where they don't go to the gym much or at all . . . um . . . now and then I like a big portly guy to have sex with . . . maybe a taller guy.

The interviews with Bathhouse B patrons revealed a sense that patrons go there for a variety of reasons including to meet "regular" types of guys.

Sexual and condom using behaviors. Most patrons did not say that anal sex was common at Bathhouse B among other patrons. When asked when they use condoms, patrons at Bathhouse B most frequently stated that they always use condoms for anal intercourse. For instance, one patron of Bathhouse B named Jeff shared his condom using behaviors there:

> I: How do you decide when to use them (condoms) for particular acts or partners? And you say you always use them.
> R: Yea . . . I always use them for anal sex.

Bathhouse B patrons tended to state that they always use condoms for anal sex and none said that they hated condoms or never used them.

Substance use. Bathhouse patron respondents reported that substances were used at both bathhouse locations. However, the type of substances used varied by site. Marijuana and poppers were the most frequently reported substances used at Bathhouse B. James, a patron interviewed at Bathhouse B, shared this perspective of substance use behaviors there:

> R: What I think? I mean like I know like some people in here use poppers and I'm not sure . . .
> I: Okay, like the percentage, what would you guess?
> R: Yea. I'd probably use the poppers, thirty percent, thirty percent, but maybe forty . . .
> I: Okay. And what about other drugs? How about alcohol? What percentage of people . . .
> R: They do, I've seen people bring like beer or whatever, or mixed drinks in like juice bottles. And I'd probably say maybe twenty percent of them that come here . . .
> I: What about other drugs like crystal meth, marijuana . . .
> R: I've never seen, I've seen like marijuana, like on the roof on occasions. I've seen guys when they smoke a little weed. I'd probably say probably twenty, twenty percent of some the guys that come here . . .
> R: Well a lot of guys say the poppers; you know, turn them on and get their dick harder. And they say it makes them go longer, so they, you know, get the little bottle of poppers and they sniff that.

If patrons and workers interviewed at Bathhouse B are correct, the clientele there is primarily Latino and black and quite diverse in terms of sexual orientation and body type; some may also be closeted or married men. According to patrons interviewed, anal sex does happen at Bathhouse B, but oral sex is more common.

Summary of Behavioral and Demographic Similarities and Differences

Similarities and differences were apparent between the behavioral patterns of the patrons from the two bathhouses. Similarities included the perception that patrons were more likely to use condoms for anal sex compared to oral sex; the perception that nonverbal communication about sex is the most common method for showing sexual interest and negotiating sex; the perception that HIV status was mostly not discussed with sexual partners; and perceptions that both bathhouses had rules prohibiting sex in public places and substance use in the bathhouses, that were inconsistently enforced. Patrons at both bathhouses described a top/bottom typology for making assumptions about the HIV status of their sexual partners in which tops were perceived as being less likely to contract HIV during unprotected sex. When asked how they decide to use condoms (if at all), the most common response of patrons at both sites was they allowed their partners to make that decision. Minimal verbal communication tends to be the rule in initiating sexual activities at both bathhouses and all decision-making about what happens during a sexual encounter may be determined by non-verbal cues.

Differences were noted regarding reports of bathhouse rules. Although the patrons and workers interviewed stated that rules regarding safer sex and substance use were present at each location, the degree to which such rules were noticed and enforced varied within and across the bathhouses examined. For instance, bathhouse workers claimed that safer sex information in the form of posters and other promotional materials were prevalent, but patrons did not identify these materials. While some patrons did state that management expelled offenders of the "no substance use" rules at one site (Bathhouse A), the efficacy and consistency of bathhouse "rule" enforcement across bathhouses remains unclear. Some patrons even stated that no rules existed. Overall, there is varying awareness of the bathhouses' efforts to regulate sexual behavior and substance use and these efforts have unknown degrees of success.

Important differences in norms and rules guiding sexual practices at each site were also identified. Bathhouse B patrons and workers were likely to state that patrons were straight, bisexual, closeted, or married; patrons at Bathhouse B were commonly perceived as being primarily Latino and African American. Patrons at Bathhouse A perceived their fellow patrons to be very interested in anal sex and were likely to state a dislike for condoms as the reason for not using them. Patrons at Bathhouse B were commonly perceived to make no assumptions about the HIV status of their sexual partners, while patrons at Bathhouse A were likely to assume that their partners were HIV-negative. Substance use was prevalent at both bathhouses. However, different substances were used at each site and patrons described more extensive substance use at Bathhouse A. Perhaps, as a consequence, patrons at Bathhouse A commonly cited both the rules and the enforcement of rules about substance use. The use of substances to lower inhibitions and enjoy sex was also a major theme reported by patrons at Bathhouse A.

DISCUSSION

This analysis suggests that differences exist between bathhouse behavioral risk patterns located within the same city. The differences between the sites examined here suggest that bathhouses are quite varied by a number of dimensions that may apply to such analyses of other bathhouses. Each site may promote a self-selection among patrons who organize around domains like race and ethnicity, body type of clientele (muscular or "regular"), the type of sex practiced by patrons, assumptions about HIV status, bathhouse rules and enforcement of rules, and the recreational drugs of choice used therein. Efforts to develop prevention strategies at bathhouses must take into account these differences. Due to these variations, approaches that work at one bathhouse may not be successful at another. The differences in substance use between Bathhouse A and Bathhouse B are one example. For example, interventions that address the on-site use of poppers and marijuana at Bathhouse B may not address Bathhouse A patrons' use of crystal methamphetamine and ecstasy.

These results reveal key considerations for developing prevention and harm reduction strategies responsive to specific HIV risk factors at particular bathhouse sites. The patrons describe patterns of sexual risk taking, lack of verbal communication, nondisclosure of HIV status, and frequent substance use among patrons regardless of the specific bathhouse location or racial/ethnic composition of its patrons. For instance, the top/bottom belief regarding HIV status of sexual partners described by patrons from both bathhouses suggests that bathhouse patrons may be making erroneous judgments about partner risk. The idea that men who are willing to engage in insertive anal sex with them are less at risk for HIV infection and are HIV-negative may be used as a rationale to practice unprotected sex without talking about HIV. The attribution of HIV status (rather than communication about it) may further increase opportunities for HIV transmission, particularly if patrons perceive their sexual partners to be HIV-negative when they are not. Such opportunities for HIV transmission may be more prevalent in bathhouses where patrons make more erroneous assumptions about HIV status.

These findings suggest that some bathhouses may be more risk-conducive than others. For instance, interviewees reported more perceived sexual risk behaviors (noncondom use, assumptions about HIV status, and substance use activities) at one of the sites. Such varied perceptions of norms regarding sexual practices, communication about sex and

HIV, substance use, and safer sex rules across bathhouses suggests that HIV transmission risks exist at varying levels and that patrons naïve to the norms driving sexual behavioral patterns at particular bathhouses may be at particular risk of HIV infection.

Patrons at both bathhouses observed sexual risk behaviors that are known to transmit HIV and other STDs among MSMs. Some patrons were perceived to be married, closeted, or bisexual at both sites; such perceptions were more evident in the perceptions of patrons at one of the sites. The implications for the female sexual partners of patrons from some sites may be more pressing than for other sites. If condoms are not being used for oral sex, as perceived by patron respondents at both bathhouses, then the opportunities for transmission of sexually transmitted diseases (STDs) are evident at both sites. Since communication about HIV status does not happen, it may also be true that communication about STDs does not happen. These themes highlight the importance of understanding the bathhouse environments and the roles they may play in the spread of sexually transmitted infections (such as the syphilis outbreak in Los Angeles County) to partners outside the bathhouse.

The assumption that bathhouses attract many MSM who do not identify as being gay and, therefore, offer unique access to hard-to-reach populations should be continually examined. Even among racial minorities interviewed, the majority of patrons identified as being gay. Patrons and workers interviewed stated that straight and bisexual men were active at both bathhouses, yet one of the sites appears to draw a larger proportion of clientele from such populations. These findings provide a starting point to better understand the nexus of sexual orientation, sexual behavior, and sexual risk activities among men who attend bathhouses and who do not identify as gay. These data also suggest further research questions regarding how, if at all, sexual risk behaviors are associated with race/ethnicity and class status.

The image of the good-looking, muscular type appeals to the patrons of Bathhouse A, while homoerotic videos and "regular" guys are important components of the erotic draw of Bathhouse B. Both features suggest potential means of reinforcing safer sex practices with patrons such as prevention strategies that incorporate idioms, themes and images from the repertoire of gay behavioral patterns. The explicit gay self-consciousness of these clubs might be the optimal basis for planning and implementing interventions. Still, little is known about what attracts closeted or bisexual men to particular bathhouses for sex with men. It is possible that they cluster themselves into sites that are less explicitly gay-identified where they can seek sexual fantasies with other men without associating themselves with an explicitly gay experience.

The use of recreational drugs by a substantial number of the men interviewed remains a perplexing challenge to encouraging sexual behaviors that promote enjoyment and maintain health. The differences between the recreational drugs of choice of patrons at the two sites suggest another example of self-selection that may be helpful in narrow casting interventions to promote harm reduction. If patrons use choice of drugs to cluster themselves into specific sites, then prevention strategies can be developed around particular patterns of drug use and related risky sexual behaviors. For example, if one bathhouse is characterized by patrons who use ecstasy, cocaine, GHB and crystal methamphetamine, then a combination of strongly enforced rules prohibiting use of these drugs, staff training in the symptoms of drug intoxication, and tailored marketing messages may impact unsafe behaviors driven by substance misuse. Given the unique odors associated with marijuana and poppers, a more aggressive and visible staff presence may positively impact these behaviors and how they interact with sexual risk activities in another bathhouse site. More research is needed to learn how substance use choices are associated with sexual risk behaviors within the context of bathhouses in order to further understand how sexual risk is differentiated by bathhouse sites.

The use of drugs and alcohol by patrons before entering both bathhouses remains a significant prevention challenge with no easy or apparent solution. The patrons' perceptions that their fellow patrons use substances, albeit different ones, at each site also highlight the potential for HIV risk behaviors across bathhouses. The finding that some patrons may be arriving at the bathhouses already intoxicated further supports the need to explore associations among sexual risk behaviors and the effects of alcohol and drugs on bathhouse patrons' sexual decision-making processes.

Bathhouses remain important sites for sexual exploration for significant numbers of men. Patrons may be perceived or actually be more likely to be straight, married, closeted, bisexual, or gay depending on the particular bathhouse being considered. However, all patrons seek to fulfill male-to-male sexual fantasies in settings that bill themselves as gay establishments. These data suggest that HIV interventions should seek to make use of the fantasy element by incorporating safer sex imagery into specific sexual scenes. Drawing on Kelly's work (Kelly et al., 1992), using popular patrons at Bathhouse A to diffuse safer sex messages into erotic scenes might be useful at Bathhouse A, while incorporating such messages in other sexual scenes (e.g., videos, sex shows, etc.) through the diffusion of innovations (Rogers, 2000) might be more useful at Bathhouse B.

This project demonstrates that qualitative studies of bathhouse sexual behavioral patterns are possible. However, there are limitations to this study. For instance, these data are based on self-reported sexual risk behaviors among a small sample that was not randomly selected. This study of bathhouse sexual behavioral patterns differs from those conducted in public sex environments because bathhouses are private businesses. As such, gatekeepers at particular bathhouses may limit access to participants. In the bathhouses we studied, public sex is not officially allowed. Although the rules at both establishments require that patrons have sex in rented rooms that are private, ethnographic research involving participant observation methodologies may yield more detailed information regarding the sexual and social structures of bathhouse sexual behavioral patterns. Such research may provide more information to determine if and where social diffusion interventions like Kelly's popular opinion leader model may work and which other interventions may be warranted for particular bathhouse sites.

The heuristic value of these findings is that HIV prevention programs targeting bathhouses must be tailored to unique sexual risk behavioral patterns. Differences may be detected among other bathhouses in the sexual behavioral pattern domains identified here. In all cases, these findings suggest that formative research should be conducted in each to inform targeted HIV prevention programs for individual bathhouse intervention sites. Given the solid position that bathhouses hold within gay sexual cultures, there is a compelling obligation to understand them and to use these unique environments to promote health and safety among their patrons.

ACKNOWLEDGMENTS

The authors wish to thank the bathhouse workers, patrons, and management for their participation, which made this study possible. Also essential to this study were the efforts of the interviewers, Craig King, Andy Diaz, Alex Truong, and David Bronstein; the qualitative data coders, Deborah Schwartz, Daphne Cobb, and Stephanie Macari; the data manager, Ilya Pearlman; and the LA study coordinator, Alan Brown. Helpful comments on earlier drafts of this manuscript were provided by Jim Carey, Ron Stall, George Ayala, and Uyen Bui. M. Summra Shariff provided essential support preparing the manuscript. Jim Carey also coordinated the interviewer training, along with Bryan Kim. In addition, Wes Ford, Bill Reidy, Mark Weber, and Linda Valleroy provided important input during the early stages of the study. Finally, Olga Grinstead, Dennis Osmond, Jay Paul and Greg Rebchook provided useful feedback on later drafts of the manuscript.

REFERENCES

Alexander, P. (1996). The bathhouses and brothels: Symbolic sites in discourse and practice. In E. G. Colter & W. Hoffman (Eds.), *Policing Public Sex: Queer Politics and the Future of AIDS Activism* (pp. 221-247). Boston: South End Press.

Bérubé, A. (1996). The history of gay bathhouses. In E. G. Colter & W. Hoffman (Eds.), *Policing Public Sex: Queer Politics and the Future of AIDS Activism* (pp. 187-219). Boston: South End Press.

Binson, D., Woods, W., Pollack, L., Paul, J., Stall, R., & Catania, J. (2001). Differential HIV in bathhouses and public cruising areas. *American Journal of Public Health, 91*(9), 1482-1486.

Buroway, M., Burton, A., Ferguson, A. A., Fox, K. J., Gamson, J., Cartrell, N., Hurst, L., Kurzman, C., Salzinger, L., Schiffman, J., & Ui, S. (1991). *Ethnography Unbound: Power and Resistance in the Modern Metropolis.* Berkeley: University of California Press.

Carey, J., Morgan, M., & Oxtoby, M. (1996). Inter-coder agreement in analysis of responses to open-ended interview questions: Examples from tuberculosis research. *Cultural Anthropology Methods Journal, 8*(3), 1-5.

Carey, J., Wenzel, P., Reilly, C., Sheridan, J., & Steinberg, J. (1998). Software for management and analysis of semistructured qualitative data sets. *Cultural Anthropology Methods Journal, 10*(1), 14-20.

CDC. (2001). Outbreak of syphilis among men who have sex with men–Southern California, 2000. *MMWR Weekly, 50*(07), 117-120.

Elwood, W., & Williams, N. (1998). Sex, drugs, and situation: Attitudes, drugs use, and sexual risk behaviors among men who frequent bathhouses. *Journal of Psychology & Human Sexuality, 10*(2), 23-45.

Goldbaum, G., Perdue, T. R., & Higgins, D. (1996). Non-gay-identifying men who have sex with men: Formative research results from Seattle, Washington. *Public Health Reports (Suppl. 1)*, 36-40.

HIV/AIDS Surveillance Report. (1999). Atlanta, GA: Centers for Disease Control and Prevention.

HIV/AIDS Surveillance Report. (2000). Atlanta, Georgia: Centers for Disease Control and Prevention.

Kelly, J., Lawrence, J. S., Stevenson, L., Hauth, A., Kalichman, S., Diaz, Y., Brasfield, T., Koob, J., & Morgan, M. (1992). Community AIDS/HIV risk reduction: The effects of endorsements by popular people in three cities. *American Journal of Public Health, 82*(11), 1483-1489.

Kuzel, A. (1992). Sampling in qualitative inquiry. In B. F. Crabtree, Miller, W. L. (Ed.), *Doing Qualitative Research* (pp. 31-44). Newbury Park, California: Sage.

MacQueen, K., McLellan, E., Kay, K., & Milstein, B. (1998). Codebook development for team-based qualitative analysis. *Cultural Anthropology Methods Journal, 10*(2), 31-36.

Miles, M., & Huberman, A. (1994). *Qualitative Data Analysis* (2nd ed.). Thousand Oaks, California: Sage.

Patton, M. (1990). *Qualitative Evaluation and Research Methods.* Newbury Park, California: Sage.

Richwald, G., Kyle, G., Gerber, M., Morisky, D., Kristal, A., & Friedland, J. (1988). Sexual activities in bathhouses in Los Angeles County: Implications for AIDS prevention education. *The Journal of Sex Research*, 169-181.

Rogers, E. M. (2000). Diffusion theory: A theoretical approach to promote community-level change. In J. I. Peterson & R. J. DiClemente (Eds.), *Handbook of HIV Prevention* (pp. 57-66). New York: Kluwer Academic.

Sey, K., & Harawa, N. (2001). *High-risk behavior among individuals diagnosed with acute/primary or recent HIV infection. HIV epidemiology program, Los Angeles, CA.* Paper presented at the 8th Conference in Retroviruses and Opportunistic Infections, Chicago, Illinois.

Shilts, R. (1987). *And The Band Played On: Politics, People, and the AIDS Epidemic.* New York: Penguin Books.

Stall, R., Hays, R., Waldo, C., Ekstrand, M., & McFarland, W. (2000). The Gay '90s: A review of research in the 1990s on sexual behavior and HIV risk among men who have sex with men. *AIDS, 14*(Suppl. 3), S1-S14.

Strauss, A. (1987). *Qualitative Analysis for Social Scientists.* New York: Cambridge University Press.

Wolitski, R., Valdiserri, R., Denning, P., & Levine, W. (2001). Are we headed for a resurgence of the HIV epidemic among men who have sex with men? *American Journal of Public Health, 91*(6), 883-888.

Contributors

Allan Bérubé is a MacArthur Fellow currently operating a bed and breakfast and writers' retreat in the Catskills. He is working on a history of gay men who worked as cooks and stewards on luxury ocean liners from the 1920s to the 1950s. He is the author of *Coming Out Under Fire: The History of Gay Men and Women in World War Two.*

Trista Bingham is Chief of the Seroepidemiology Unit at the Los Angeles County Department of Health, HIV Epidemiology Program. She is currently conducting epidemiological research to estimate HIV incidence rates and risk factors for infection among men who have sex with men (MSM) in a variety of settings, including bathhouses, STD clinics, HIV testing sites, and in community- and field-based settings in Los Angeles. Her current writing and analyses focus on the disproportionate burden of HIV among African American and Latino MSM compared to white MSM.

Diane Binson is an assistant adjunct professor in the Department of Medicine, Center for AIDS Prevention Studies, at the University of California San Francisco. Her research interests center on the contextual determinants of HIV-related sexual risk behavior among gay men, particularly men who go to public sex environments. She has written several articles related to bathhouses, sex clubs and public cruising areas, as well as on methodological issues related to assessing sexual behavior in surveys.

Bernard M. Branson is Chief of the HIV Diagnostics and Surveillance Methods section in the Division of HIV/AIDS Prevention, National Center for HIV, and TB Prevention at the Centers for Disease Control and Prevention. He is currently engaged in evaluations of rapid HIV tests and of other diagnostic techniques that are feasible for monitoring HIV and antiretroviral therapy in resource-poor settings. He has pub-

http://www.haworthpress.com/store/product.asp?sku=J082
© 2003 by The Haworth Press, Inc. All rights reserved.
10.1300/J082v44n34_11

lished several papers on operational research related to HIV counseling and testing.

Scott Burris is a professor at Temple University Beasley School of Law and Associate Director of the Center for Law and the Public's Health at Georgetown and Johns Hopkins Universities. His research focuses on the influence of law on public health.

Miguel A. Chion is a research and evaluation specialist in the Research and Evaluation Core at AIDS Project Los Angeles. He is currently engaged in evaluating several prevention interventions to reduce risk of HIV and sexually transmitted infections (STI) among young men, men who have sex with men and men who have sex with men and women.

Christopher Disman is an independent scholar in San Francisco. He has also researched patrol organizations that worked in San Francisco from the 1970s to the 1990s to prevent and intervene in homophobic street violence, and he has published one article about them in *Our Stories*, the newsletter of the Gay, Lesbian, Bisexual, Transgender Historical Society of Northern California. He has written another article about the patrols which is under consideration for the *Journal of the History of Sexuality*.

Gary M. Goldbaum is Chronic Disease and Injury Control Officer for Public Health–Seattle and King County and Associate Professor in the School of Public Health and Community Medicine at the University of Washington. He is currently engaged in studies of new technology to estimate the incidence of HIV infection. He has published several papers on behavioral risks associated with HIV and community level interventions to prevent HIV.

Michael J. Helquist is currently writing an historical novel set in the early 20th century with several characters defining their sexual identities in the midst of great cultural change. He is retired from his position as Director of the AIDS Health Communication Project, a U.S. Government program to assist developing countries with AIDS prevention. He has edited several books on health communication and AIDS mental health issues and was one of the first journalists to cover AIDS.

Richard A. Jenkins is a behavioral scientist in the Division of HIV/AIDS Prevention at the Centers for Disease Control and Prevention in Atlanta,

GA. He has been involved in community studies of HIV risk, behavioral aspects of HIV vaccine trials, and cross-cultural HIV prevention research. He is currently involved in studies of behavioral factors related to recent HIV infection and research regarding the use of behavioral data in HIV public policy.

Lee E. Klosinski is Director of Programs at AIDS Project Los Angeles. In addition to directing all client service, education and media and marketing programs, he has been involved in diverse research and interventions focusing on commercial sex venues.

Ann Kurth is an epidemiology STD Fellow at the University of Washington Center for AIDS and STDs. She is trained as a nurse-midwife and has 15 years of experience with sexual health research and practice in hospital, clinic, community-based, and public health agency settings. Her current research includes an audio computer-assisted self-interviewing sexual risk assessment study involving 600 clients of the Seattle public STD Clinic.

Matt G. Mutchler is the manager of Research and Evaluation at AIDS Project Los Angeles. He has conducted community level studies of HIV risk behaviors among multiple populations. Dr. Mutchler is forging an applied research agenda and is currently involved in investigating HIV prevention, substance use, and treatment issues among HIV-positive individuals. He manages a staff responsible for HIV-related program evaluations and evaluation trainings in community-based settings across Los Angeles County.

Rick Osmon is a realtor in San Francisco. He writes for his business and occasionally for local fundraising campaigns.

Gina M. Secura is an epidemiologist in the Division of HIV/AIDS Prevention, National Center for HIV/STD/TB Prevention, Centers for Disease Control and Prevention. She is currently conducting research on HIV and STD prevalence and associated risk behaviors among young minority women, young men who have sex with men, and men who attend bathhouses. She has published papers on HIV/STD prevalence and risk behaviors among young men who have sex with men.

Freya Spielberg is an assistant professor in the Department of Family Medicine and The Center for AIDS and STDs at the University of Washington in Seattle. In her research, she has had 15 years of experience evaluating new HIV testing technologies, and for the past 6 years has been conducting studies to identify more acceptable and effective HIV counseling and testing strategies to overcome barriers to testing among people at high risk, including men who have sex with men (MSM) in bathhouse venues. She is currently engaged in several studies to reduce risk of HIV and sexually transmitted infections (STI) among substance using populations and MSM.

Daniel P. Tracy lives, works, and loves in San Francisco. He is currently employed by the University of California San Francisco where he works on two epidemiological research studies, one looking at oral sex and HIV transmission and the other at hepatitis C prevalence amongst prison populations. He also facilitates support groups for HIV-negative men who are specifically concerned about their risks of becoming infected with HIV.

Robert W. Wood is Director, HIV/AIDS Control Program, Public Health–Seattle and King County and Associate Professor of Medicine and of Health Services (adjunct) at the University of Washington. Dr. Wood was the Seattle Principal Investigator for the CDC's AIDS Community Demonstration Project and for NIDA's National AIDS Demonstration Research. He is currently PI of Seattle's Viral Hepatitis Integration Project. He has written on HIV/AIDS clinical care, epidemiology, and prevention.

William J. Woods is an assistant adjunct professor in the Department of Medicine, Center for AIDS Prevention Studies, at the University of California San Francisco. He is currently engaged in several prevention intervention trials to reduce risk of HIV and sexually transmitted infections among young men leaving prison and men who have sex with men. He has published several papers related to HIV/STI prevention in bathhouses and sex clubs.

Index

Abrams, Don, 91,110
Abrams, Harry, 82
Academic literature, gay bathhouses
    in, 56-57
Agnost, George, 87-88,96,97
AIDS (Acquired Immune Deficiency
    Syndrome), 3. *See also* HIV
    (human immunodeficiency virus)
    awareness, in gay bathhouses,
        159-161
    awareness, in San Francisco
        bathhouses, 78-79
    early aspects of, in San Francisco,
        76-78
    prevention of, in gay bathhouses,
        161-164
    San Francisco Chronicle's stories
        about, 82-85
    San Francisco Department of Public
        Health's evidence on, 99-101
    spread of, and gay bathhouses, 8,9
    suggestions for bathhouses to halt
        spread of, 50-53
Altman, Dennis, 85,113
Andrews, Rick, 91
And the Band Played On (Shilts), 72,
    75,76
Animals bathhouse, 93,94,116
Arcara v. Cloud Books Inc., 144,145

Barracks, 40
Bathhouse owners, health
    professionals and, 3
Bathhouses. *See* Gay bathhouses;
    Sex-facilitating businesses
    (SFBs)

Bay Area Physicians for Human
    Rights (BAPHR), 79,97,
    98,101
Bay Area Reporter (B.A.R.), 86,
    105-106
Bayer, Ronald, 100,107,132
Bérubé, Allan, 33-53,74,75-76,243
Bingham, Trista, 221-242,243
Binson, Diane, 1-21,23-31,55-70,243
Bookstores, 184. *See also* Sex-facilitating
    businesses (SFBs)
    First Amendment and, 144-145
    prevention education by, 180-181
    in San Francisco, 178-184
Bottom/top myth, and HIV status, 230
Bowers v. Hardwick, 115,144
Branson, Bernard M., 203-220,
    243-244
Britt, Harry, 75,82,83,86,88,93
Broadway Books, Inc. v. Roberts, 141,
    142
Brown, Willie, 39,98
Bulldog Baths, 40
Burris, Scott, 131-151,244
Burtle, Meriel, 112

Caen, Herb, 83
Caldron, 93
Campbell, Bobbi, 89,97,99
Carfagni, Arthur, 99
Catacombs, 92-93
Chion, Miguel A., 221-242,244
Circle J Club, 184-185
*City News and Novelty, Inc. v. City of
    Waukesha,* 136

City of Colorado Springs v. 2354 Inc.,
    136
City of New York v. New St. Mark's Baths, 142
Civil liberties, closure of bathhouses
    and, 86
Closure policies, 3,16
    civil liberties and, 86
    courts and, 132-133
    early San Francisco, 46-49
    social/financial costs of, 49-50
Club Baths, 93
Club San Francisco, 93
Club Turkish Baths, 38,39
Coalition for Healthy Sex, 12
Collaborations, 3
Collaborative policy, 11-16
    institutional context for, 11-12
    physical settings for, 12-13
Collins, Daniel, 105,114
Commercial sex environments (CSEs), 4
Community based organizations
    (CBOs), 3
Conant, Marcus, 83,91,110
Concurrency, 9
Consenting-Adults Bill (California), 98
Counseling. *See* HIV (human
        immunodeficiency virus)
        counseling and testing
Curran, James, 82,83

Damron Address Book, 58
Dana case (New York), 145
Darrow, William, 100
Dave's Baths, 39,40
Denver Principles, 77
Disman, Christopher, 71-129,244
Doe v. City of Minneapolis, 144
Domains of bathhouse environments,
    27-28

Echenberg, Dean, 100
Ehrlich, Dorothy, 95

Ellwest Stereo Theater, Inc. v. Bonner,
    136,143-144,144,146-147
Enlow, Roger, 111
Environments, of gay bathhouses,
        studying, 6-10,24-25
Epidemiological studies, of gay
        bathhouses, 56-57
Eradication policy, 10-11
Ethnographic studies, of gay
        bathhouses, 56

Fannin, Shirley, 111
Fantasy environments, 40
Feinstein, Dianne, 82,88,93,103,104,
        114,116. *See also* San
        Francisco, Ca.
    community responses to police
        surveillance of bathhouses,
        94-96
    orders police surveillance of
        bathhouses, 93-94
    position of, on closure of baths, 90
    position of, on Dan White, 96
Feldman, Mark, 77
Ferels, Jim, 108
Films, about bathhouses, 40
First Amendment, bookstore and
        theater cases and, 144-145
Fitzgerald, Frances, 102
Friedman-Kein, Alvin, 78
FW/PBS, Inc. v. City of Dallas, 136

Gain, Charles, 39
Gaspar, Louis, 78
Gay bathhouses, 2. *See also* HIV
        (human immunodeficiency
        virus) counseling
    and testing; San Francisco, Ca.; Sex
        clubs
    in academic literature, 56-57
    advantages of, 37
    AIDS awareness in, 159-161

AIDS prevention in, 161-164
alternative counseling strategies
  for, 205-206
amenities in, 169-171
developing prevention
  partnerships to, 215-216
differences in behavior of
  patrons between, 224-225
discussion of study results
    for, 237-240
methodology for studying,
    225-228
study results for, 228-237
early history of, 34-36
environmental domains of,
  27-28
environments of, 6-10
as erotic environment, 155-159
facilitative role, for men having
  larger numbers of partners, 9
health education in, 24
HIV transmission and, 9-10
individual and private sex in,
  165-169
personal conclusions about,
  171-173
personal recommendations for,
  173-175
person-environment theoretical
  model of, 25-27
preparing for HIV counseling
  and testing in, 206-207
prevention policy and, 6
for promoting health education
  and prevention programs, 24
public and group sex in, 162-165
and public sex environments,
  4-6
raids on, 41-46
rapid testing for HIV in, 207,
  213,215-216
as resource for promoting safe
  sex, 51-52
review of effectiveness of
  interventions for, 29-30

role of, and sexual behavior, 223
San Francisco Department of
  Public Health's evidence on,
  99-101
sex in, 7-8
social climate of, 26,27-28
spread of AIDS and, 8,9
stages of early, 36
structural interventions for,
  28-29
study enumerating
  discussion of, 66-68
  methodology for, 58-61
  results for, 61-66
studying environments of, 24-25
suggestions for, to halt spread of
  AIDS, 50-53
as venues for prevention
  interventions, 205
Gay press, 41
Glory holes, 40
Goldbaum, Gary M., 203-220,244
Griswold v. Connecticut, 143
Group sex, in gay bathhouses, 162-165
Gyms, gay, 4

Harvey Milk Lesbian & Gay
  Democratic Club, 13
5H CLUB, 192
Health departments, 3
Health education, gay bathhouses for
  promoting, 24
Health professionals, bathhouse
  owners and, 3
Helquist, Michael, 77,87,101,104,
  153-175,177-201,244
Highly active antiretroviral therapy
  (HAART), 222
HIV Alternative Testing Strategies
  (HATS), 205-206
HIV (human immunodeficiency virus).
  See also AIDS (Acquired
  Immune Deficiency
  Syndrome)

incidence rates for, 222
role of gay bathhouses, and
    transmission of, 9-10
top/bottom myth, and status of, 230
HIV (human immunodeficiency virus)
    counseling and testing. *See
    also* Gay bathhouses
    clients of, 209-211
    keys to success for, 217
    logistics of, 211-215
    and men who have sex with men,
        204-205
    preparing for, 206-207
    staffing for, 208
    techniques for offering, 208-209
Hongisto, Richard, 97
Horstman, William, 99
Hughes, Sally Smith, 87,101
Human Rights Commission (San
    Francisco), 101-102

Individual sex, in gay bathhouses,
    165-169
Institutional context, for collaborative
    policy, 11-12

Jack-off clubs, 192-197. *See also* Sex
    clubs
    future directions for, 197-199
Jack's Baths, 38,39
    in 1930s and 1940s, 47
Jaguar Bookstore, 184
Jenkins, Richard A., 221-242,244-245
Jones, Bill, 93
Jordan, Frank, 117
Judicial fact-finding, 139-142

Kinsella, James, 109
Klosinski, Lee E., 221-242,245
Kraus, Bill, 86,98
Kurth, Ann, 203-220,245

Law
    as education, 148
    as effective regulatory tool, 148
    politics and, 147
    public sex and, 142-146
    sex-facilitating business and, 133
Leap, William, 117
Liberty Baths, 41
    closure of, 92
    raid on, 39
Lifelong AIDS Alliance, 206
Littlejohn, Larry
    community responses to petition of,
        86-87
    debate with Mervyn Silverman and,
        79-82
    dropping of petition by, 92
    petition of, 85-86
Lorch, Paul, 95
Lourea, David, 112

McBride, Laurie, 108
McKusick, Leon, 99
Mass, Lawrence, 78
Masturbation, 40
Maupin, Armistead, 74-75
Men who have sex with men (MSM)
    HIV counseling and testing for,
        204-205
    risk behavior and transmission for,
        222-223
Midler, Bette, 40
Migden, Carole, 86
Milk, Harvey, 95
*Mitchell v. Commission on Adult Entertain-
    ment Establishment*, 146
Moos, Rudolf, 25-28
Morin, Steve, 99
Moscone, George, 95
Mount Morris Baths, 12
Movies. *See* Films; Theaters
*Movie & Video World v. Board of
    Commissioners of Palm
    Beach County*, 141

Mullins, William, 110-111
Murray, Stephen, 102
Mutchler, Matt G., 221-242,245

National Gay and Lesbian Task Force
    (NGLTF), closure of
    bathhouses and, 89-90
New York City, NY, public policies
    for bathhouses in, 12-13
North West AIDS Foundation
    (NWAF), 206
Nuisance law, 137

O'Connell, John, 99
"Open-booth" cases, 136
Open-booth ordinances
    challenges to, 140
    litigation over, 138
OraQuick rapid finger-stick test,
    207,213-214
Orgy rooms, 39
Osmon, Rick, 87,101,104,153-175,
    177-201,245
Owen, Bob, 104

Palace Baths, 38,39
Palko v. Connecticut, 144
Paris Adult Theatre I v. Slayton,
    143,144
Payne, Kenneth, 102
People v. Owen et al., 109-112,116
People With AIDS (PWA), 77
    closure of baths and, 89
Peretti, Tom, 91
Person-environment theory, 25-27,30
Police power, 137
Politics, law and, 147
Prevention education
    in bookstores, 180-181
    in safe sex clubs, 193
    in sex clubs, 190-191
    in theaters, 187

Prevention interventions
    developing partnerships with
        bathhouses for, 215-216
    gay bathhouses and, 205
Prevention policies, gay baths and, 6
Prevention programs, gay bathhouses
    for promoting, 24
Privacy, right, of, and sex-facilitating
    businesses, 132
Private sex, in gay bathhouses,
    165-169
Proposition 64,115-116
Public health departments
    in New York City, 12-13
    in San Francisco, 12-13
Public health policy, 10
    collaborative policy, 11-16
    eradication policy, 10-11
    services and, 13-16
Public sex
    in gay bathhouses, 162-165
    legal doctrine and, 142-146
Public sex environments (PSEs)
    distinguishing characteristics of, 4-6
    types of, and sex space, 5-6
Raids, on gay bathhouses, 41-46
Rapid blood testing, 207,213
    bringing, to bathhouses, 215-216
Renton v. Playtime Theaters Inc.,
    142,146
Richter, Steven, 91
Risk behavior, public sex
    environments and, 5-6
Risk guidelines
    by Bay Area Physicians for Human
        Rights, 79,81
    chart for, by San Francisco AIDS
        Foundation, 79,80
Ross, Bob, 95
Ruffing, Bob, 47

Safe sex, bathhouses as resource for
    promoting, 51-52. *See also*
    Sex

Safe sex social clubs, prevention
    education in, 193. *See also*
    Sex clubs
Sandmire, Rev. James, 91-92
San Francisco, Ca. *See also* Feinstein,
    Dianne; Gay bathhouses
  changes in gay bathhouses in,
    during 1960s and 1970s,
    39-41
  AIDS awareness in gay bathhouses
    in, 78-79
  bathhouse battles of 1984 in,
    introduction, 72-74
  bathhouses after 1984 in, 115-118
  changes in gay bathhouses in,
    during 1980s, 41
  bookstores in, 178-184
  closure of gay bathhouses in,
    46-50,104
  court case over closure of
    bathhouses and, 109-112
  early aspects of AIDS in, 76-78
  early gay bathhouses in, 35-36
  early history of gay bathhouses in,
    37-41
  gay bathhouse closure attempts in,
    46-49
  history of baths in, 1970s to
    1984,74-76
  Human Rights Commission
    investigations in, 101-102
  Judge Wonder's first ruling on
    closure of bathhouses in,
    111-112
  Judge Wonder's second ruling on
    closure of bathhouses in,
    114-115
  positions on closure from activists
    and mayor in, 88-90
  public policies for bathhouses in,
    12-13
  reaction of bathhouse owners to
    closure in, 104-105
  response by, on Judge Wonder's
    ruling, 113-114

  Silverman's first press conference
    on baths in, 87-88
  Silverman's second press
    conference on baths in, 90-92
  theaters in, 184-186
San Francisco AIDS Foundation
    (SFAF), 79,97,105,115
San Francisco Baths on Ellis, 39
San Francisco Chronicle, AIDS stories
    by, 82-85
San Francisco Department of Public
    Health, evidence on AIDS
    and bathhouses of, 99-101
San Francisco Police Department
  community responses to
    surveillance of bathhouses
    by, 94-96
  gay community and, 95-96
  surveillance of bathhouses by,
    93-94
Saunaguide, 57-58
Savages, 185
Secura, Gina, 221-242,245
Sex. *See also* Safe sex
  in gay bathhouses, 7-9
  group, in gay bathhouses, 162-165
  individual, in gay bathhouses,
    165-169
  privacy and, 144
Sex clubs. *See also* Gay bathhouses;
    Jack-off clubs; San
    Francisco; Sex-facilitating
    businesses (SFBs)
  after 1984, in San Francisco,
    116-117
  environments of, 7
  prevention education in, 190-191
  for safe sex, 193
Sex emporiums. *See* Bookstores
Sex-facilitating businesses (SFBs). *See
    also* Bookstores; Gay
    bathhouses; Sex clubs;
    Theaters
  explanations for case outcomes for,
    137-146

law and, 133
legal bases for regulating, 137
legal doctrine and, 132-133
owners of, and social responsibility, 186-192
personal conclusions and recommendations for, 199-201
public knowledge, attitudes, and beliefs and, 147-148
right of privacy and, 132
survey of case law for, 133-136
Sex spaces, types of public sex environments and, 5-6
Sexually transmitted infections (STIs), 2-3
SF JACKS, 192,197
Shilts, Randy, 3,72,75,76-77,82-85, 86,94,106,107,108,113-114
Silverman, Mervyn, 77,192,194
closure of San Francisco baths controversy and, 92-93
closure order of, 108-109
debate with Larry Littlejohn and, 79-82
evidence on AIDS and bathhouse sand, 99-101
first press conference on bathhouses by, 87-88
hiring of investigators by, 105-107
public opinion and, 102-104
resignation of, 114
response to Littlejohn's petition by, 86
second press conference on bathhouses by, 90-92
on Shilts's articles, 83-85
Single Use Diagnostic System (SUDS) for HIV-1,207,213
Sisters of Perpetual Indulgence, 13
Slate, Hal, 93
Slot sex club, 116
Social climate, 26
Spielberg, Freya, 203-220,246
St. Marks Baths, 12,142

Stanley v. Georgia, 143
Steel, Thomas, 111,113,114,115
Structural interventions, bathhouse policy and, 28-29
Structural policy, 10. *See also* Public health policy
Suburban Video, Inc. v. City of Delafield, 136,142
Sutro Baths, 78,93

Tales of the City (Maupin), 74-75
Testing. *See* HIV (human immunodeficiency virus) counseling and testing
Theaters, in San Francisco, 184-186. *See also* Sex-facilitating businesses (SFBs)
Top/bottom myth, and HIV status, 230
Tracy, Daniel P., 55-70,246
21st Street Baths, 116

Volberding, Paul, 110

Ward, Philip, 105,113
Ward v. Rock Against Racism, 145,146
White, Dan, 95
White Night Riot (1979), 95-96
Wonder, Roy, 111,112,116
Wood, Robert W., 203-220,246
Woods, William J., 1-21,23-31, 55-70,246

YMCA, 49-50

Love Letters Between a Certain Late Nobleman and the Famous Mr. Wilson, edited by Michael S. Kimmel, PhD (Vol. 19, No. 2, 1990). *"An intriguing book about homosexuality in 18th Century England. Many details of the period, such as meeting places, coded language, and 'camping' are all covered in the book. If you're a history buff, you'll enjoy this one." (Prime Timers)*

Homosexuality and Religion, edited by Richard Hasbany, PhD (Vol. 18, No. 3/4, 1990). *"A welcome resource that provides historical and contemporary views on many issues involving religious life and homosexuality." (Journal of Sex education and Therapy)*

Homosexuality and the Family, edited by Frederick W. Bozett, PhD (Vol. 18, No. 1/2, 1989). *"Enlightening and answers a host of questions about the effects of homosexuality upon family members and the family as a unit." (Ambush Magazine)*

Gay and Lesbian Youth, edited by Gilbert Herdt, PhD (Vol. 17, No. 1/2/3/4, 1989). *"Provides a much-needed compilation of research dealing with homosexuality and adolescents." (GLTF Newsletter)*

Lesbians Over 60 Speak for Themselves, edited by Monika Kehoe, PhD (Vol. 16, No. 3/4, 1989). *"A pioneering book examining the social, economical, physical, sexual, and emotional lives of aging lesbians." (Feminist Bookstore News)*

The Pursuit of Sodomy: Male Homosexuality in Renaissance and Enlightenment Europe, edited by Kent Gerard, PhD, and Gert Hekma, PhD (Vol. 16, No. 1/2, 1989). *"Presenting a wealth of information in a compact form, this book should be welcomed by anyone with an interest in this period in European history or in the precursors to modern concepts of homosexuality." (The Canadian Journal of Human Sexuality)*

Psychopathology and Psychotherapy in Homosexuality, edited by Michael W. Ross, PhD (Vol. 15, No. 1/2, 1988). *"One of the more objective, scientific collections of articles concerning the mental health of gays and lesbians. . . . Extraordinarily thoughtful. . . . New thoughts about treatments. Vital viewpoints." (The Book Reader)*

Psychotherapy with Homosexual Men and Women: Integrated Identity Approaches for Clinical Practice, edited by Eli Coleman, PhD (Vol. 14, No. 1/2, 1987). *"An invaluable tool. . . . This is an extremely useful book for the clinician seeking better ways to understand gay and lesbian patients." (Hospital and Community Psychiatry)*

Interdisciplinary Research on Homosexuality in The Netherlands, edited by A. X. van Naerssen, PhD (Vol. 13, No. 2/3, 1987). *"Valuable not just for its insightful analysis of the evolution of gay rights in The Netherlands, but also for the lessons that can be extracted by our own society from the Dutch tradition of tolerance for homosexuals." (The San Francisco Chronicle)*

Historical, Literary, and Erotic Aspects of Lesbianism, edited by Monica Kehoe, PhD (Vol. 12, No. 3/4, 1986). *"Fascinating . . . Even though this entire volume is serious scholarship penned by degreed writers, most of it is vital, accessible, and thoroughly readable even to the casual student of lesbian history." (Lambda Rising)*

Anthropology and Homosexual Behavior, edited by Evelyn Blackwood, PhD (cand.) (Vol. 11, No. 3/4, 1986). *"A fascinating account of homosexuality during various historical periods and in non-Western cultures." (SIECUS Report)*

Bisexualities: Theory and Research, edited by Fritz Klein, MD, and Timothy J. Wolf, PhD (Vol. 11, No. 1/2, 1985). *"The editors have brought together a formidable array of new data challenging old stereotypes about a very important human phenomenon . . . A milestone in furthering our knowledge about sexual orientation." (David P. McWhirter, Co-author, The Male Couple)*

Homophobia: An Overview, edited by John P. De Cecco, PhD (Vol. 10, No. 1/2, 1984). *"Breaks ground in helping to make the study of homophobia a science." (Contemporary Psychiatry)*

Bisexual and Homosexual Identities: Critical Clinical Issues, edited by John P. De Cecco, PhD (Vol. 9, No. 4, 1985). *Leading experts provide valuable insights into sexual identity within a clinical context-broadly defined to include depth psychology, diagnostic classification, therapy, and psychomedical research on the hormonal basis of homosexuality.*

Bisexual and Homosexual Identities: Critical Theoretical Issues, edited by John P. De Cecco, PhD, and Michael G. Shively, MA (Vol. 9, No. 2/3, 1984). *"A valuable book . . . The careful scholarship, analytic rigor, and lucid exposition of virtually all of these essays make them thought-provoking and worth more than one reading." (Sex Roles, A Journal of Research)*

Homosexuality and Social Sex Roles, edited by Michael W. Ross, PhD (Vol. 9, No. 1, 1983). *"For a comprehensive review of the literature in this domain, exposure to some interesting methodological models, and a glance at 'older' theories undergoing contemporary scrutiny, I recommend this book." (Journal of Sex Education & Therapy)*

Literary Visions of Homosexuality, edited by Stuart Kellogg, PhD (Vol. 8, No. 3/4, 1985). *"An important book. Gay sensibility has never been given such a boost." (The Advocate)*

Alcoholism and Homosexuality, edited by Thomas O. Ziebold, PhD, and John E. Mongeon (Vol. 7, No. 4, 1985). *"A landmark in the fields of both alcoholism and homosexuality . . . a very lush work of high caliber." (The Journal of Sex Research)*

Homosexuality and Psychotherapy: A Practitioner's Handbook of Affirmative Models, edited by John C. Gonsiorek, PhD (Vol. 7, No. 2/3, 1985). *"A book that seeks to create affirmative psychotherapeutic models. . . . To say this book is needed by all doing therapy with gay or lesbian clients is an understatement." (The Advocate)*

Nature and Causes of Homosexuality: A Philosophic and Scientific Inquiry, edited by Noretta Koertge, PhD (Vol. 6, No. 4, 1982). *"An interesting, thought-provoking book, well worth reading as a corrective to much of the research literature on homosexuality." (Australian Journal of Sex, Marriage & Family)*

Historical Perspectives on Homosexuality, edited by Salvatore J. Licata, PhD, and Robert P. Petersen, PhD (cand.) (Vol. 6, No. 1/2, 1986). *"Scholarly and excellent. Its authority is impeccable, and its treatment of this neglected area exemplary." (Choice)*

Homosexuality and the Law, edited by Donald C. Knutson, PhD (Vol. 5, No. 1/2, 1979). *A comprehensive analysis of current legal issues and court decisions relevant to male and female homosexuality.*